Historic Collection
edited by
transplant pioneer
Fritz Bach, specializing in
transplant immunology
Score

AF870259

IMMUNOBIOLOGY OF TRANSPLANTATION

The Histocompatibility Systems

IMMUNOBIOLOGY OF TRANSPLANTATION

The Histocompatibility Systems

Edited by

Fritz H. Bach

Professor of Medical Genetics and Surgery
University of Wisconsin
Madison, Wisconsin

GRUNE & STRATTON
New York and London
A Subsidiary of Harcourt Brace Jovanovich, Publishers

IMMUNOBIOLOGY OF TRANSPLANTATION: The Histocompatibility Systems is the hardcover edition of the *Proceedings of the Second International Symposium on CELLULAR ASPECTS OF TRANSPLANTATION.* It was originally published in the December 1973 issue (Volume V, Number 4) of the quarterly journal *Transplantation Proceedings*, an official publication of the Transplantation Society.

Library of Congress Cataloging in Publication Data

[International Symposium on Cellular Aspects of Transplantation, 2d, London and St. Paul, 1973]
Immunobiology of transplantation.

Proceedings of the symposium.
Originally published in 1973 as v. 5, no. 4, of Transplantation proceedings.
1. Transplantation immunology—Congresses.
I. Bach, Fritz H., ed. II. Transplantation proceedings. III. Title. [DNLM: 1. Histocompatibility testing—Congresses. 2. Transplantation immunology—Congresses. W3 IN916R 1973i / W068 I59 1973i]
RD120.7.I57 1973 617'.95 74-2019
ISBN 0-8089-0840-5

© *1973, 1974 by Grune & Stratton, Inc.*

All rights reserved. No part of this publication may be reproduced or transmitted in any form or by any means, electronic or mechanical, including photocopy, recording, or any information storage and retrieval system, without permission in writing from the publisher.

Grune & Stratton, Inc.
111 Fifth Avenue
New York, New York 10003

Library of Congress Catalog Card Number 74-2019
International Standard Book Number 0-8089-0840-5
Printed in the United States of America

CONTENTS

PART I. THE RECOGNITION PHASE—MLC

PART II. THE DESTRUCTION PHASE—CML

PART III. IN VIVO CORRELATES

PART IV. CELL MEMBRANE SURFACES

PROLEPSIS

THE immunobiology of transplantation has had as one central focus the understanding and application of immunogenetics. Few of those of us interested in the problem in man could have foreseen 10 years ago the vast array of biological phenomena that would be brought into the arena of histocompatibility testing and thus be linked to the HL-A chromosomal region, the major histocompatibility complex (MHC) in man. Not only have the fundamental scope and lore of transplantation biology been expanded, but endeavors in treating the patient with kidney disease or uniformly fatal immunologic deficiency disorders have been given a sounder basis in medical therapeutics. In part, the pleasure and excitement of being involved in this burgeoning area of endeavor have been based on perhaps unprecedented international cooperation between many investigators bound together in a spirit of friendship and competitive pursuit of the same intellectual and iatric goals.

Whenever it appeared during the past decade that the basic tenets of HL-A immunogenetics had been established, some one of the many colorful personalities in the field would either reinterpret old data in a heuristically valuable manner or bring new findings to light that prevented premature codification of apparently attractive constructs, rekindled the blaze, and pushed the field forward. One, and only one, such developing thrust is based on a series of experiments performed in both man and mouse between 1968 and the present—although primarily in the last three years. I choose this one example with obvious personal bias, but also to give some rationale for the organization of the Second International Symposium on Cellular Aspects of Transplantation, presented in this volume.

A decade ago, both typing for the MHC serologically defined (SD) antigens and matching with mixed leukocyte culture (MLC) were considered approaches for the study of histocompatibility in man. After the initial demonstration that these two methodologies measured disparity for the same chromosomal region, HL-A, the tests were regarded by many as alternative assays for the same antigens. The findings in man, in a series of investigations by Amos, Bach, Ceppellini, and co-workers culminating in the studies of Yunis and Amos, as well as those of Eijsvoogel, van Rood, and their colleagues, that the HL-A chromosomal products so important for MLC, the LD antigens, are different from the SD antigens, set a new springboard in the field. The immediate, liberal, and wide dissemination by these latter authors of their information, obviating the delays of formal publication, allowed rapid experimental fortification of the scaffold they had erected.

On more than one occasion workers in HL-A have benefited from the broad base of knowledge of H-2 immunogenetics in mice, which dates back almost 40 years and for which we owe so much to the giants in this field such as Gorer, Snell, and their students, as HL-A discoveries have broadened our concept of major histocompatibility systems. Widmer thus turned to the mouse, and working with Klein as well as Bailey and Stimpfling, he used well-characterized strains to look for LD components of H-2. In a large series of studies, Widmer developed a story supporting the existence of LD components of the MHC in mice essentially similar to the story in man but allowing a formal genetic demonstration of the existence of at least two MHC LD regions of differing strengths. Once again, because of international communication and interest, this story could be transmitted to Shreffler, on sabbatical with Ceppellini in Europe, months before publication, and thus facilitate the confirmation by Meo, Shreffler, and co-workers of the existence of such H-2 LD loci.

Thus LD was established as a separate entity from the SD antigens of the MHC in both mouse and man. However, a still closer union between LD and SD was to follow. The finding that some H-2 SD-identical but H-2 LD-different mouse strains (i.e., whose cells activated in MLC) did not reject skin or did so only extremely slowly presaged the realization that LD components would not necessarily account for the entire allograft reaction. Further, Trinchieri, Ceppellini, and co-workers found that despite the importance of LD for MLC activation, the SD phenotype correlates well with cell-mediated lympholysis (CML) cytotoxicity, thus suggesting a possible difference in genetic control for MLC and CML. It remained for Eijsvoogel and his collaborators, also working in man, to show unequivocally that LD differences that activated cells in MLC did not act as target in CML and that the targets for CML were either the SD antigens or molecules determined by genes closely linked to those determining the SD antigens. This finding, communicated by Eijsvoogel, once again long before publication, was rapidly confirmed in the mouse by Alter, Schendel, and collaborators. The in vitro LD–SD interaction has perhaps been most elegantly demonstrated in the subsequent parallel three-cell experiments of Schendel in mouse and Eijsvoogel in man.

Simultaneously, the continuing investigations by Festenstein have established that his M-locus alleles segregate independently of H-2 and have demonstrated the very strong lymphocyte-activating determinants controlled by this locus. The more recent in vivo studies, including those that were a major component of the London workshop summarized in this volume, provide an interesting comparative story.

So many diverse questions that have begged for attention regarding these findings are being brought rapidly into focus. The role of H-2 LD differences in graft-vs.-host reactions studied by Livnat, Klein, Elkins, and Kavathas in our laboratory and the correlation between MLC matching and secondary disease in H-2 SD-identical mouse strains studied by Rodey, Bortin, and collaborators have been brought to light in a span of only a few months. Further, preliminary correlations between LD matching in skin and kidney graft survival, already indicated in studies by Hamburger and colleagues several years ago, have given further insight into the possible biological relevance of LD. Rapid progress in our understanding of the genetics of LD is promised by the use in MLC of cells of HL-A SD phenotypically homozygous donors by Mempel, Albert, and others and the genotypically homozygous typing cells of van Rood. This latter group's serologic approach to the identification of the LD alleles, as well as the more precise mapping of LD and SD genes in the MHC of mouse, man, and now monkey by Balner, are also contributing to our overall picture.

Progressing simultaneously as individual fields of endeavor are new and more extensive studies of the puzzling patterns of MLC reactivity in families in which the parents share an HL-A SD haplotype, as first described by Dausset et al.; advances in possible clinical applicability of MLC by the standard stimulating cells of Segall, Osoba, and Falk; the dissection of cell populations possibly responding to LD and SD with concurrent in vivo analyses; the possible linking of immune-response genes to disease susceptibility in man; preliminary data from Rapaport suggesting an association between HL-A and developmental abnormalities; and the general area of physiological genetics of transplantation antigens, as Ceppellini has called it. Most important, however, just as for the marriage of LD and SD, salient biological interactions and thus critical bridges in our understanding are being established.

As I read through the above I am appalled at the number of omissions, even in this one restricted area on which I have tried to focus—omissions of both names and facts. Perhaps the most important names not present are those of some of the younger contributors in the area, whose defense mechanisms against infection with the enthusiasm of this field have fortunately failed. So many facts and so many parts of the experimental scenario as it has developed have been left out. I did not, however, mean to be all-inclusive, but rather to provide a general introduction to the conferences at which many of the new areas of effort mentioned above were first presented and discussed in depth.

We all feel deeply privileged to be a part of this field, to play a role in a little corner of the biomedical scene, which offers such enormous potential for scholarly endeavor and at the same time the promise of possibly contributing to the therapy of human disease.

It would not be proper to conclude this introduction to the volume without drawing attention to the enormous amount of energy that so many individuals have devoted to the planning of the conference. I am immensely indebted, first and foremost, to Prof. Jean Hamburger, who conceived the idea leading to the First International Symposium on Cellular Aspects of Transplantation held in Paris last year. The value of the advice received from members of the Organizing Committee for the second symposium meeting, including J. F. Bach, Ceppellini, Eijsvoogel, Lance, Thorsby, van Rood, and others, cannot adequately be documented here. Our deepest gratitude also goes to the French Direction Générale de Recherches Scientifiques et Techniques and the Foundation for Research in Biology and Medicine, under the presidency of Dr. John Marquis Converse, who generously provided financial support.

The purpose of this volume is to bring together a collection of papers that provide both perspective and incentive for the investigator or student interested in this field. I am grateful to the authors and to the editors and publisher of *Transplantation Proceedings* for establishing deadline dates for the conference that permitted the inclusion of manuscripts received as late as August, 1973, for December publication. The attempt has been to present a maximally informative and challenging volume; in this, I hope that we have succeeded.

Fritz H. Bach
Laboratory of Genetics
University of Wisconsin, Madison
August, 1973

Part I

The Recognition Phase—MLC

Genetic Mapping of H-2 LD Loci

By Michael B. Widmer, Ammon B. Peck, and Fritz H. Bach

LYMPHOCYTES from inbred strains of mice that differ genetically for all or part of the major histocompatibility complex (MHC), designated H-2, react in the mixed lymphocyte culture (MLC) test.[1,2] A great deal of attention has recently been focused on the problem of determining which MHC components are important to the MLC reaction. A genetic map of the mouse MHC is shown in Fig. 1. The H-2 region is composed of two serologically defined (SD) loci, H-2K and H-2D, separated by a recombination frequency of approximately 0.5%.[3] Between the two SD loci are (ordered from left to right) at least two genetically separable immune-response (Ir) genes, Ir-1[4] and Ir-IgG,[5] and the Ss-Slp locus controlling a serum protein.[6]

We have recently demonstrated, using intra-H-2 recombinant strains, that loci genetically separable from H-2K and H-2D are primarily responsible for MLC activation.[7,8] These results were subsequently confirmed by others using different strains.[9] The genes whose products cause MLC reactivity are referred to as lymphocyte-defined (LD). A further description of the LD loci, with regard to number and location, is the subject of the present report.

It should be emphasized that the SD, Ir, and Ss-Slp genes are used solely as regional markers in the MLC studies. For example, strains B10.A(2R) and B10.A(4R), which stimulate in MLC,[7] differ for only the Ir-IgG and Ss-Slp markers, but could in addition differ for any genes in the chromosomal segment between but not including Ir-1 and H-2D. It is not implied that the gene products of the MHC markers themselves are the MLC stimulatory entities. On the contrary, we will show here that loci separate from but closely linked to the present MHC markers can cause MLC reactivity.

Previous studies have shown that disparity at either the H-2K or H-2D end of H-2 results in reactivity.[10] After the demonstration that SD-loci differences appear to play a relatively minor role in MLC activation,[7,8] the existence of at least two LD loci, one at each end of the complex, was obvious. The precise location of an LD locus at the D end of H-2 comes from studies involving strains B10.A(1R) and B10.A(2R). The $H\text{-}2^{h\text{-}Sg}$ and $H\text{-}2^{h\text{-}2Sg}$ chromosomes present in 1R and 2R, respectively, are the products of independent recombinational events that occurred between Ss-Slp and H-2D in identical ($H\text{-}2^a/H\text{-}2^b$) heterozygotes.[11] The crossovers were indistinguishable with respect to the presently known MHC markers. Both 1R and 2R carry the H-2K, Ir-1, and Ss-Slp alleles of the $H\text{-}2^a$ and the H-2D allele of the $H\text{-}2^b$ chromosomes and are congenic on the C57BL/10 background.[12]

In previous studies,[8] occasionally significant but nonreproducible MLC reactivity between 1R and 2R was noted. Testing these strains in the sensitive serum-free or mouse-serum-supplemented micromethod of Peck and Bach[13] produced significant stimulation of 1R splenic lymphocytes by those of 2R in each of three experiments. No stimulation was seen in the reverse direction. Results of one experiment are presented in Table 1. Stimulation of 1R by 2R is highly significant ($p < 0.001$) by a t test performed on $\log_{10}$-converted data.

From the Departments of Medical Genetics and Surgery, University of Wisconsin, Madison, Wisc.

A. B. Peck is a Research Fellow of the Wisconsin Heart Association.

Supported by NIH grants AI-08439, AI-06525, and GM-15422; ONR grant N00014-67-A-0128-0003; and NF-MOD grant CRBS 246.

This is paper No. 1701 from the Laboratory of Genetics, University of Wisconsin, Madison, Wisc.

©1973 by Grune & Stratton, Inc.

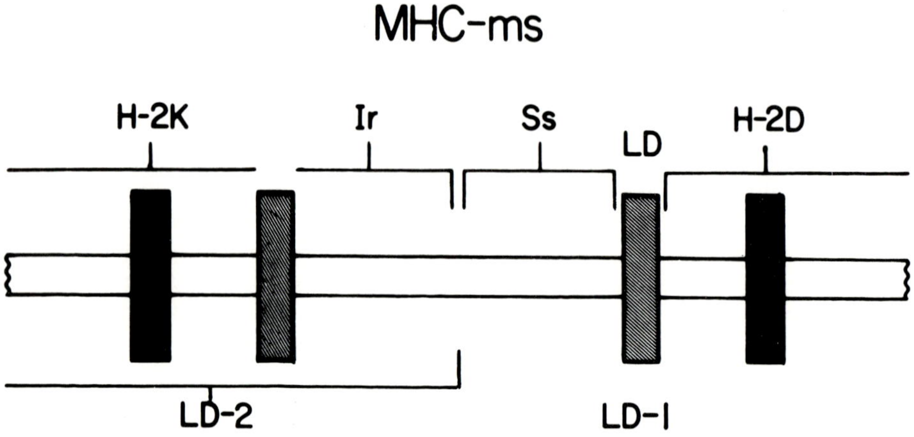

Fig. 1. A genetic map of the H-2 complex of the mouse. The black vertical bars refer to the two SD loci, H-2K and H-2D. These loci are used as the markers for the H-2K and H-2D regions, as indicated by the horizontal lines above the loci. The Ir and Ss-Slp regions are also included, although the respective loci themselves are not indicated. The striped vertical bars refer to the LD loci. LD-1 is formally mapped by studies in the B10.A(1R)–B10.A(2R) combination; LD-2 has not been genetically mapped and could be anywhere in the region indicated. (We have placed it to the right of H-2K based on preliminary and presently inconclusive data.) Where possible, the boundaries of regions are indicated. Thus H-2D and Ss-Slp are separated from LD-1; on the other hand, if LD-2 is in the position indicated, we have no evidence that it is separated from Ir-1 (in the Ir region) or from H-2K. The Ir region is separable from H-2K. We have not indicated the left and right boundaries of the H-2 complex since we feel this is a problem that cannot be resolved at present.

This finding allows the first formal mapping of an LD locus solely on the basis of MLC reactivity. Thus we refer to the locus as LD-1. Presumably the independent crossover events from which 1R and 2R originated recombined the LD-1 locus of $H\text{-}2^a$ into the resultant chromosome in one case, and LD-1 from $H\text{-}2^b$ in the other. Another possibility consistent with the one-way reactivity is that unequal crossing over occurred in the interval between Ss-Slp and H-2D such that either 1R lacks determinant(s) present in 2R or there is a quantitatively different density of similar determinants that can be recognized in MLC. This is not to imply that LD-1 will not eventually be a marker for a cluster of LD genes.

The exact location of other LD loci within the MHC has thus far been impos-

Table 1. MLC Reactivity With Identity for MHC Markers*

Responding Cells	Stimulating Cells		
	B10.A(1R)	B10.A(2R)	B10.A(5R)
B10.A(1R)	395 ± 48†	1341 ± 125 $p < 0.001$‡	12157 ± 2475 $p < 0.001$
B10.A(2R)	371 ± 54 $p < 0.01$	620 ± 55	3435 ± 1212 $p < 0.005$
B10.A(5R)	1765 ± 318 $p < 0.005$	7165 ± 1294 $p < 0.001$	329 ± 156

*MLCs were performed in the serum-free micromethod of Peck and Bach.[13] Stimulating cells were x-irradiated with 1750 rad. Strains B10.A(1R) and B10.A(2R) are identical for known MHC markers. The control B10.A(5R) strain differs from both B10.A(1R) and B10.A(2R) at H-2K, Ir, and H-2D.

†Mean counts per minute (c.p.m.) of triplicate cultures ± standard deviation.

‡Indicates significance level of stimulation.

sible to establish. Previous studies involving 173 strain combinations indicated that strong MLC reactivity is associated with Ir-1 differences.[8,14] No strain combination is yet available that differs for only the Ir-1 marker; that is, disparity at Ir-1 in the presently available combinations is always accompanied by disparity at H-2K or Ss-Slp.

Combinations that differ at H-2K and Ir, with identity at Ss-Slp and H-2D (LD-1 compatibility), react strongly in MLC. The stimulation indices (allogeneic c.p.m./isogeneic c.p.m.) for 11 such combinations range from 3.2 to 18.3, with a mean of 6.6.[8,14] While these results indicate that there is a locus or LD region determining strong reactivity (designated LD-2 in Fig. 2) that is genetically separable from LD-1, they do not determine whether LD-2 lies between H-2K and Ss-Slp or to the left of H-2K. We favor the positioning of LD-2 between H-2K and Ss-Slp for the following reasons: (1) Combinations with only an H-K difference should show strong reactivity if LD-2 is to the left of but close to H-2K; however, the one such combination available to us (AQR–B10.A)[7,8] and another tested by Meo et al.[9] exhibit minimal reactivity. (2) Strong reactivity occurs between the H-2K-identical, Ir-, Ss-Slp-different strains AQR–B10.T(6R),[7,8] as well as strains A.TH–A.TL.[9] Although this could be due to the effects of LD-1, the average ratio of stimulation between 11 Ss-Slp-, H-2D-different combinations tested one to four times ranges from 0.7 to 4.7 with a mean of 2.0, suggesting that stimulation due to LD-1 is relatively weak and probably does not entirely account for the stronger stimulation between AQR and B10.T(6R) (average ratio = 5.8, range = 2.7 to 12.8) tested five times in the same series of experiments.[8,14]

There is as yet no conclusive evidence that separates LD-2 from the Ir region. However, two congenic strains that may be important in this regard are B10.S(7R) and B10.HTT. The derivation of their H-2 chromosomes is depicted diagrammatically in Fig. 2. The H-2th chromosome present in B10.S(7R) is the product of a recombinational event between either Ir-1 and Ss-Slp or Ss-Slp and H-2D that occurred in an H-2^{a}/H-2^{s} heterozygote;[12] the exact position of the crossover cannot be determined, since the Ss-Slp allele is identical in H-2^{a} and H-2^{s}.[15] Recombination in an (H-2^{al}/H-2^{s}) heterozygote resulted in the H-2^{tl} chromosome,[16] which was backcrossed to the C57BL/10 background in the production of B10.HTT. The Ir-1 allele of B10.HTT is *provisionally* designated as Ir-1^{k} (originating from H-2^{al}), although B10.-HTT has yet to be typed for Ir-1. However, strain A.TL, which was derived from the same initial H-2^{tl} recombinant chromosome,[16] carries the Ir-1^{k} allele.[9]

An experiment testing the MLC reactivity between B10.S(7R) and B10.HTT in the human-plasma-supplemented system[8] is presented in Table 2. Cells from B10.S(7R) and B10.HTT stimulate each other only slightly compared to the strong stimulation of either strain by B10.BR (H-2^{k}). Two additional experiments, one performed in human plasma and the other in the mouse-serum-supplemented system,[13] gave similar results. If B10.HTT has the Ir-1^{k} allele, these findings indicate that Ir-1 disparity is not always associated with strong MLC reactivity, thus separating LD-2 from Ir-1. The low-level reactivity between B10.HTT and B10.S(7R) could be due to the LD-1 locus.

H-2^{a}	K^{k}	Ir-1^{k}	Ss-Slp^{d}	D^{d}
H-2^{s}	K^{s}	Ir-1^{s}	Ss-Slp^{s}	D^{s}
H-2^{al}	K^{k}	Ir-1^{k}	Ss-Slp^{k}	D^{d}
H-2th	K^{s}	Ir-1^{s}	Ss-$Slp^{d(s)}$	D^{d}
H-2^{tl}	K^{s}	Ir-1^{k}	Ss-Slp^{k}	D^{d}

Fig. 2. H-2th was derived from an H-2^{a}/H-2^{s} heterozygote.[12] The exact position of the crossover with respect to Ss-Slp cannot be determined since Ss-Slp^{d} and Ss-Slp^{s} are identical.[15] H-2^{tl} was derived from an H-2^{al}/H-2^{s} heterozygote.[16] H-2th and H-2^{tl} differ for the Ir and Ss-Slp regions.

Table 2. MLC Reactivity Between B10.S(7R) and B10.HTT*

Responding Cells	Stimulating Cells		
	B10.S(7R)	B10.HTT	B10.BR
B10.S(7R)	4699 ± 861†	5290 ± 1537 NS‡	51581 ± 2896 $p < 0.001$
B10.HTT	6460 ± 1702 NS	4236 ± 1048	35537 ± 2256 $p < 0.001$
B10.BR	18465 ± 1183 $p < 0.001$	28876 ± 3085 $p < 0.001$	3853 ± 1645

*MLCs were performed in RPMI-1640 supplemented with 5% human plasma, as previously described.[8] Stimulating cells were treated with mitomycin C. The derivation of these strains is described in the text.

†Mean counts per minute (c.p.m.) of quadruplicate cultures ± standard deviation.

‡Indicates significance level of stimulation; NS, not significant.

Preliminary results from a separate experiment indicate that B10.S(7R) responds strongly in MLC to A.AL (stimulation index in mouse serum for B10.S(7R)–$(A.AL)_{x\text{-irradiated}}$ = 8.5, compared with B10.S(7R)–$(B10.HTT)_x$ stimulation ratio of 2.5). That this reactivity is not due to non-H-2 differences between the A and C57BL/10 backgrounds is suggested by minimal reactivity between the H-2-identical A and B10.A strains, which presumably differ for the same non-H-2 genes as B10.S(7R) and A.AL. Since the crossover from which B10.HTT was derived presumably included the Ir-1, Ss-Slp, and H-2D but not the H-2K markers of A.AL, the weak and strong response, respectively, of B10.S(7R) to B10.HTT and A.AL suggests the presence of a strong LD region to the left of Ir-1. It must be stressed that the aforementioned evidence can be interpreted in this manner only if B10.HTT carries the $Ir\text{-}1^k$ allele. Should it possess $Ir\text{-}1^s$, a separation of LD-2 from Ir-1 would not be supported. Meo et al. in this same symposium suggest that the H-2 chromosome of B10.HTT may have been involved in a second, undetected recombinational event, with respect to LD-2, during its history of heterozygosity with $H\text{-}2^s$. Their suggestion is based on the observation that B10.HTT and A.TL (which would be identical for the MHC markers provided B10.HTT has $Ir\text{-}1^k$) are highly reactive toward each other in MLC.[17] Our findings are consistent with this interpretation.

We use the term locus in reference to LD-1 or LD-2 for purely descriptive purposes. There may actually be many LD loci in the LD-1 region between Ss-Slp and H-2D or in the LD-2 region to the left of Ss-Slp. This possibility has previously been discussed.

In previous MLC studies testing H-2D-different strains, stimulation was detected with some combinations but not with others.[8,14] Some of those that did not stimulate have been retested and found to be reactive in the sensitive mouse-serum-supplemented system.[13,18] These findings are consistent with the suggestion that those H-2D-different combinations that stimulate do so because of an LD-1 difference. Alternatively, the H-2D antigens themselves, or LD loci to the right of H-2D, might be involved. We have tested the latter possibility by examining the MLC behavior of two strain combinations derived from ostensibly reciprocal recombination between H-2D and the H-2D-linked Tla locus.[19] Although no reactivity between these combinations was obtained, the possibility that there are LD loci to the right of H-2D cannot be excluded.

The observation that strong stimulation occurs between LD-1-identical, K-, Ir-1-different strains permits the positioning of LD-2 to the left of Ss-Slp. More indirect evidence presented here suggests that this strong LD locus may lie between H-2K and Ir-1. A formal demonstration of the type used to map LD-1 will require the isolation from identical F_1 heterozygotes of H-2K/Ir-1 recombinants that either stimulate each other or react differentially with the H-2K-different parental chromosome from which they were derived.

Note added in proof: It has been determined that B10.HTT carries the Ir-1^s allele[20] and is therefore Ir-1-compatible with B10.S(7R) and Ir-1-incompatible with A.AL. Thus LD-2 has not as yet been separated from Ir-1.

ACKNOWLEDGMENT

We are grateful to Drs. Jan Klein, Jack Stimpfling, and Donald Shreffler for providing us with breeding pairs of several mouse strains used in these studies.

REFERENCES

1. Dutton RW: J Exp Med 123:655, 1966
2. Rychliková M, Démant P, Iványi P: Nature [New Biol] 230:271, 1971
3. Klein J, Shreffler DC: Transplant Rev 6:3, 1971
4. McDevitt HO, Benacerraf B: Adv Immunol 2:31, 1969
5. Lieberman R, Paul WE, Humphrey W, Jr, Stimpfling JH: J Exp Med 136:1231, 1972
6. Passmore HC, Shreffler DC: Biochem Genet 4:351, 1970
7. Bach FH, Widmer MB, Segall M, et al: Science 176:1024, 1972
8. Bach FH, Widmer MB, Bach ML, Klein J: J Exp Med 136:1430, 1972
9. Meo T, Vives J, Miggiano V, Shreffler D: Transplant Proc 5:377, 1973
10. Klein J, Widmer MB, Segall M, Bach FH: Cell Immunol 4:442, 1972
11. Stimpfling JH, Richardson A: Genetics 51:831, 1965
12. Stimpfling JH, Reichert AE: Transplant Proc 2:39, 1970
13. Peck AB, Bach FH: J Immunol Meth (in press)
14. Widmer MB, Omodei-Zorini C, Bach ML, Bach FH: Tissue Antigens (in press)
15. David CS, Shreffler DC: Tissue Antigens 2:241, 1972
16. Shreffler DC, David CS: Tissue Antigens 2:232, 1972
17. Meo T, David CS, Nabholz M, et al: Transplant Proc 5:1507, 1973
18. Peck AB: unpublished data
19. Widmer MB, Schendel DJ, Bach FH, Boyse EA: Transplant Proc 5:1663, 1973
20. Deak B, McDevitt HO: personal communication

Demonstration by MLR Test of a Previously Unsuspected Intra-H-2 Crossover in the B10.HTT Strain: Implications Concerning Location of MLR Determinants in the Ir Region

By Tommaso Meo, C. S. David, M. Nabholz, V. Miggiano, and D. C. Shreffler

SEROLOGIC detection of antigens genetically controlled by the Ir region (the H-2K–Ss-Slp interval) of the H-2 gene complex was recently reported.[1,2] David et al.[1] used antisera produced by reciprocal immunizations between intra-H-2 recombinant strains A.TL and A.TH. These strains are identical in the H-2K and H-2D regions, but differ in Ir and Ss-Slp regions. When these antisera were tested against cells from strain B10.HTT, it was found that not only the A.TH anti-A.TL but also the A.TL anti-A.TH serum reacted strongly. This was unexpected because both strain A.TL and strain B10.HTT were derived from the same intra-H-2 recombinant animal and should have identical H-2 haplotypes. To explain this discrepancy, it was postulated that the H-2 chromosome of B10.HTT may have undergone a later, second intra-H-2 crossover that brought in a segment of the Ir region from the $H\text{-}2^s$ haplotype.[1]

Since A.TH and A.TL stimulate each other very strongly in MLR, due to the difference in their Ir regions (A.TH is Ir^s and A.TL is Ir^k)[3,4] and since the H-2 haplotypes of A.TL and B10.HTT would be predicted a priori to be identical in the MLR, we undertook to test the relationship of the serologic inconsistency to MLR reactivity. This paper presents results that support the hypothesis that the B10.HTT haplotype represents the product of a secondary intra-H-2 crossover. This apparent intra-Ir crossover may yield important information on the position and genetic structure of the MLR determinants in the H-2K–Ss-Slp interval relative to specific Ir genes.

MATERIALS AND METHOD

MLR Assay. Unidirectional assays were conducted according to the modified conditions previously described.[4] Levels of significance of differences in mean c.p.m. incorporated between experimental and control were determined by Student's t test on log-transformed data.

Animals. Strains A.TH and A.TL have been described previously.[5] Strain B10.HTT was developed by Démant in Prague by backcrossing onto the C57BL/10Sn (B10) strain background the H-2 haplotype of strain HTT. The HTT strain was derived by Shreffler from the progeny of recombinant ♂22,[6] the original $H\text{-}2^{tl}$ recombinant. Strain A.TL was also derived from the progeny of ♂22 by backcrossing the recombinant haplotype onto the A.CA strain background.[5] However, the HTT and A.TL strains were separated from each other in the first generation of ♂22 progeny. For two generations the $H\text{-}2^{tl}$ haplotype was heterozygous with $H\text{-}2^s$; therefore a recombination between the $H\text{-}2^{tl}$ and $H\text{-}2^s$ haplotypes could have occurred in the HTT line in either generation. However, the B10.HTT strain has been shown to be identical to the A.TL strain in H-2K and H-2D antigens and in Ss-Slp type.[8]

RESULTS AND DISCUSSION

We have previously shown that when strains A, A.AL, A.TL, A.TH, and A.SW are tested in MLR in all possible combinations the strongest activations are due to genetic differences in the Ir region.[3,4] To allow a direct comparison of the different patterns of MLR incompatibilities of strains A.TL and B10.HTT, an experiment

---

From the Basel Institute for Immunology, Basel, Switzerland, and the Department of Human Genetics, University of Michigan, Ann Arbor.

Supported in part by USPHS program project grant GM-15419 and USPHS career development award K3-HL-24980.

©1973 by Grune & Stratton, Inc.

Table 1. MLR Incompatibility of A.TL and A.TH

Responding Cells	Stimulating Cells: A	A.AL	A.TL	A.TH	A.SW
A	10,019	Ss† / 11,562‡	K,Ss / 25,719*	K,Ir,Ss / 147,014***	H-2 / 148,347***
A.AL	Ss / 7,505	7,505	K / 14,413	K,Ir,Ss / 78,288***	H-2 / 165,412***
A.TL	K,Ss / 54,748**	K / 48,592	30,353	Ir,Ss / 225,204***	Ir,Ss,D / 259,503***
A.TH	K,Ir,Ss / 349,947***	K,Ir,Ss / 246,538***	Ir,Ss / 239,330***	9,111	D / 27,976**
A.SW	H-2 / 348,528***	H-2 / 410,556***	Ir,Ss,D / 429,063***	D / 51,032**	19,258

*$p < 0.05$.
**$p < 0.01$.
***$p < 0.001$.
†H-2 region(s) in which responding and stimulating cells differ.
‡c.p.m. ^{3}H-thymidine incorporated, mean of three replicates.

with the five A strains is shown in Table 1. These data demonstrate (1) a strong MLR incompatibility between A.TH and A.TL, (2) a strong incompatibility between A.TL and A.SW, and (3) a weak incompatibility between A.TL and A or A.AL. Thus A.TL is predominantly H-2^k-like in its MLR determinants.

In Table 2 it is seen that strains B10.HTT and A.TL stimulate each other strongly. This stimulation is not entirely due to the known M-locus differences between the B10 and A strains,[7] since B10.HTT stimulates A.TL much more strongly than does B10.A. B10.HTT gives approximately equal levels of stimulation with B10.S and B10.A, as either responder or stimulator, in contrast with the strong A.TL vs. A.SW and weak

Table 2. MLR Reactivity of B10.HTT With A.TL and A.TH

Responding Cells	Stimulating Cells: B10.HTT	A.TL	B10.A	B10.S
B10.HTT	20,552†	?,M / 75,832**	K,Ss‡ / 97,752**	Ir,Ss,D / 109,607***
A.TL	?,M / 472,084***	17,446	K,Ss,M / 44,330*	Ir,Ss,D,M / 491,692***
B10.A	K,Ss / 114,796***	K,Ss,M / 71,821***	3,724	H-2 / 161,019***
B10.S	Ir,Ss,D / 132,499***	Ir,Ss,D,M / 265,356***	H-2 / 241,333***	20,075
(A.TH × B10.D2) F_1§	Ir,Ss / 27,100*	Ir,Ss / 92,161***	K,Ir / 166,612***	D / 87,622***

*$p < 0.05$.
**$p < 0.01$.
***$p < 0.001$.
†c.p.m. ^{3}H-thymidine incorporated, mean of three replicates.
‡H-2 region(s) in which responding and stimulating cells are expected to differ. M indicates M-locus difference.[7]
§c.p.m. with autologous cells = 9,635.

Table 3. MLR Reactivity of B10.HTT With A.TL and A.TH in F_1 Hybrid Combinations

	Stimulating Cells			
Responding Cells	Autologous Cells	A.TL	B10.HTT	B10.AKM
(A.TL × B10.D2) F_1	7,643†	8,816	? / 102,719***	K,D‡ / 70,883***
(A.TH × B10.D2) F_1	11,562	Ir,Ss / 41,632***	Ir,Ss / 11,366	H-2 / 213,875***
(A.TH × B10.HTT) F_1	4,131	? / 21,926***	4,511	K,D / 156,293***

***$p < 0.001$.
†c.p.m. ^{3}H-thymidine incorporated, mean of four replicates.
‡H-2 region(s) in which responding and stimulating cells are expected to differ.

A.TL vs. A or A.AL reactions (Table 1). The (A.TH × B10.D2) F_1 responds quite weakly to B10.HTT but strongly to A.TL. (Note that the F_1 combination eliminates any M-locus or other non-H-2 incompatibilities.)

The three F_1 hybrid responders in Table 3 likewise show that A.TL and B10.HTT are strongly incompatible, while A.TH and B10.HTT have minimal incompatibility. (The F_1 combinations again eliminate any background incompatibilities.) In this experiment, the (A.TH × B10.D2) F_1 gave no response to B10.HTT stimulating cells. In other experiments, e.g., Table 2, weak but significant stimulation was observed, depending upon the relative levels of stimulating cells and responding cells.

The data in Tables 2 and 3 demonstrate that strain B10.HTT is MLR-incompatible with both strain A.TL and strain A.TH. However, in the MLR test, B10.HTT appears to be more compatible with A.TH than with A.TL. These data reveal a major MLR incompatibility between B10.HTT and A.TL—almost as great as that between A.TH and A.TL. The results with F_1 hybrids (Tables 2 and 3) show that this difference is specifically associated with H-2 haplotype. Consistent with the relative

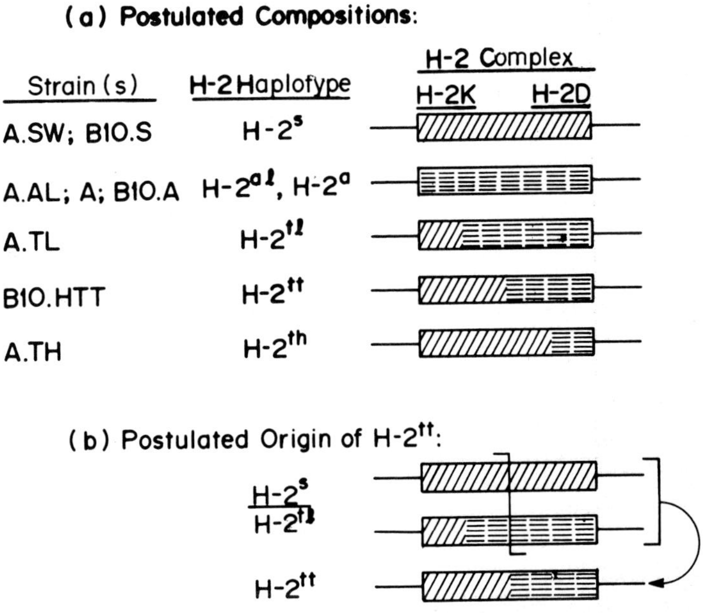

Fig. 1. Schematic representation of H-2 haplotype compositions of key strains. The H-2 haplotypes of A and B10.A differ from A.AL in the Ss-Slp region, but are otherwise identical. $H-2^{tt}$ is proposed provisionally as the symbol for the H-2 haplotype of B10.HTT.

compatibility of B10.HTT with A.TH is the approximately equal stimulation of B10.HTT with H-2^a and H-2^s strains, compared with the strong incompatibility of A.TL with H-2^s strains and minimal incompatibility with H-2^a or H-2^{al} strains. All of these observations indicate that B10.HTT has a different H-2 haplotype than A.TL and that the MLR determinants of the B10.HTT haplotype are more H-2^s-like than those of A.TL.

These results in the MLR test are consistent with previous serologic findings on Ir-region-associated antigens.[1,8] In particular, the serologic data indicate that the Ir region of strain B10.HTT is more like H-2^s than any other H-2 haplotype but also has some specificities associated with the Ir region of H-2^k.

To account for the MLR and serologic findings, it is postulated that the H-2 chromosome of B10.HTT is rather intermediate between those of A.TL and A.TH in relative amounts of H-2^k and H-2^s genetic information. This is represented diagrammatically in Fig. 1a. (In this figure, no attempt has been made to relate these chromosome compositions specifically to the Ir-1, Ir-IgG, and Ss-Slp regions.) The secondary recombination that is thought to have given rise to this condition is illustrated diagrammatically in Fig. 1b. This is the simplest model consistent with the data. Other explanations—mutation in A.TL or B10.HTT, secondary recombination in A.TL with the H-2^f (strain A.CA) haplotype or in B10.HTT with the H-2^b (strain B10) haplotype—have been considered but are either incompatible with the data or require multiple improbable events.

Thus far, strain B10.HTT has not been typed for the various H-2-associated immune responses. This information will, of course, be most useful. If B10.HTT is like A.TL in its responses, a significant dissociation of Ir genes from MLR and Lna genes will be indicated. This would support an interpretation of the organization of MLR genetic determinants that we have previously proposed.[4] Even if B10.HTT is like A.TH in its immune responses, the MLR and serologic data indicate that there are still additional MLR and Lna genetic determinants outside the segment of Ir region putatively shared by B10.HTT and A.TH (Fig. 1a). It seems clear that in the long run B10.HTT may yield important new information about the genetic organization and function of the Ir region.

ACKNOWLEDGMENTS

We wish to thank Dr. Peter Démant (Institute for Experimental Biology and Genetics, Prague) for having supplied the strain B10.HTT. The skilled assistance of Miss A. M. Reynbeck is gratefully acknowledged.

REFERENCES

1. David CS, Shreffler DC, Frelinger JA: PNAS (in press)

2. Hauptfeld V, Klein D, Klein J: Science 181:167, 1973

3. Meo T, Vives J, Miggiano V, Shreffler DC: Transplant Proc 1:377, 1973

4. Meo T, Vives J, Rijnbeek AM, et al: Transplant Proc 5:1339, 1973

5. David DC, Shreffler DC: Tissue Antigens 2:241, 1972

6. Shreffler DC: in Palm J (ed): Isoantigens and Cells Interactions. Philadelphia, Wistar Institute Press, 1965, pp 11–19

7. Festenstein H, Abbasi K, Sachs JA, Oliver RTD: Transplant Proc 2:219, 1972

8. David CS, Shreffler DC: unpublished data

Mixed Lymphocyte Cultures (MLC) Between Serologically HL-A-identical Parent and Child and Between HL-A Homozygous and Heterozygous Individuals

By J. Dausset, M. Sasportes, and A. Lebrun

THE observation by Amos and Bach[1] and Yunis and Amos[2] that the MLC reaction could be governed by a gene closely linked to the second HL-A locus has been confirmed by several laboratories.[3-6] That this locus is distinct from the second HL-A locus and is not situated between the two HL-A loci is suggested by positive reactions observed between some HL-A-identical siblings and negative reactions between some HL-A-haploidentical siblings.[2,7,8] In order to clarify the relationship between MLC and HL-A loci, several laboratories have systematically studied the MLC reactions between pairs of serologically HL-A-identical unrelated individuals.[2,9,18] We have undertaken similar study in families where both parents[2,4,9,10,13,15,19-25] share a serologically identical HL-A haplotype.

In this simplified genetic situation, some of the offspring are heterozygous and possess the common haplotype, i.e., they are phenotypically HL-A-identical with one of their parents. Some other siblings are homozygous and serologically HL-A-compatible with both parents. In the present survey, we have pooled our 10 families with 22 other similar families reported in literature.

MATERIALS AND METHOD

Our material of HL-A genotyped families includes 10 families in which the parents share an HL-A haplotype. Four families (0110, 0325, 0225, and 0341) present the following situation: both parents are heterozygous for an identical HL-A haplotype with at least one heterozygous and one homozygous child for this particular haplotype. Families 0110, 0325, and 0225 have been reported earlier.[24,25] In five families (0222, 0308, 0226, 0221, and 0334), at least one parent was serologically identical with at least one child. In another family (No. 0343), there were three homozygous children but no heterozygous siblings. MLC reactions were performed in all possible combinations in the one- and two-way directions. They were repeated at least twice with different blood samples from each donor. The technique of the MLC test and criteria for positive reactions have been described in detail elsewhere.[7]

RESULTS

MLC Between Parent–Child Serologically HL-A-identical Situations

This situation was observed here in 9 families and in 22 other families in the literature. In our material, 4 were negative and 3 were positive in both directions. Three were nonreciprocal (Table 1). Of the 34 pairs studied in the literature[1,3,6,8,9,12,14,17-19,21-24] from 32 families, 15 were reciprocally negative and 9 were nonreciprocal with the nonresponding cells, including five times with the parent and four times with the child (Table 2).

MLC Between HL-A-heterozygous and -homozygous Cells (Parents or HL-A-haploidentical Siblings)

In these families, the reactions of the heterozygous cells (parents or HL-A-haploidentical siblings) against the homozygous cells are informative. The reactions observed in our families, as well as in those of the literature[4,7,10,18,21-25] are shown in Table 3. Among the 82 MLC of heterozygous cells responding against homozygous cells, 35 were weak and 1 was negative. In contrast, among the 78 MLC in the reverse

From the Institut de Recherches sur les Maladies du Sang, INSERM U93, Hôpital Saint-Louis, Paris, France.

Supported in part by NIH grant AI-9293.

©1973 by Grune & Stratton, Inc.

Table 1. MLC Between Phenotypically HL-A-identical Parent–Child Combinations (Nine Families)

Parent-shared HL-A Haplotypes	Father or Mother	One-Way MLC (Index) Parent → Child$_m$	Child → Parent$_m$
1, 8	F	1.8; 2.4	1.7; 2.9
1, 8	M	13	1.8
3, 7	F	1.0	1.2
3, 7	F	1.0	0.7
2, 5	F	1.2	8.5
	M	4.5	17.5
2, 12	F	11.3; 7.8	9.0; 16.6
	M	9.4; 13.0	9.0; 11.6
W24, W21	F	0.9	4.5
W30, W18	F	8.9	4.1
W29, 12	M	1.2	1.4

Table 2. Further Parent–Child MLC Results

	Parent-shared Haplotype	Number of Families With: Asymmetrical MLC Negative P → C	Asymmetrical MLC Negative C → P	Reciprocal Negative	Positive
Δ_+	1, 8	2	2	6 (43 ± 26)	4
Δ_+	1, x			1	
Δ_+	3, 7	1	2	4	1
Δ_+	W29, 12			1	
Δ_+	2, 12	1			2
	2, 7			1	
	2, W5			1	1
	W24, W21			1	
	2, 5	1			
	2, W15				1
	W30, W18				1

Δ = Gametic association or linkage disequilibrium between the two HL-A loci.

direction, only 3 were weak and 1 was negative.

MLC Reaction of the Same Parental Cell Responding Against Children Respectively Heterozygous and Homozygous for the Common Haplotype

In three families (Nos. 0110, 0325, and 0225), the reactions between serologically identical parent and child were negative. In contrast, the reactions of the same cells responding against the homozygous child were positive. In family No. 0341 the father did not react against his serologically identical child, but he reacted weakly against his homozygous children. The mother of family No. 0341 reacted against both heterozygous and homozygous children. Other cases published in the literature[10,18,23–25] are gathered in Table 4. Among the 18 cases studied there were instances where the reactions against the homozygous cells were clearly stronger than against the heterozygous cells.

DISCUSSION

The families in which the parent shared an HL-A haplotype are of particular interest for the understanding of the genetics and physiology of the MLC gene(s); 32 such families (including our 10) were studied. The probable linkage disequilibrium between the MLC locus and the second HL-A locus was suggested by the negative results sometimes observed between unrelated serologically HL-A-identical individuals; 158 pairs were studied by several au-

Table 3. MLC Reactions Between HL-A-homozygous and -heterozygous Cells in 17 Families

Homozygous Haplotypes	No Families	Homozygous → Heterozygous: Strong	Weak	Negative	Heterozygous → Homozygous: Strong	Weak	Negative
HL-AI, 8	6	29	0	0	13	15	1
HL-A3, 7	7	23	3	1	19	10	0
HL-A2, 7	1	4	0	0	4	0	0
HL-A2, 12	1	—	—	—	2	0	0
HL-A2, 5	1	12	0	0	8	4	0
HL-A3, W5	1	6	0	0	0	6	0
Totals	17	74	3	1	46	35	1

Table 4. Parents Responding Against Children Heterozygous and Homozygous for an HL-A Haplotype Shared by Parents

Shared Haplotype		Against Heterozygous	Against Homozygous
HL-A1, 8*	F	865 c.p.m.	795 c.p.m.
	M	2150; 949 c.p.m.	1440; 1761 c.p.m.
HL-A1, 8‡	F	1.8; 2.4	4.4†
HL-A3, 7‡	F	1.0†	21.7
HL-A3, 7‡	F	1.0	3.0; 6.4
HL-A2, 5‡	F	1.2	2.1; 1.5; 1.7; 2
	M	4.5	4.8; 5.9; 4.4; 5
HL-A3, 7§	M	290 c.p.m.	1,444 c.p.m.
HL-A3, 7§	F	506 c.p.m.	1,483 c.p.m.
	M	180 c.p.m.	768 c.p.m.
HL-A1, 8¶	F	2.0; 2.1	10.7
	M	0.4	1.9
HL-A1, 8¶	F	27	25; 38
HL-A3, 7¶	F	39	404
	M	31; 12	30
HL-A2, 7¶	M	15	213; 537
HL-A3, 7¶	M	91; 72	75

*Reference 9; †Index.
‡Reference 24 and this article.
§Reference 17.
¶Reference 22.

thors.[2,9-18] The total of negative results is 6.9%; however, when HL-A1, 8 individuals are analyzed separately, this figure rises to 10% (Table 5).

The same approach was possible using serologically identical parent–child combinations; 34 pairs* were studied where 15 combinations were reciprocally negative, mostly when the HL-A1, 8 or 3, 7 haplotypes were involved. These haplotypes are known for their high degree of linkage disequilibrium in caucasoid between the two HL-A SD loci (Table 2). For HL-A1, 8 haplotype the percentage of reciprocal negative reactions was 43 ± 26.

The comparison of the two figures 10% and 43% is suggestive of a strong linkage disequilibrium between the MLC locus and the second HL-A locus of about the same order as the linkage disequilibrium between the two HL-A loci.

When heterozygous cells respond against HL-A-compatible homozygous cells, a positive reaction is almost always observed (only 1 negative reaction out of 82); however, this reaction is frequently weak (35 reactions). A positive reaction in such a compatible situation has also been found in mice[26,27] and in pigs,[28] but not in rats.[29] By contrast, in the reverse incompatibility situation the reactions are almost always strongly positive (74 of 78) (Table 3).

The most paradoxical observation is the reaction of one same parental cell responding in most of the cases (10 of 17 combinations) more strongly against the homozygous-compatible cells of one offspring than against the heterozygous serologically identical cells of other siblings. This fact is now well established. There are several possible interpretations. The existence of a recessive MLC gene is possible but unlikely in view of the usual codominant character of the alloantigens. An allelic gene interaction is a variant of the recessive hypothesis. The intervention of another gene not closely linked to HL-A appears to be unlikely, since most HL-A-identical siblings

*The MLC between one parent and several HL-A-identical siblings is considered as only one pair.

Table 5. MLC Between Unrelated HL-A Pheno-identical Individuals

HL-A Phenotypes	No. Individuals Studied	No. Pairs Studied	No. Negative Reciprocal MLC	Percent
1, 8, 3, 7	32	89	9	10.1
1, 8, 2, 12	16	19	2	10.5
1, 8 and 2 other antigens	17	17	0	
3, 7 and 2 other antigens	24	15	0	0.0
5 other phenotypes	14	18	0	
Total	103	158	11	6.9

are MLC negative. It has also been suggested that the mitomycin-treated stimulating cells in contact with incompatible cells may release a mitogenic factor that induces the division of the responding cells.[30] Another suggestion is that the heterozygous AB cells, deprived of anti-B alloreceptors, reacted against this receptor, which was present on the cell surface of the homozygous AA cells.[31]

We have proposed[24,25] an alternative interpretation based on these paradoxical observations, as well as on the hybrid effect of Snell[31] and the numerous anomalies of the MLC (and GvH) when considered as an immunologic reaction. According to this hypothesis, the MLC may be a recognition gene (AB recognizing AA as non-self, either by complementary structures or by cytoplasmic components), analogous to those that are known in plants[33-35] or in lower animals.[33,36,37] Eijsvoogel's observation[8] that MLC activation is a prerequisite for lymphocyte killing is in keeping with the possibility that the immunologic machinery currently present developed during evolution from such an archaic form of defense.

The MLC genes would act as a starter to mount as rapidly as possible a vigorous response against the easiest and most dangerous parasitic, which are the other individuals of the same or close species. This conception would explain that the number of cells responding corresponds rather to a secondary than to a primary response.

REFERENCES

1. Amos DB, Bach FH: JEM 128:623–637, 1968
2. Yunis EJ, Amos DB: PNAS 68:3031, 1971
3. Dupont B, Nielsen LS, Svejgaard A: Lancet 2:1336, 1971
4. Gatti RA, Meuwissen HJ, Terasaki PI, Good RA: Tissue Antigens 1:239, 1971
5. Lebrun A, Sasportes M, Lebrun D, Dausset J: C R Acad Sci (Paris) 273:2130, 1971
6. Eijsvoogel VP, Koning L, de Groot-Kooy L, et al: Transplant Proc 4:199, 1972
7. Sasportes M, Lebrun A, Rapaport FT, Dausset J: Transplant Proc 4:209, 1972
8. Eijsvoogel VP, Van Rood JJ, Du Toit ED, Schellekens PTA: Eur J Immunol 2:413, 1972
9. Meuwissen HJ, Terasaki PJ, Rodey G, et al: in Histocompatibility Testing 1970. Copenhagen, Munksgaard, 1970, p 423
10. Eijsvoogel VP, Schellekens PTA, Breur-Vriesendorp B, et al: Histocompatibility Testing 1970, Copenhagen, Munksgaard, 1970, p 523
11. Van Rood JJ, Eijsvoogel VP: Lancet 1:698, 1970
12. Eijsvoogel VP, Schellekens PTA, Breur-Vriesendorp B, et al: Transplant Proc 3:85, 1971
13. Sorensen SF, Staub-Nielsen L: Acta Pathol Microb Scand 78B:719, 1970
14. Kissmeyer-Nielsen F, Svejgaard A, Sorensen LS, et al: Nature 228:63, 1970
15. Sengar DPS, Mickey MR, Myhre BA, et al: Transfusion 2:251, 1971
16. Bach ML, Day E, Myhre BA, et al: Tissue Antigens 1:39, 1971
17. Koch CT, Frederiks E, Eijsvoogel VP, Van Rood JJ: Lancet 2:1334, 1971
18. Mempel W, Grosse-Wilde H, Albert E, Thierfelder S: Transplant Proc 5:401, 1973
19. Bach JH, Amos DB, Science 156:1506, 1967
20. Seigler HF, Ward FE, Amos DB, et al: J Exp Med 133:411, 1971
21. Rudolph RH, Mickelson EM, Thomas ED: Transplantation 13:434, 1972
22. Thompson JS, Parmely MJ, Flink RJ, Severson CD: J Exp Med 135:596, 1972
23. Thompson JS, Flink RJ, et al: Transplant Proc 5:1763, 1973
24. Dausset J, Lebrun A, Sasportes M: C R Acad Sci (Paris) 275D:2279, 1972

25. Lebrun A, Sasportes M, Dausset J: Transplant Proc 5:363, 1973
26. Adler WH, Takiguchi T, Marsh B, Smith RT: J Immunol 105:984, 1970
27. Huemer RP, Keller LG, Lee Kyung-Dong, Transplantation 6:706, 1968
28. Vaiman M, Arnoux A, Nizza P: Tissue Antigens 3:3, 1973
29. Wilson DB: J Exp Med 126:625, 1967
30. Kennedy JC: personal communication
31. Ramseier H, Lindermann J: Transplant Rev 10:57, 1972
32. Snell GD: J Natl Cancer Inst 21:843, 1958
33. Burnet FM: Nature 232:230, 1971
34. Lewis D: Proc Roy Soc 140B:127
35. Rizet G, Esser K: C R Acad Sci (Paris) 237:760, 1953
36. Theodor JL: Nature 227:690, 1970
37. Oka H: in: Profiles of Japanese Science and Scientists. Tokyo, Kodanska, 1970, p 198

MLR in Families With an HL-A Haplotype Shared by Parents: Recombination Between SD2 and LD2 and Possible Evidence for an LD3 Locus

By M. Sasportes, C. Mawas, A. Bernard, Y. Christen, and J. Dausset

STUDIES of two families already published[1,2] with an HL-A haplotype common to both parents gave the following results in macro-MLR: a negative MLR between two HL-A-heterozygous cells, a positive MLR with a heterozygous cell reacting against a homozygous one. This paradoxical response was also observed on a weaker scale in micro-MLR and will be discussed mainly on the basis of the peculiar state of immunization of these families, and on the possible existence of an LD3 locus, involved in MLR, in at least one of these families, where an LD2 recombinant outside the SD2 locus can clearly be considered from the results.

MATERIALS

(1) Family Co (No. 0110): the father A and the mother B share the same haplotype HL-A1, 8; D and E are SD-identical children and no serologic incompatibility between them and their father A exists, since the mother has transmitted the common HL-A haplotype to both children. The child C is homozygous for this haplotype. In addition, the father received skin grafts from D, E, and C in 1968;[3] the allografts were performed according to the standard methods of Rapaport et al;[4] they were accorded survival times of 15, 18, and 15 days, respectively. Nineteen months after the grafts, the father was immunized by 5 leukocyte injections (50×10^6 each) from D, producing a leukoagglutinating antibody that reacted positively with 89 unrelated cells of 108 tested. The HL-A specificity of this antibody has not been detected so far. The micro-MLR were performed 40 mo after the last immunization.

(2) Family Le (No. 0225): the haplotype HL-A3, 7 is common to both parents. Two siblings are SD-identical with their parents: E with the father, F with the mother; C and D, who inherited the common specificities HL-A3, 7 from the parents, are homozygous for this haplotype. The father received skin grafts from C and F that survived 19 and 5 days, respectively, after one leukocyte injection (15×10^6) from the mother. The micro-MLR were performed 45 mo after the skin graft rejections.

METHOD

The micro-MLR technique used was that of Hartzman et al.[5] with slight modifications. Heparinized blood (liquemine: 50 U/ml of blood) drawn in sterile flasks is half diluted with physiological water and then layered over a Ficoll Angiocontrix* gradient according to the method of Thorsby and Bratlie[6] in glass centrifuge tubes; one part of Ficoll Angiocontrix* is used for two parts of diluted blood. The tubes are spun at 18°C for 15 min providing 800 g at the interface. Mononuclear cells are removed with plasma above, at the interface, pooled and centrifuged at 300 g 10 min in conic glass tubes; the supernatant is poured off, the cell pellet resuspended in medium 199 Hepes (Gibco); this suspension is divided according to ratio of responding cells (RC) to stimulating cells (SC), as needed; mitomycin C (25 μg/ml) is added to the SC, which are incubated at 37°C for 30 min. RC and SC are then washed twice by centrifugation at 300 g and 180 g for 10 min. The cells, resuspended in the final medium RPMI-1640 (Gibco) with 20% human heat-inactivated pooled plasma from nonimmunized male donors, are counted (monos and polys separate); they are adjusted at the following concentrations: 10^6 monocytes/ml for the RC, 4×10^6 leukocytes/ml for the SC, and are distributed in microplates (Linbro ISFB 96 TC); 0.1 ml/each RC and SC/well using a Hamilton syringe with a repeating dispenser for distribution.

The cultures are incubated for 5 days at 37°C in a 5% CO_2 humidified incubator. On the fifth day, two μCi of ^{3}H-thymidine (SA, 1 Ci/mM) are added to each microplate well; 16 to 18 hr later the reaction is stopped by placing the microplates in a 4° refrigerator. The cultures are finally precipitated on a microprecipitator (Otto Hiller, Madison, Wisc.); the filters (Whatman) are put into glass tubes. After 1 hr at 45°C, 3 ml of scintillation liquid (toluene, PPO,

---

*Lotalamate de sodium, Laboratoires A. Guerbet, France.

From the Laboratoire d'Immuno-Hématologie, INSERM U93, Institut de Recherches sur les Maladies du Sang, Hôpital Saint-Louis, Paris, France.

Supported in part by grant A1-CA-9293, National Institutes of Health, Bethesda, Md.

©1973 by Grune & Stratton, Inc.

Table 1. Family Co (No. 0110); Heterozygous vs. Homozygous Combinations

EXPERIMENTS	1		2		3	
	CPM	I	CPM	I	CPM	I
AAm	2220 ± 559		537 ± 115		581 ± 210	
ACm	11029 ± 1581	5.0	11387 ± 1600	21	6010 ± 80	10. 3
BBm	637 ± 470		353 ± 156		764 ± 54	
BCm	882 ± 36	1.4	1144 ± 479	3.0	2363 ± 143	3.1
DDm	780 ± 250		374 ± 63		2171 ± 422	
DCm	2762 ± 169	3.5	721 ± 204	2.0	4897 ± 292	2.2
EEm	489 ± 112		788 ± 50		1291 ± 477	
ECm	1914 ± 74	3.9	2939 ± 259	3.7	3305 ± 145	2.6

GENOTYPES : A = 1,8/W32, W10 ; B = 1,8/W23,12; C = 1,8/1,8 ; D and E = W32,W10/1,8

I = index = MLR / CONTROL ; m = mitomycin treated cells

POPOP) are added; the tubes are placed in plastic counting vials that are processed in an Intertechnic liquid scintillation counter (model SL 36). The results are expressed as counts per minute (c.p.m.) and represent mean values obtained from quadruplicate cultures for each test. Family Co was tested three times and family Le two times on separate occasions.

The criteria for the interpretation of an MLR as negative or positive are based upon the results of MLR performed between 44 pairs of SD-identical siblings in whom the mean stimulation index was less than 2 in the one-way MLR. Values less than 2 are therefore negative; between 2 and 5, they are considered as borderline positive and above 5 as positive.

RESULTS

Family Co (No. 0110): two types of unexpected results were obtained. As can be seen in Table 1, in all the combinations where the homozygous C is the stimulating cell and the heterozygous cells of the family are the responding cells (ACm, BCm, DCm,

Table 2. Family Co (No. 0110): Heterozygous vs. Heterozygous Combinations

EXPERIMENTS	1		2		3	
	CPM	I	CPM	I	CPM	I
AAm	2220 ± 559		537 ± 115		581 ± 210	
ADm	4690 ± 620	2.0	2047 ± 328	3.8	1744 ± 309	3.0
AEm	302 ± 82	0.1	714 ± 215	1.4	1742 ± 270	2.9
DDm	780 ± 250		374 ± 63		2171 ± 422	
DAm	2715 ± 550	3,5	465 ± 76	1.2	5221 ± 315	2.4
EEm	489 ± 112		788 ± 50		1291 ± 477	
EAm	3046 ± 474	6.2	1349 ± 273	1.7	1194 ± 421	0.9
EDm	935 ± 800	1.9	822 ± 200	1.0	1144 ± 414	0.9
DEm	938 ± 290	1.2	458 ± 90	1.2	520 ± 190	0.2

GENOTYPES : A = 1, 8/ W32, W10 ; D and E = W32, W10/ 1, 8

I = index = MLR / CONTROL ; m = mitomycin treated cells

Table 3. Family Le (No. 0225): Heterozygous vs. Homozygous Combinations

EXPERIMENTS	1 CPM	I	2 CPM	I
AAm	368 ± 57		991 ± 86	
ADm	1428 ± 427	4	10571 ± 79	10
ACm	530 ± 176	1.4	1222 ± 126	1.2
BBm	350 ± 152		266 ± 46	
BCm	664 ± 164	1.8	452 ± 62	1.7
BDm	637 ± 25	1.8	1168 ± 120	4.3
EEm	376 ± 67		374 ± 40	
ECm	835 ± 46	2.2	1081 ± 169	2.8
EDm	1880 ± 85	5	4730 ± 520	12
CCm	366 ± 32		1413 ± 152	
CDm	2684 ± 998	7	5645 ± 662	4
DDm	370 ± 88		2000 ± 189	
DCm	607 ± 185	1.6	3394 ± 440	1.7

GENOTYPES : A = 2, 12/3,7 B = W24, X/3,7 C and D = 3,7/3,7 E = 2,12/3,7

I = index = $\frac{\text{MLR}}{\text{CONTROL}}$ m = mitomycin treated cells

ECm), a positive MLR response occurs; however, only with A as responding cell is the MLR clearly positive in three successive experiments; the other reactions are borderline positive according to our criteria. Table 2 shows that the two siblings D and E, phenotypically SD-identical to the father, behave differently as stimulating cells against the father responding cells in the three experiments performed: ADm is always slightly positive, while AEm is negative. Conversely DAm, EAm, and EDm, as well as DEm, are negative.

Family Le (No. 0225): As can be seen in Table 3, the heterozygous father A reacts differently against the siblings C and D, both homozygous for the haplotype HL-A3, 7: ADm is positive in two experiments, while ACm is negative. The other heterozygous members of the family are either negative or slightly positive toward the two homozygous cells C and D. Sibling E, phenotypically SD-identical to the father A, responds differently toward the two identical sibs C and D: ECm is slightly positive, while EDm is clearly positive. Furthermore, between the two homozygous cells C and D, a unilateral MLR is found: CDm is positive, while DCm is negative. As shown in Table 4, F, although phenotypically SD-identical to the mother, reacts positively against B, but does not react against the homozygous cell C, while FDm is slightly positive. In addition, F behaves as a stimulating cell like the 3, 7-homozygous cell C, but not like D toward the other allogeneic cells of the family. The combinations BFm, CFm, and DFm are clearly negative. Therefore in all combinations involving D as stimulating cell, D behaves as if it may possess an additional factor relevant to the MLR.

DISCUSSION

These families present two peculiarities: (1) The parents share the same haplotype HL-A1, 8 in one case, HL-A3, 7 in the other case; the frequencies for these haplotypes in the French population are, respectively: expected 0.0546, 0.0294; observed 0.0505, 0.0349.[7] Apparently in these two families the LD2 locus on the shared haplo-

Table 4. Family Le (No. 0225): Combinations With F as Responding or Stimulating Cell Against the Other Family-Member Cells

EXPERIMENTS	1 CPM	1 I	2 CPM	2 I
FFm	374 ± 56		577 ± 62	
FBm	17777 ± 3721	47	13575 ± 224	23
FCm	377 ± 50	1.0	ND	
FDm	1248 ± 298	3.3	ND	
CCm	366 ± 32		1413 ± 152	
CFm	561 ± 112	1.2	1997 ± 210	1.4
DDm	370 ± 88		2000 ± 189	
DFm	681 ± 36	1.8	4343 ± 610	2.2
AFm	1079 ± 303	3.0	1630 ± 230	1.6
BFm	561 ± 112	1.2	ND	
EFm	731 ± 146	1.9	1122 ± 94	3.0

GENOTYPES = A = 2, 12/3,7 B = W24,X/3,7 C and D = 3,7/3,7 E = 2, 12/3,7

F = W24, X/3,7.

I = index = $\frac{\text{MLR}}{\text{CONTROL}}$; m = mitomycin treated cell.

type is identical in both parents, since the MLR performed between at least one of the phenotypically SD-identical individuals are negative. These results can be explained by the existence of a strong linkage disequilibrium between the SD2 and LD2 loci, as already suggested by negative MLR obtained either between SD-identical unrelated individuals[8–10] or among SD-identical parent–child combinations, especially with the haplotypes HL-A1, 8 and HL-A3, 7 (see reference 11). (2) The fathers have been immunized by skin grafts and leukocyte injections.

The results will be discussed in view of these two peculiarities. The micro-MLR results in family Co (No. 0110) confirm the paradoxical reaction already described with the macrotechnique: the heterozygous cell A gives a clear positive MLR with the homozygous cell C as stimulating cell and a negative MLR with the phenotypically SD-identical cell E; these results cannot be due to an LD2 activation, since we have to assume an LD2 identity of the paternal and maternal shared haplotype to explain the negative MLR in combination AEm. Besides, the combinations BCm, DCm, and ECm are borderline positive. There is no way to determine whether these positive or borderline positive results have a biological meaning. The immunization of A may only account for the higher intensity of the MLR response seen in ACm, but it is generally admitted that the immunization does not increase the level of the MLR response when the test is performed in standard conditions. The immunization definitely cannot account for the borderline positive responses obtained in BCm, ECm, or DCm. The fact that the supernatant removed from CmAm, added to cells A, induces the transformation of A, while the supernatant from Cm alone does not (unpublished data), could be relevant to the hypothesis of a blastogenic factor released from the mitomycin-treated homozygous cells C leading to the proliferation of the responding incompatible cells A; this cannot exclude other possibilities such as recessive gene, allelic interaction, or recognition by cytoplasmic incompatibility.[11]

The response of A toward D and E is also unexpected since both D and E have received the same haplotype HL-A1, 8 from the mother and are therefore phenotypically SD-identical to the father A: AEm is negative, while ADm is slightly positive. An antigenic determinant probably serologically defined independent from SD1 and SD2, located on the HL-A chromosome at a recombinant distance or on another chromosome, could lead to an antigenic-like response in MLR, since A has been repeatedly immunized by leucocyte injections from D. The same determinant present on C could also partially explain the ACm-positive MLR. This concept is supported by the CML data presented by Mawas et al.[12] The complete demonstration of this hypothesis requires the in vivo immunization of E by D or C.

Two types of unexpected results can be seen in family Le (No. 0225): the first concerns sib F: although F is phenotypically SD-identical to the mother B but SD-different from sibs C and D, the combination FCm is MLR negative and FDm is borderline positive. These results can be explained if F is considered as an LD2 recombinant where the d haplotype has acquired the LD2 from the a^m haplotype through a maternal crossing-over. Other laboratories,[13–17] as well as ours,[1] have already reported similar examples of LD2 recombinants.

Furthermore, three other unexpected responses are present in this family: (1) the positivity of ADm contrasting with the ACm-negative MLR; (2) the slight positivity of FDm contrasting with the negativity of FCm; (3) the unilateral MLR between the SD-identical sibs C and D, CDm being positive. Thus D seems to possess something coming from the mother that C does not possess.

The following explanation can be proposed (Fig. 1): besides LD1 situated between SD1 and SD2 and LD2 located outside SD2, one can postulate a third LD

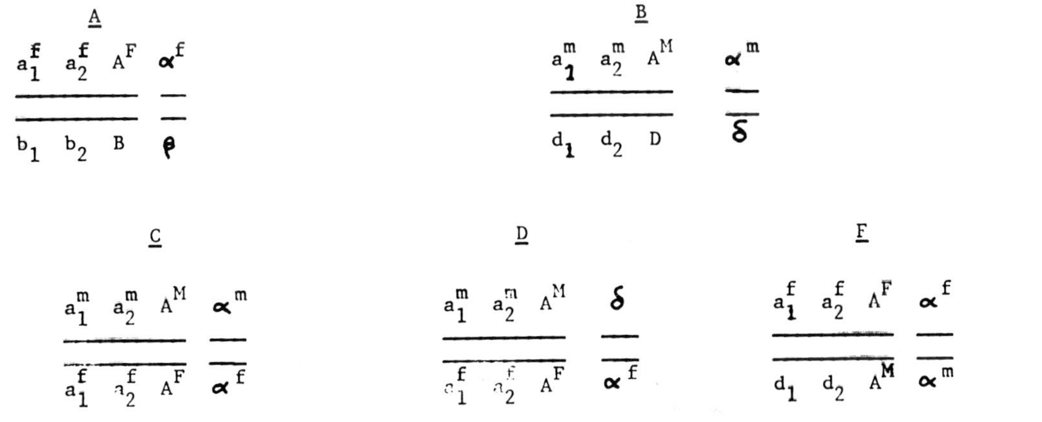

- SD_1 SD_2 ALLELES : $A = a_1^f\, a_2^f / b_1\, b_2$, $B = a_1^m\, a_2^m / d_1\, d_2$, C and $D = a_1^m\, a_2^m / a_1^f\, a_2^f$
  $F = a_1^f\, a_2^f / d_1\, d_2$.
- LD_2 ALLELES : $A = A^F/B$, $B = A^M/D$, C and $D = A^M/A^F$, $F = A^F/A^M$
- LD_3 ALLELES : $A = \alpha^f/\beta$, $B = \alpha^m/\delta$, $C = \alpha^m/\alpha^f$ $D = \delta/\alpha^f$, $F = \alpha^f/\alpha^m$

Fig. 1. F as an LD2 recombinant; D as possible evidence for an LD3.

locus tentatively named LD3, weaker than LD2. This LD3 locus could be located either on the HL-A complex at a recombinant distance or on another chromosome. The former hypothesis needs to suppose a maternal recombination on the HL-A chromosome but is more likely than the latter in view of the necessary identity of the LD3 genes α^f and α^m situated in this case on the shared HL-A complex. The location of LD3 would be, then, outside SD2 and close to LD2, as indicated by the common segregation of A^M and α^m in sib F after recombination between SD2 and LD2.

In conclusion, the extensive study of the MLR in two familes in which both parents shared an HL-A haplotype (1) confirms a weak MLR positivity when an SD heterozygous cell reacts against an SD homozygous cell, (2) gives some indications that in vivo immunization can induce a positive or borderline positive MLR without apparent LD2 differences, (3) brings a new example of SD2/LD2 recombination, and (4) favors the existence of a third LD3 locus possibly situated on the HL-A complex close to the LD2 locus and outside SD2.

ACKNOWLEDGMENTS

We wish to express our gratitude to the volunteer families who have generously given of themselves to make possible the investigations described in this report. We also wish to acknowledge Dr. and Mrs. A. Lebrun for their dedicated work with these families, Mrs. J. Roullier and A. Soulie for the excellence of their technical assistance, and the secretaries, Mrs. M. Marceau and A. Touboulic, for their kind help.

REFERENCES

1. Sasportes M, Lebrun A, Rapaport FT, Dausset J: Transplant Proc 4:209, 1972
2. Lebrun A, Sasportes M, Dausset J: Transplant Proc 1:363, 1973
3. Dausset J, Rapaport FT, Legrand L, et al: in Terasaki PI (ed): Histocompatibility Testing, 1970. Copenhagen, Munksgaard, 1970, p 381
4. Rapaport FT, Lawrence HS, Thomas L, et al: J Clin Invest 41:2166, 1962
5. Hartzman RJ, Segall M, Bach ML, Bach FH: Transplant Proc 3:268, 1970
6. Thorsby E, Bratlie A: in Terasaki PI (ed): Histocompatibility Testing, 1970. Copenhagen, Munksgaard, 1970, p 655
7. Dausset J, Colombani J, Legrand L, et al: in Dausset J, Colombani J (eds): Histocompatibility Testing, 1972. Copenhagen, Munksgaard, 1973
8. Eijsvoogel VP, Schellekens PTA, Breur-Vriesendorp B, et al: in Terasaki PI (ed): Histocompatibility Testing, 1970. Copenhagen, Munksgaard, 1970, p 523
9. Bach FH, Day E, Bach ML, et al: Tissue Antigens 1:39, 1971
10. Mempel W, Grosse-Wilde H, Albert E, Thierfelder S: Transplant Proc 5:401, 1973
11. Dausset J, Sasportes M, Lebrun A: Transplant Proc 5:1511, 1973
12. Mawas C, Sasportes M, Christen Y, et al: Transplant Proc 5:1683, 1973
13. Amos DB, Bach FH: J Exp Med 128:623, 1968
14. Bach FH, Albertini RJ, Amos DB, et al: Transplant Proc 1:339, 1969
15. Plate JM, Ward FE, Amos DB: in Terasaki PI (ed): Histocompatibility Testing, 1970. Copenhagen Munskgaard, 1970, p 153
16. Yunis EJ, Plate JM, Ward FE, et al: Transplant Proc 3:118, 1970
17. Eijsvoogel VP, Van Rood JJ, Toit ED, Schellekens PTA: Eur J Immunol 2:413, 1972

A Second Locus Determining Human MLC Response: Separate Lymphocyte Populations Recognize the Products of Each Different MLC-Locus Allele in Allogeneic Combinations

By E. Thorsby, H. Hirschberg, and Astri Helgesen

RECENT reports suggest that antigenic products other than HL-A are responsible for a positive mixed lymphocyte culture (MLC) response.[1,2] The most important products seem to be determined by a locus (or loci) closely linked to the second HL-A locus, the MLC locus.[3,4] Recently a second MLC locus has also been proposed.[4,5] The following results, from a family we have studied, also strongly suggest the existence of a separate second locus (or loci) of importance for allogeneic cell interactions in vitro. This second MLC locus also seems to be part of the major histocompatibility system (MHS) chromosomal region.

MATERIALS AND METHOD

HL-A Typing. HL-A typing[6] was performed with a battery of 54 highly selected lymphocytotoxic antisera whereby 10 antigens from the first and 21 antigens from the second segregant series could be identified.

Micro-MLC Tests. Our method has been described in detail elsewhere.[7] Briefly, 0.15 × 10^6 responding lymphocytes prepared by Ficoll Isopaque flotation are mixed with an equal amount of mitomycin-treated stimulating cells in 0.2 ml of medium 199 supplemented with antibiotics and 20% pooled AB serum in the wells of microtiter plates. The cultures are set up in triplicate, labeled with ^{14}C-thymidine after 96 hr, and harvested 24 hr later by suction on glass-fiber filters.

Tritiated Thymidine Hot-Pulse Technique. Details of this method have been presented.[8] In short, 1.5 × 10^6 responding cells and 3 × 10^6 mitomycin-treated stimulating cells are mixed in 2 ml of supplemented medium 199. 5 μCi of ^{3}H-thymidine is added to each culture after 48 and 72 hr of incubation. Lymphocytes proliferating in response to initial stimulating cells incorporate a lethal dose of ^{3}H-thymidine and are eliminated from the culture. 24 hr after the last pulse the cultures were washed and resuspended in fresh medium. The remaining cells were subsequently used as responding cells in secondary micro-MLC tests, employing additional mitomycin-treated cells from the initial stimulating cell donor or different third-party donors. The degree of proliferation was measured by uptake of ^{14}C-thymidine added 72 hr later and the secondary cultures were harvested 96 hr after initiation.

Responding cells used in control cultures were first incubated with ^{3}H-thymidine for 48 hr, but in the absence of stimulating cells. This was followed by secondary stimulation identical to the test cultures.

RESULTS

Ordinary MLC Tests

Family G.O. was investigated because one of the children (C_1) is a candidate for kidney transplantation. The results of two different MLC tests performed with an interval of 3 mo, are given in Table 1. HL-A typing data of the family are also shown in the table. The father is dead, but his most probable HL-A types are indicated in parentheses. Children 2, 3, and 5 are MHS-identical, as witnessed by HL-A identity and reciprocal MLC nonstimulation. Children 1 and 4 are also HL-A-identical, but nevertheless show strong MLC stimulation toward each other. In addition, mitomycin-treated cells from child 4 were not able to stimulate cells from child 2, 3, or 5. The most likely explanation is a paternal recombination between the HL-A and the strong MLC loci, whereby child 4 inherited the paternal haplotypic HL-A combination 3,7 together with MLC-locus allele designated x. He would, therefore, have the

---

From the Tissue Typing Laboratory, Rikshospitalet University Hospital, Oslo, Norway.

Supported by grants from the Norwegian Research Council for Science and the Humanities, and Anders Jahre's Fund for the Promotion of Science.

©1973 by Grune & Stratton, Inc.

Table 1. Recombination Between HL-A and MLC and Possible Evidence for Second MLC Locus

Stimulating Cells	Responding Cells						MLC Alleles	
	M	C_1	C_2	C_3	C_4	C_5	First	Second
[F 2,W15/(3,7)]							x/y	a/b
Mm 3,7/28,W10	86–130	1652– 846	1511	617	1730–1828	1311–1160	z/v	b/c
C_1m (3,7)/3,7	1954–781	233– 415	1765	1663	4864–1347	3034–1614	y/z	b/b
C_2m 2,W15/3,7	564	1818	329	239	598	159	x/z	a/b
C_3m 2,W15/3,7	888	2387	257	202	558	215	x/z	a/b
C_4m (3,7)/3,7	1456–613	2262–2034	413	228	106– 112	175– 159	x/z	b/b
C_5m 2,W15/3,7	1204–921	2707–2919	221	156	763–1058	64– 157	x/z	a/b

All values are c.p.m.; first and second entries are results from separate experiments.
SE; usually $<10\%$.
Mitomycin controls: Mm, C_1m: 109; C_4m, C_5m: 5.

MLC-locus alleles designated x/z and thus be MLC-locus-identical to children 2, 3, and 5 (see right part of Table 1). However, responding cells from child 4 were clearly stimulated by mitomycin-treated cells from child 2, 3, or 5. This indicates the effects of other antigenic structures than those determined by the strong MLC locus. These structures could be products of a second MLC locus, situated somewhere else in the MHS chromosomal region. To explain the lack of reciprocal stimulation between cells from C_4 on the one hand and cells from C_2, C_3, or C_5 on the other, one has further to postulate that the father and mother share one allele (b) at this second MLC locus. Child 4 thus becomes homozygous b/b and children 2, 3, and 5 heterozygous a/b. This highly theoretical explanation is outlined at the extreme right of the table.

Hot-Pulse MLC Tests

In order to test this hypothesis, ^{3}H-thymidine hot-pulse MLC experiments were employed. We first investigated whether it was possible to eliminate the proliferating responding cells with specificity for the products of the strong or first MLC locus. Families were selected in which the members unambiguously differed for one or two complete MHS haplotypes, as revealed by HL-A typing data and ordinary MLC tests. In these experiments, the whole MHS haplotypes in a family are designated a, b, c, and d. The results from one of our experiments are depicted in Fig. 1. It can be seen that eliminating, in a hot-pulse MLC, the responding cells from C_1 (haplotypes a/c) toward C_2 (a/d) also eliminated the secondary stimulation response toward C_3 (c/d). More important, the secondary stimulation response toward C_4 (b/d), who thus only shares one haplotype (d) with the initial stimulating cell donor C_2, was reduced to about 50% of control values. Studies in other families gave similar results. It appears that separate populations of lymphocytes recognize the antigenic products of each MHS haplotype. This was further corroborated in other experiments where we were able to completely eliminate the response of C_1 (a/c) toward C_4 (b/d) by using a mixture of stimulating cells from two sibs (b/c and a/d) in the initial hot-pulse MLC. Details of these studies are presented elsewhere.[9]

Similar experiments were then performed in family G.O. We investigated whether it was possible to eliminate the responding cells with specificity for products of the first MLC locus and still obtain a response in MLC tests with cells that differ for the hypothetical second MLC locus. Figure 2 shows that lymphocytes from child 1 (tentatively designated by/bz at his MLC loci) are clearly stimulated with mitomycin-treated cells from children 4 and 5, the mother, and unrelated control donor X (open columns). After stimulation of responding cells from C_1 with mitomycin-

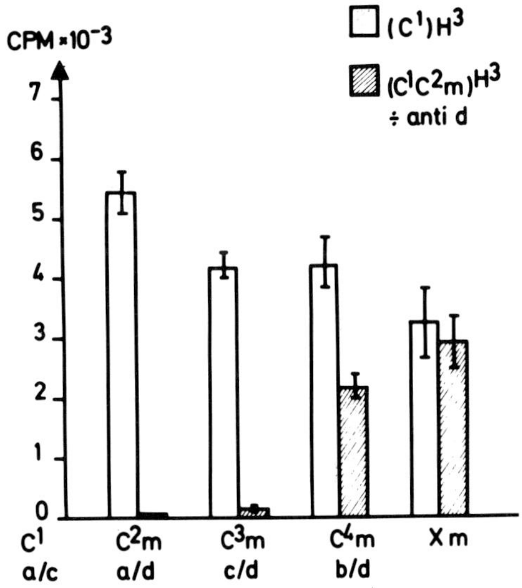

Fig. 1. Hot-pulse MLC experiments in a family; a, b, c, and d designate the whole MHS haplotype as determined by HL-A typing and ordinary MLC tests. The mean response against different mitomycin-treated cells before (white bars) and after (cross-hatched bars) a hot-pulse MLC involving responding cells from C_1 (a/c) and stimulating cells from C_2 (a/d) is shown in c.p.m. ± SE. Autologous controls have been subtracted before plotting [$(C_1)^{3H}$ = 248 ± 35; $(C_1C_4m)^{3H}$ = 397 ± 43].

treated cells from C_4 in a hot-pulse MLC (shaded columns in the figure), the response toward products of MLC allele x was eliminated, as shown by the lack of a restimulation response with new mitomycin-treated cells from C_4. The response toward cells from C_5 is reduced but not eliminated, in clear contrast to the results obtained in the other families. The structures on cells from C_5, which can possibly cause stimulation of C_1, after elimination of the responsive cells to products of allele x, are the products of allele a at a second MLC locus or HL-A incompatibility. The result, therefore, supports the assumption that products of other loci than those determined by the first (or strong) MLC locus cause MLC stimulation in this family.

As mentioned above, if a second MLC locus is responsible for the odd results obtained in this family, it was necessary to postulate that the mother and father had one identical second-locus allele b. Experiments were, therefore, constructed to test this assumption.

Children 4 and 5 are assumed to share one complete MHS haplotype (bz) and to differ with respect to antigenic products determined by a second MLC locus on the other (ax and bx respectively; see left part of Fig. 3). The bx product is paternal, while the bz product is assumed to be maternal.

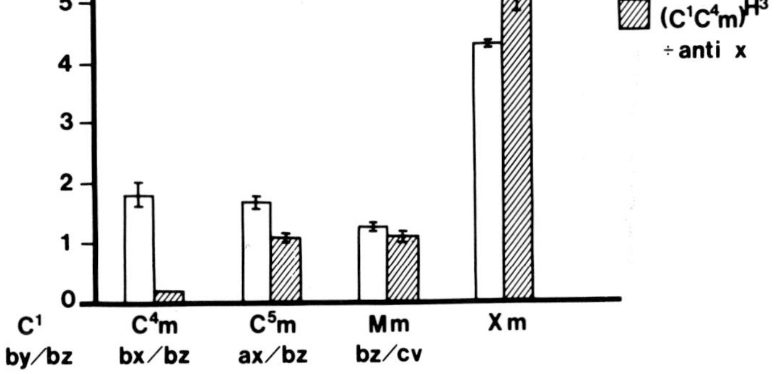

Fig. 2. Hot-pulse MLC test in family G.O.; x, y, z, and v are used to assign different alleles at the strong MLC locus; a, b, c, and d designate different alleles at another MHS locus responsible for MLC activation. The mean response against different mitomycin-treated cells before (open columns) and after a hot-pulse MLC (shaded columns) between responding cells from C_1 and stimulating cells from C_4 is shown in c.p.m. ± SE. The autologous controls have been subtracted before plotting [$(C_1)^{3H}$ = 72 ± 2; $(C_1C_4m)^{3H}$ = 352 ± 18].

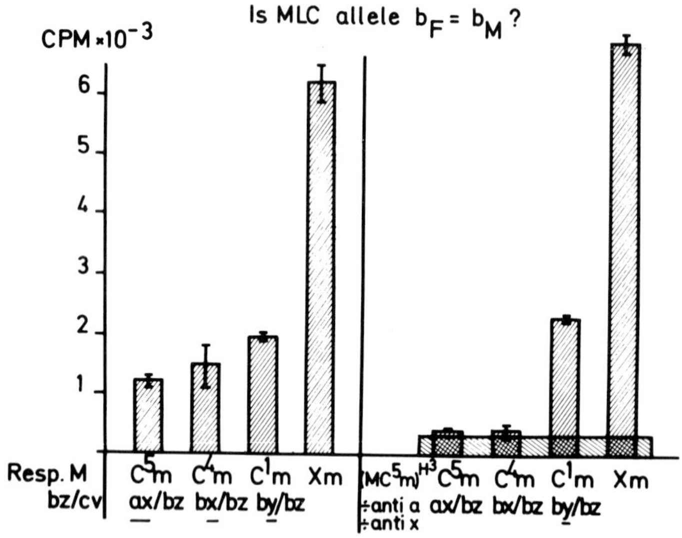

Fig. 3. MLC tests with cells from the mother in family G.O. as responding cells. The left part of the figure shows the results of normal micro-MLC tests, without ^{3}H-thymidine treatment of responding cells. On the right side of the figure is shown the result after a hot-pulse MLC between responding cells from the mother and stimulating cells from child 5. The results are given as mean c.p.m. ± SE. Autologous controls have not been subtracted and are indicated as the shaded area just above the abscissa.

Are the b alleles identical for these two different haplotypes?

Cells from the mother (bz/cv) were confronted with cells from C_5 (ax/bz) in a hot-pulse MLC, abolishing the response toward products of MLC alleles a and x (right part of Fig. 3). The ^{3}H-thymidine-treated culture was also confronted in a secondary MLC test with stimulating cells from C_4. No restimulation response was obtained, indicating that the b allele of the father (on the bx haplotype) is identical to the b allele of the mother (on the bz haplotype). As a control, the ^{3}H-thymidine-treated culture was also stimulated with cells from C_1 (incompatible for products of the MLC allele y) and third-party control cells X, each of which gave a normal response.

Since it was found possible to eliminate the response toward a product (x) of the first MLC locus without eliminating the response toward a product (a) of the possible second MLC locus carried by the same haplotype (Fig. 2), separate cell populations most probably recognize the different MLC-loci products of a given haplotype, as well as the products of each haplotype (Fig. 1).

DISCUSSION

One of the children (C_4) in family G.O. most probably represents a paternal recombination between the HL-A loci and the strong MLC locus outside the HL-A region proper. Furthermore, our studies indicate that structures other than those determined by the strong MLC locus can cause stimulation in some allogeneic combinations.

Eijsvoogel et al.,[4] from studies of families where a parental recombination between the two HL-A loci has taken place, and Mempel et al.,[5] from studies of unrelated combinations, have suggested that a second, weaker MLC locus is situated between the two HL-A loci. The existence of a second MLC locus is also a satisfactory explanation for our results in family G.O. This locus is also most probably situated in the MHS chromosomal region. If not, MLC stimulation in HL-A/MHS-identical sib combinations should be a phenomenon occurring much more often than observed. In family G.O., cells from C_2, C_3, and C_5 are reciprocally nonstimulatory toward each other, and they all stimulate C_4. Possibly HL-A incompatibility is necessary in order for an effect of this second MLC locus to be expressed. The reason why this second MLC locus is not easily detectable could be that disparity (either alone or together with HL-A) usually gives rise to a relatively weak MLC response. Another explanation could be a lesser degree of polymorphism displayed at this locus compared to the first MLC locus.

An alternative explanation for the results obtained in this family could be that the HL-A antigens themselves are able to cause stimulation in MLC. The mother and father most probably share the haplotypic information for a set of HL-A antigens, HL-A3, 7. This renders C_4 (and C_1) fully HL-A-compatible toward C_2, C_3, and C_5, while these three individuals are HL-A-incompatible toward C_4 (and C_1). Accordingly, C_2, C_3, and C_5 stimulate C_4, while the reversed combinations are MLC-negative.

Objections to this interpretation can, however, be raised. Several groups have recently reported HL-A-incompatible combinations that are MLC-negative.[2,3,5] Since child 4 in this family has not previously been immunized, we can also exclude proliferation of HL-A-reactive clones of lymphocytes because of presensitization of the responding cell donor.[10]

Our studies in family G.O. thus indicate the possible existence of at least two MLC loci. Separate lymphocyte populations seem to have receptors for products of these two loci; the response toward the product of the strong MLC locus could be eliminated without abolishing the response toward the other products of the same MHS haplotype (see Fig. 2). From our other family studies (Fig. 1) it can also be concluded that separate lymphocyte populations are responsive to the antigenic products determined by each MHS haplotype.[9] Thus in random allogeneic combinations, at least four different populations or clones of lymphocytes are usually proliferating. When responding cells from immunized donors are used in MLC tests, proliferation of HL-A-antigen-reactive lymphocyte populations may add to the response.[10]

The antigenic structures causing the MLC response demonstrate an extensive polymorphism, as witnessed by a positive MLC response in almost all random combinations. The finding that 1 to 3% (or even more) of the total lymphocytes proliferate initially in a given allogeneic combination[11] has been difficult to reconcile with a uniclonal restriction on the responding cells. If only one MLC locus is responsible for the corresponding antigenic structures, far too many lymphocytes would apparently have receptors for a particular set of allogeneic histocompatibility antigens. Our observations indicate that multiple separate but specific clones of lymphocytes most probably respond in concert in a particular allogeneic combination. This, taken together with the assumption that some of the many different histocompatibility structures causing MLC activation may be shared between individuals,[12,13] would greatly reduce the theoretically large number of lymphocytes that need receptors for alloantigenic structures.

REFERENCES

1. Amos DB, Bach FH: J Exp Med 128:623, 1968

2. Yunis E, Amos DB: Proc Natl Acad Sci 68:3037, 1972

3. Dupont B, Staub-Nielsen L, Svejgaard A: Lancet 2:1336, 1971

4. Eijsvoogel VP, van Rood JJ, du Toit ED, Schellekens PTA: Eur J Immunol 2:413, 1972

5. Mempel W, Grosse-Wilde H, Albert E, Thierfelder S: Transplant Proc 5:407, 1973

6. Kissmeyer-Nielsen F, Thorsby E: Transplant Rev 4, 1970

7. Thorsby E, Helgesen A: Symp Ser Immunobiol Stand (Karger, Basel) 18:141, 1973

8. Hirschberg H, Thorsby E: J Immunol Methods (in press)

9. Hirschberg H, Rankin B, Thorsby E: Cell Immunol. (in press)

10. Bondevik H, Thorsby E: Transplant Proc 5:1477, 1973

11. Wilson DB, Blyth JL, Nowell PC: J Exp Med 128:1157, 1968

12. Bach FH, Bach ML, Sondel PM, Sundharadas G: Transplant Rev 12:30, 1972

13. Hirschberg H, Thorsby E: Transplantation (in press)

Population Genetics of the MLC Response: Typing for MLC Determinants Using Homozygous and Heterozygous Reference Cells

By W. Mempel, H. Grosse-Wilde, P. Baumann, B. Netzel, I. Steinbauer-Rosenthal, S. Scholz, J. Bertrams, and E. D. Albert

AFTER the demonstration of clearly separated but closely linked systems governing the expression of HL-A antigens and MLC determinants,[1-9] the genetic and biologic interrelationships of these two systems required further investigation.

Four different approaches were followed: (1) the investigation of the MLC reactivity in relation to the HL-A typing in 922 combinations of 461 unrelated healthy individuals; (2) cross-testing in large groups of full-house HL-A-identical unrelated individuals in all possible combinations; (3) studies in families in which both parents share one HL-A haplotype and selection of HL-A-homozygous persons who could be shown to be homozygous also for one MLC determinant; (4) typing for MLC determinants using HL-A/MLC-homozygous cells and cells belonging to groups of HL-A-identical, unrelated, mutually nonstimulatory persons.

MATERIALS AND METHOD

HL-A typing[10] and MLC tests[11] were performed as previously described.

RESULTS

Population Studies

The comparison of the MLC stimulation ratios in relation to varying numbers of HL-A incompatibilities is shown in Fig. 1. As one can clearly see, growing numbers of HL-A differences result in increased MLC stimulation ratios. All observed differences are statistically significant ($p < 0.001$).

If the groups with one or two antigens difference are broken down (Fig. 2) according to the I and II HL-A loci, it is evident that incompatibilities for antigens of the I HL-A locus generally produce lower mean stimulation ratios than incompatibilities for the II HL-A locus.

HL-A-identical unrelated individuals show significantly lower mean stimulation ratios than persons who are identical for antigens of the II HL-A locus but differ in one or two antigens of the I HL-A locus, thus requiring the assumption of at least one additional MLC locus (provisionally named LD-1) more closely linked to the I HL-A locus.

HL-A-identical Unrelated Persons

Three different groups of full-house HL-A-identical unrelated persons were tested in all possible combinations. Figure 3 shows the number and size of nonstimulatory groups within each HL-A phenotype. In the largest group (HL-A1, 3, 7, 8) there were two pairs and one group of five mutually nonstimulatory persons, thus indicating the existence of at least three different MLC determinants. Four persons of the HL-A1, 3, 7, 8 nonstimulatory group were cross-tested with four nonstimulatory persons with the HL-A1, 2, 7, 8 phenotype (Fig. 4). With few exceptions this cross-test shows nonstimulation between the HL-A1, 3, 7, 8 and 1, 2, 7, 8 groups, thus suggesting identity at least for the MLC determinants (of the LD2 locus) linked to the II HL-A locus.

From the Institut für Hämatologie, Abt. Immunologie der GSF München; Kinderpoliklinik der Universität München: Klinikum der Universität Essen; and Sonderforschungsbereich 37 München, West Germany.

Supported in part by Deutsche Forschungsgemeinschaft, grant AL 92/7.

©1973 by Grune & Stratton, Inc.

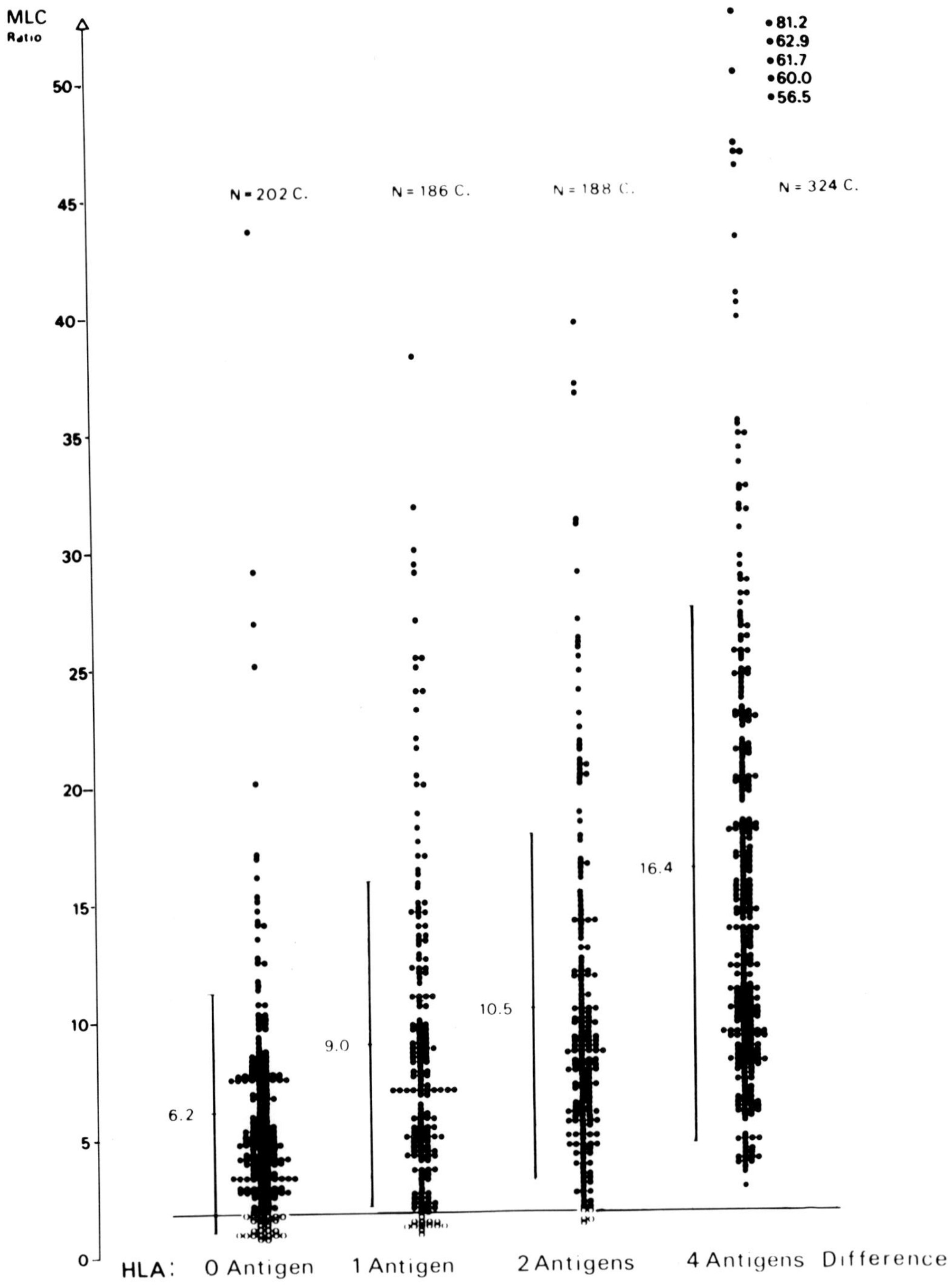

Fig. 1. MLC stimulation ratios in relation to HL-A incompatibilities. MLC ratio = ABm/AAm.

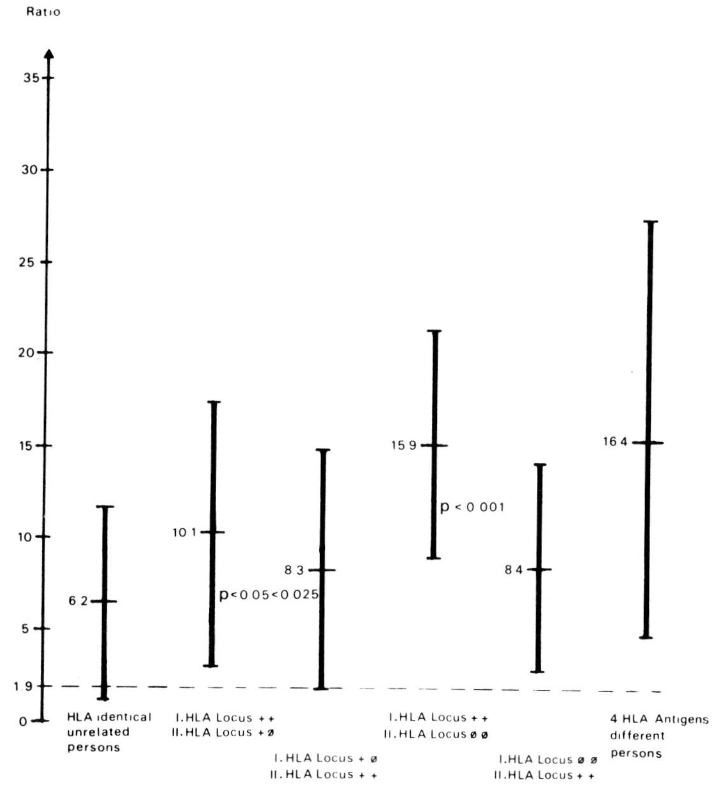

Fig. 2. MLC stimulation ratios in relation to HL-A incompatibilities at the different loci: +, identity; ø, incompatibility. Ratio = ABm/AAm.

HLA – Phenotype	Number of tested Persons	MLC Nonstimulation
1-3-7-8	19	5-2-2
1-2-7-8	14	5
1-2-8-12	11	3

Fig. 3. Groups of MLC-identical persons among HL-A-identical unrelated individuals.

	Am	Bm	Cm	Dm	Em	Fm	Gm	Hm	Ym
A		1.6	1.2	1.2	0.9	1.6	1.7	1.5	10.8
B	1.5		1.2	2.0	2.8	1.0	1.9	4.4	17.2
C	0.8	1.0		1.3	0.9	0.9	n.d.	n.d.	10.6
D	0.7	0.9	0.8		0.8	0.7	6.9	1.8	64.3
E	1.2	1.7	2.0	2.6		1.7	1.4	1.7	5.1
F	0.7	1.0	0.8	1.0	1.0		0.9	1.4	4.9
G	0.8	1.5	n.d.	2.9	1.2	1.4		2.5	11.9
H	0.5	1.0	1.8	4.2	1.5	1.9	2.2		15.7
Y	11.3	16.6	11.1	19.8	10.4	11.0	12.3	12.1	

MLC Crosstest (Results in Stimulation Ratio) between unrelated persons with the phenotype HLA 1-2-7-8 (A-D) and HLA 1-3-7-8 (E-H). Control person (Y).

Fig. 4. MLC cross-tests between unrelated persons with the phenotype HL-A1,2,7,8 (A–D) and HL-A1,3,7,8 (E–H). Ratio = ABm/AAm.

Family Studies

Among nine families in which parents share one HL-A haplotype, we found three instances in which it could be shown by two-way nonstimulation of HL-A-identical parent–child combinations that the shared haplotypes are also identical for the MLC determinant. Unfortunately only two of these three families had HL-A3, 7/MLC-homozygous children. Interestingly enough, the homozygous children from each family did not stimulate each other, suggesting identity for their MLC determinants. As we have previously reported, some but not all of the expected one-way nonstimulations within the families could be clearly demonstrated,[12] although in all these instances the homozygotes stimulated far less than they were stimulated by the heterozygotes.

TYPING FOR MLC

Frozen lymphocytes from these homozygous children defining the MLC determinant Pi were tested against the above-described HL-A1, 3, 7, 8 and HL-A1, 2, 7, 8 nonstimulatory groups (Fig. 5). One-way nonstimulations with all members of both groups revealed that these individuals are all heterozygous for the MLC type Pi. Their mutual nonstimulation allows the assumption that these HL-A1, 3, 7, 8 and HL-A1, 2, 7, 8 individuals were identical also for the second MLC allele X coupled with HL-A8. Therefore these heterozygous Pi/X cells could also be used as a reference for MLC typing.

Two groups of unrelated individuals were typed with the HL-A3, 7/Pi homozygous cells. In a group of 67 persons positive for HL-A7 (most of them had either HL-A3, 7 or HL-A2, 7), 24 individuals showed one-way nonstimulation with Pi and were therefore assumed to possess this MLC determinant in a heterozygous state. One individual with HL-A3, 10, 7, W18 showed a bidirectional nonstimulation, indicating homozygosity for Pi. A similar observation involving the HL-A3, 10, 7, W18 phenotype is reported by Dupont et al. in this issue.[13] A second group of 48 random individuals included six persons positive for Pi, of which four were HL-A7-positive upon typing.

DISCUSSION

The results of the population studies are in full agreement with the assumption of one MLC locus (provisionally designated as LD2) in the proximity of the second HL-A locus, a concept derived from crossing-over families.[1,4,6,7,9,14] In the same way, these population data lend further support to the hypothesis of a second MLC locus (provisionally called LD1) closer linked to the I HL-A locus causing generally lower

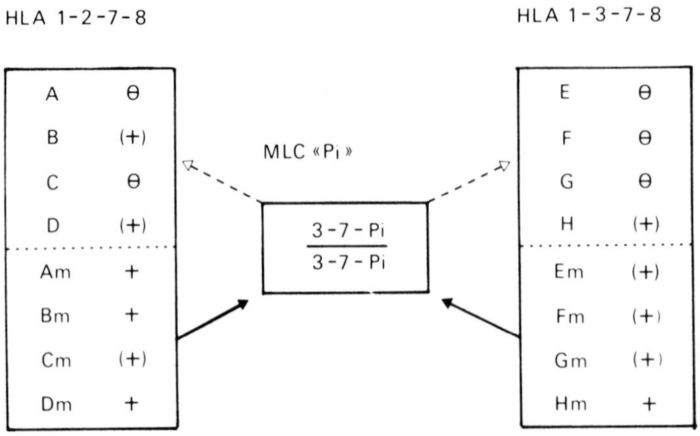

Fig. 5. MLC typing for the Pi specificity in HL-A/MLC-identical unrelated individuals with the phenotypes HL-A1,2,7,8 and HL-A1,3,7,8: solid arrow, positive stimulation; dashed arrow, negative stimulation.

MLC stimulation. Evidence for this locus was obtained in families with crossover between the I and II HL-A loci by Eijsvoogel[15] and more recently by Thorsby et al.[16] and Revillard et al.[17]

In families in which HL-A-identical parent–child combinations show bidirectional nonstimulation, one would expect that homozygous children stimulate neither parents nor heterozygous siblings. However, in some of these combinations a low but definite stimulation by the homozygous cell has been observed.[12,18] The reasons for this paradoxical MLC (Dausset) are presently not known. One possible explanation could be the production of a blastogenic factor by the mitomycin-C-treated homozygous cells.[19] The analysis of the karyotypes of a two-way MLC between a homozygous brother and his heterozygous sister showed 21 male vs. 7 female mitoses, indicating that this paradoxical reaction is a biological phenomenon rather than a laboratory artifact caused by mitomycin C. Another possible explanation is that the paradoxical stimulation could reflect differences that were acquired during the ontogeny.

At the present time none of these explanations can be considered satisfactory. In spite of the unexplained paradoxical low-grade stimulation by homozygotes, one can use these cells for MLC typing provided that the homozygosity for MLC can be deduced from an HL-A-identical and MLC-negative parent-child combination in the family of the homozygote. In order to eliminate a low stimulation of cells from unrelated individuals that could be due either to the above discussed paradoxical stimulation or to differences at the LD1 locus, we have used a ratio derived by the following formula:

$$\frac{(AB_m - AA_m) \cdot (BX_m - BB_m)}{(AX_m - AA_m) \cdot (BA_m - BB_m)}$$

where A is the typing cell and X is the highest stimulating cell of the unrelated controls. The subscript m stands for the mitomycin-treated stimulating cells. A ratio of greater than 3.0 indicates a possible one-way nonstimulation.

In a preliminary experiment it was attempted also to use for MLC typing, in addition to the MLC-homozygous cells, cells that had been shown to be heterozygous for certain defined MLC specificities. As expected, a medium MLC stimulation was observed in the critical combinations, possibly indicating identity for one MLC allele. It must be stressed, however, that with present techniques the distinction between a one- or a two-MLC-allele difference in unrelated individuals is extremely difficult.

To overcome this problem one can use two or more heterozygous reference cells that have been shown to be MLC-identical by nonstimulation. Using this procedure it is possible to define three MLC specificities with reference cells taken from the various nonstimulatory groups among the HL-A1, 3, 7, 8 phenotype. It should be borne in mind that at this time it seems impossible to distinguish by the degree of stimulation between incompatibility for one MLC haplotype (consisting of one LD1 and one LD2 determinant) and one or more incompatibilities at either MLC locus. It is equally disturbing that a LD1 difference might result in the same kind of low stimulation as the above-mentioned paradoxical stimulation observed with MLC homozygotes. The typing for MLC using homozygous reference cells was also performed in dogs. Two different types of MLC specificities, one associated with DL2, 4 and a second one with DL2, 5, could be defined by the above-mentioned criteria.[20] Interestingly enough, in 26 instances the paradoxical stimulation by the homozygous cells could never be observed. Since these dogs originate from a closely bred beagle colony, it is difficult to distinguish whether the lack of paradoxical stimulation is due to the close genetic relationship of these dogs or to the fact that x-irradiation rather than mitomycin treatment was used to inactivate the stimulating cells.

Using the above-described limitations, it can be stated that it is possible to type an unrelated population by homozygous[12] and heterozygous reference cells.[13,21]

The preliminary results about the distribution of the MLC specificity Pi indicate a frequency of about 14% in the Munich population and a frequency of 36% among individuals selected for the presence of HL-A7, suggesting a rather strong linkage disequilibrium between Pi and HL-A7, which will be discussed in the article in this issue by Albert et al.[22]

REFERENCES

1. Bach FH, Albertini RJ, Amos DB, et al: Transplant Proc 1:339, 1969

2. Eijsvoogel VP, Konig L, de Groot-Kooy L, et al: Transplant Proc 4:199, 1972

3. Gatti RA, Meuwissen HJ, Terasaki PI, Good R: Tissue Antigens 1:239, 1971

4. Lebrun A, Sasportes A, Lebrun D, Dausset J: C R Acad Sci 273D:2130, 1971

5. Plate JM, Ward FE, Amos DB: Histocompatibility Testing, 1970. Copenhagen, Munksgaard pp 531–535

6. Yunis EJ, Plate GM, Ward FE, et al: Transplant Proc 3:118, 1971

7. Mempel W, Albert E, Burger A: Tissue Antigens 2:250, 1972

8. Eijsvoogel VP, Schellekens PTA, Breur-Vriesendorp B, et al: Transplant Proc 3:85, 1970

9. Eijsvoogel VP, van Rood JJ, du Toit ED, Schellekens PTA: Eur J Immunol 2:413, 1972

10. Albert E, Scholz S, Rosenthal J, et al: Histocompatibility Testing, 1972. Copenhagen, Munksgaard (in press)

11. Bach ML, Solliday S, Stambuk M: Histocompatibility Testing, 1970. Copenhagen, Munksgaard, pp 643–653

12. Mempel W, Grosse-Wilde H, Baumann P, et al: Transplant Proc 5:1529, 1973

13. Dupont, et al: Transplant Proc 5:1543, 1973

14. Dupont B, Nielsen LS, Svejgaard A: Lancet 2: 1336, 1971

15. Eijsvoogel VP, du Bois MJGJ, Melief CJM, et al: Histocompatibility Testing, 1972. Copenhagen, Munksgaard, 1973, p 501

16. Thorsby et al: Transplant Proc 5:1523, 1973

17. Cordier G, Betuel H, Revillard JP: Transplant Proc 5:1855, 1973

18. Lebrun A, Sasportes M, Dausset J: Transplant Proc 5:363, 1973

19. Kasakura S: Nature 227:507, 1970

20. Grosse-Wilde et al: Transplant Proc 5:1567, 1973

21. van den Tweel et al: Transplant Proc 5:1535, 1973

22. Albert et al: Transplant Proc 5:1551, 1973

Typing for MLC (LD): I. Lymphocytes From Cousin-Marriage Offspring as Typing Cells

By J. G. van den Tweel, A. Blussé van Oud Alblas, J. J. Keuning, E. Goulmy, A. Termijtelen, M. L. Bach, and J. J. van Rood

WHEN it was observed that the majority of SD-identical unrelated individuals stimulated each other in the MLC test, it was postulated in agreement with earlier suggestions by others that MLC activation might be coded by a locus separate from the LA and Four loci.[1-4] The existence of such a MLC locus is now generally accepted.[5,6] About 10% of the MLC tests between SD-identical unrelated persons are negative, indicating that a linkage disequilibrium exists between the MLC locus and the LA and Four loci. It is furthermore likely that SD-identical unrelated individuals who are also LD-identical carry MLC determinants that occur rather frequently.

In this study we tried to recognize the MLC-locus determinants. To this end we used lymphocytes from double-homozygous offspring of cousin marriages. As shown in Table 1, it is possible with these cells to indicate whether another cell carries the same MLC determinant and if so whether the determinant occurs in a homozygous or heterozygous form. We will refer to the lymphocytes obtained from the double-homozygous cousin-marriage offspring as typing cells. Typing cells are for LD the equivalent of typing sera for SD.

In this and the following paper we will describe a systematic approach to recognize the MLC (LD) determinants. This paper describes the definitions of five MLC determinants by MLC or LD testing. The basic principle of this approach is that if two individuals carry the same MLC determinants they will not stimulate in the MLC test.

MATERIALS AND METHOD

Test cells were selected from a file of more than 20,000 HL-A-typed individuals. Two suitable cell populations were used for this experiment: (1) cells of unrelated SD- and LD-identical individuals and (2) cells of children from cousin marriages that are homozygous at both HL-A loci. Both serotyping for SD and MLC testing for LD were done as described before.[7-10] The combinatorial experiment was performed in a microtechnique.[11]

RESULTS

SD-identical individuals (137 persons) were first tested within their respective SD-identical groups in bidirectional and unidirectional MLC tests; 24 persons were repeatedly MLC-negative, with 1 or 2 SD-identical individuals. From 6 MLC-negative combinations with different HL-A phenotypes, we selected 8 individuals for the test (group A). From 52 cousin marriages we were able to select 11 children homozygous at both HL-A loci, with 6 different HL-A phenotypes. From each family that had homozygous children, the lymphocytes from one homozygous child were used for the experiment (group B). In the combinatorial experiment of group A and group B, 10 of these 14 cells were informative because they were involved in a MLC-negative combination. The other 4 cells were positive with all other cells in the test. Table 2 shows the results of the uni-

---

From the Department of Immunohaematology and the J. A. Cohen Institute for Radiopathology and Radiation Protection, University Hospital, Leiden, The Netherlands.

M.L. Bach is a Faculty Research Awardee of the American Cancer Society and was a Visiting Professor in Leiden while participating in these studies.

Supported in part by the Dutch Organization for Health Research, TNO, the Dutch Organization for Pure Research (FUNGO), the Whitehall Foundation, and the National Institute of Health (contract PH 43-65-992).

©1973 by Grune & Stratton, Inc.

Table 1. Typing for MLC (LD): Description and Interpretation of MLC Results Using Typing Cells Homozygous at LA, Four, and MLC (SD and LD)

Pattern Number	Cell to Be Typed	Homozygous Typing Cell	MLC Reaction	MLC Type of X
1	X	a/a_m	neg	a/a a/b or a/c etc.
2	X	a/a_m	pos	b/c etc.
3	X_m	a/a	neg	a/a
4	X_m	a/a	pos	a/b or a/c or b/c etc.

Interpretation: 1 + 3, X = a/a; 2 + 3, should not occur; 1 + 4, X = a/b or a/c etc.; 2 + 4, X = b/c, d/e etc.

lateral MLC test between cells of these 10 informative individuals. The cells being MLC-negative between each other are surrounded by a solid line or a broken line when the cells of donor L are involved. The cells within each square share one or two MLC (LD) determinants. The determinant LD1 is shared by the cells G, H, O, and L, the weak stimulation between G and H on the one hand and O and L on the other (while O and L are mutually negative) suggests that O and L might share a determinant LD2. The determinant LD3 is shared by the cells L and K, while LD5 is present probably in a homozygous form in M and only on one chromosome in N (Table 1). The fourth LD determinant (LD4) is seen on the SD-identical cells I and F. The cells D and L might share a sixth LD determinant, but further confirmation is needed.

DISCUSSION

This study is based on the assumption that if two normal (unrelated) individuals do not stimulate each other in the MLC test, this implies that they share MLC determinants. In this manner the first three individuals were found who shared one or more MLC determinants.[3,12] The same approach was used by Mempel and Albert,[13] who not only confirmed our findings but extended them by using cells from SD and LD double-homozygous offspring of unrelated parents. We have done the same, but found that these cells were often not homozygous for LD.

For this reason we collected lymphocytes from cousin-marriage offspring which were homozygous not only for SD but also (barring crossover) for LD, as the two haplotypes came from the same great-grandparent. With this approach we were able to recognize four of the five MLC determinants of Table 2.

The reaction with the typing cell L should be considered as preliminary. Even if one assumes that a crossover in the parent or grandparents of L has occurred, it is difficult to interpret the data obtained with L without allowing for the possibility that one chromosome can carry several (even more than two) LD determinants. There is a priori nothing against this possibility, which would be in agreement with the findings for the Ir genes, but because of the basic importance of such an observation, we feel that further confirmation is needed.[14] Another explanation could be that one of the two 1,8 haplotypes was not inherited from a great-grandparent but was introduced by one of the grandparents. Especially with frequently occurring haplotypes such as 1,8, this is a possibility one should consider. Lebrun et al.[15] have reported unexpected positive unilateral MLC tests between SD-homozygous children as stimulating cells and their parents as responder cells. The mechanism by which this is brought about is as yet unclear, but the use of typing cells is only possible if this phenomenon does not interfere. Our findings so far indicate that when typing cells are used that are SD- and LD-homozygous because they are obtained from cousin marriages, this is at least in some instances not a problem. We would like to submit that just as there exist in serology poor and good sera, in LD typing we will find poor and good typing cells. Typing cells from cousin marriages seem to be better than those from

Typing for MLC (LD): II. The Selection of Nonstimulator Cells by MLC Inhibition Tests Using SD-identical Stimulator Cells (MISIS) and Fluorescence Antibody Studies

By A. van Leeuwen, H. R. E. Schuit, and J. J. van Rood

IN the preceding paper van den Tweel et al.[1] have outlined the procedure by which, in a small panel, five different MLC determinants (LD1, 2, 3, 4, and 5) could be defined. Although this procedure at this moment is probably the most reliable if one wants to recognize MLC (LD) determinants, it is also cumbersome and time-consuming.

In this paper we want to report on our findings attempting to define these MLC determinants by antibody using the MLC inhibition and immunofluorescence techniques. Ceppellini et al.[2] showed that anti-HL-A antibodies were able to inhibit the MLC reaction. We have confirmed and extended their observations and those of others[3] by using as responder cells those from the individual who made the antibody to be studied and as stimulator cells those from unrelated individuals that were SD-identical with the responder cell. This procedure will be further referred to as the MLC inhibition test using SD-identical stimulator cells, or MISIS. It was argued that if under these conditions MLC inhibition was found it could be due to an interaction of antibody with the MLC determinants, although other mechanisms cannot a priori be excluded (see discussion). This approach appears to work and to provide findings that correlate well with those of van den Tweel et al.[1] The fluorescence antibody technique furthermore seems to provide a serologic approach to the recognition of MLC determinants.

From the Department of Immunohematology, University Hospital, Leiden, and the Laboratory of Experimental Gerontology, Radiobiological Institute, TNO, Rijswijk, The Netherlands.

Supported in part by the Dutch Organization for Health Research TNO, the Dutch Organization for Pure Research (FUNGO), the J. A. Cohen Institute for Radiopathology and Radiation Protection, the National Institute of Health (contract PH 43-65-992), and the Whitehall Foundation.

© 1973 by Grune & Stratton, Inc.

MATERIALS AND METHOD

For responder cells, three men immunized by skin transplants and seven women immunized by pregnancy were selected. Stimulator cells were SD-identical with the responder cell, i.e., they carried the same LA and Four antigens. Absorptions were performed as described before.[4]

The MLC tests were performed according to a procedure modified from Schellekens et al.,[5] the MLC inhibition test as described by Ceppellini et al.[2] To demonstrate antibody on lymphocytes with the fluorescence antibody technique, 2×10^6 lymphocytes in a 0.05-ml suspension were incubated with 0.15 ml of serum for 60 min at 22°C or 37°C, washed three times, incubated for 30 min at 22°C with diluted rabbit anti-human γ-globulin serum, washed two times, and incubated with rhodamine-labeled goat anti-rabbit γ-globulin serum (Nordic, Tilburg, The Netherlands). The general procedures and precautions as described by Hijmans et al. were followed.[6]

RESULTS

MLC Inhibition Studies. The sera of 3 of the 10 individuals tested were able to inhibit in a significant and reproducible fashion the MLC test between the lymphocytes of the serum donor and SD-identical stimulator cells (Table 1). All 3 were multiparous women. One other parous woman showed a pattern that gave many dubious reactions. All other sera so far did not inhibit.

Fluorescence Antibody Studies. The percentage of fluorescent cells found with serum Sch against the SD-identical stimulator cells is indicated in Table 1. Using our procedure, the background stain is 4 to 9%, probably due to staining of.B cells. We have so far found no combinations in which

Table 1. Typing for MLC LD: MLC Inhibition and Immunofluorescence

Parous Woman Sch: HL-A2,3,7, W10				
	AB Serum (c.p.m.)	Serum Sch (c.p.m.)	AB Serum/ Serum Sch	Fluorescent (% Pos. Cells)
Sch + P_m	3,300	400	*7.3*	*17*
Q_m	14,000	8,000	1.7	4
N_m	9,700	1,100	*9.5*	*17*
R_m	10,000	6,400	1.6	9
S_m	4,200	2,800	1.7	7
T_m	5,200	700	*7.4*	7
U_m	13,500	1,300	*10.0*	*16*
V_m	26,500	1,100	*24.1*	*17*
W_m	1,800	200	*10.0*	–

All stimulator cells were SD-identical with the responder cells Sch: HL-A2,3,7,W10. The column AB Serum/Serum Sch depicts the inhibition index values obtained by dividing the c.p.m. obtained by culturing the cells in AB serum by the c.p.m. obtained when they were cultured in serum Sch. The significant inhibitions are in italics.

more than 25% of the cells were stained. Arbitrarily, 15 to 25% was considered to indicate a positive reaction. All tests shown were repeated at least twice. Reproducibility was over 90%. In Table 2 the results of the fluorescence antibody test is given of three sera (Pl, St, and Sch) against the panel of cells in which the MLC LD determinants were defined through MLC reactivity by van den Tweel et al. Serum Pl might contain an anti-LD1 + 4, serum St an anti-2, while serum Sch reacted with the cell carrying LD5 and one other cell.

Absorption Studies. Table 3 shows that the MLC-inhibiting substance in the relatively weak Pl serum could be removed by lymphocytes but not by platelets. From the much stronger Sch serum, lymphocytes removed part of the inhibiting substance but not all of it. The serum of Mrs. v. R. did not contain MLC-inhibiting substances and served as a control to demonstrate that by absorption with platelets MLC-inhibiting substances are not released.

MLC Combinatorial Experiment. When the stimulator cells shown in Table 1 were tested in an unilateral MLC test against each other, it turned out that cells P and W did not stimulate each other, thus suggesting that they carried the same MLC determinants. This would be in agreement with the inhibition studies.

DISCUSSION

Although our results are of a preliminary nature, there exists a striking agreement between the findings obtained by direct MLC testing[1] and the MLC-inhibition studies and the fluorescence antibody testing. If confirmed in a larger study, this would im-

Table 2. Typing for MLC LD

	Cells	MLC Determinant 1	MLC Determinant 4	Fluorescence Pl	MLC Determinant 2	Fluorescence St	MLC Determinant 5	Fluorescence Sch
1,2,8,W10	G	+++	–	+++	–	–	–	–
1,2,8,W15	H	+++	–	+++	–	–	–	–
1,2,8,12	O	+++	–	+++	+++	+++	–	–
1,8/1,8	L	+++	–	+++	+++	+++	–	+++
2,3,7,W10	N	–	–	–	–	–	+++	+++
1,2,8,W10	I	–	+++	+++	–	–	–	–
1,2,8,W10	F	–	+++	+++	–	–	–	–
2,12/2,12	P	–	–	–	–	–	–	–

The cells are from the same donors as those depicted in Table 2 of the previous paper, in which the MLC determinants were assigned.

Table 3. Typing for MLC LD: MLC Inhibition and Absorption

Cells:	In AB Serum	In Woman's Serum: neat	after absorption with: platelets*	lymphocytes*
Pl + Pl $husband_m$	14,600	8,400	9,900	13,000
Pl + K skin $donor_m$	13,600	–	8,100	15,100
Sch + D_m	6,800	600	400	1,200
v.R. + v.R. $husband_m$	6,200	6,000	6,000	6,200

*2×10^9 platelets and 1×10^8 lymphocytes were used to absorb 1 ml of serum.

ply that it might become possible to routinely select MLC LD-identical individuals by serotyping.

The fact that cells P and W did not stimulate each other is a first example of such a selection procedure. The practical importance for organ transplantation has been discussed before.[7-9] Although in all instances bilateral and unilateral tests have been performed, only the unilateral tests in which the antibody producer was the responder have been presented here. Inhibition in the two MLC tests showed an almost identical pattern, while the inhibition of the unilateral MLC test in which the cells of the antibody producer were the stimulator showed either no inhibition at all or an inhibition that was weak and poorly reproducible.

The finding that the MLC inhibition is observed in some combinations but not in others suggests that a polymorphism is recognized. Family studies will be necessary to exclude the possibility that the inhibition is due to an antibody directed against a non-HL-A antigen. The possibility that the inhibiting antibody is directed against a subgroup of, for instance, W10 must also be excluded. We favor the interpretation of our data that regards them as indicating that the antibodies in these sera can interact with the MLC determinant. The inhibition tests were repeated at least twice and for some combinations three times; reproducibility was over 95%. The absorption studies make it highly likely that the inhibiting substance is an antibody.

The correlation of the MLC typing results by selecting pairs that do not stimulate each other in the MLC test with the fluorescence antibody assay should be regarded as preliminary. Since with the fluorescence antibody test MLC determinants can be recognized in a single dose, it is to be expected that in some instances this test will recognize the same MLC determinant on two cells that nevertheless stimulate each other in the MLC test.

We have found that not more than maximally 15 to 25% of the cells showed specific fluorescence. Barring technical complications or weak sera (both of which seem unlikely), this finding might indicate that the MLC determinant is present only on part of the lymphocytes. This could be in agreement with recent findings of Klein et al.,[10] who were able to produce a cytotoxic antibody against the products of the gene area that carries the Ir genes and MLC genes in the mouse.

In agreement with our findings that only part of the cells are stained by fluorescent antibody, their sera killed only 40 to 50% of the lymphocytes. Carbonara[11] has demonstrated inhibition of the MLC test using a serum BNT produced against W16 by intersibling immunization. Because inhibition in the unilateral MLC test occurred only when the antibody producer was the stimulator cell (in contrast to our findings) and because this antibody inhibited the in vitro response against old tuberculin, it is possible that it is directed not against the MLC determinants but against the T-cell receptor. In this context the question may again be raised[12] whether the same molecule might carry the MLC determinants and the T-cell receptor. The MLC determinants could then be the equivalent of the immunoglobulin markers like Gm, etc., on the constant part of the immunoglobulin molecule, while the receptor would be the equivalent of the variable part.

To our knowledge this is the first time that the MLC inhibition test using SD-identical unrelated stimulator cells (MISIS) has been used systematically. The results presented here appear to indicate that it is a worthwhile adjunct to unravel the complexities of the major histocompatibility complex.

ACKNOWLEDGMENTS

The authors would like to thank Dr. W. Hijmans from the Institute of Experimental Gerontology, TNO, Rijswijk, for advice and support in setting up the immunofluorescence assay and Dr. J. Ràdl from the same institute for the monospecific rabbit anti-human IgG. Miss J. Parlevliet gave excellent technical assistance.

REFERENCES

1. Van den Tweel JG, Blussé van Oud Alblas A, Keuning JJ, et al: Transplant Proc 5:1535, 1973

2. Ceppellini R, Bonnard GD, Coppo F, et al: Transplant Proc 3:63, 1971

3. Revillard JP, Robert M, DuPont E, et al: Transplant Proc 5:331, 1973

4. Van Rood JJ: in McDevitt HO, Landy M (eds): Proceedings of the International Conference on Genetic Control of Immune Responsiveness, Brook Lodge, Augusta, May 8–10, 1972. New York, Academic, 1972, p 130

5. Schellekens PTA, Eijsvoogel VP: Clin Exp Immunol 3:571, 1968

6. Hijmans W, Schuit HRE, Klein F: Clin Exp Immunol 4:457, 1969

7. Van Hooff JP, Schippers HMA, van der Steen GJ, van Rood JJ: Lancet ii, 7792:1385, 1972

8. Van Rood JJ, Koch CT, van Hooff JP, et al: Transplant Proc 5:409, 1973

9. Van Rood JJ: Transplant Proc 5:1747, 1973

10. Klein J: unpublished data

11. Carbonara A: personal communication

12. Koch CT, Frederiks E, van Leeuwen A, et al: unpublished data

Typing for MLC Determinants by Means of LD-homozygous and LD-heterozygous Test Cells

By Bo Dupont, Casper Jersild, Grete S. Hansen, Lillian Staub Nielsen, Mogens Thomsen, and Arne Svejgaard

APPROXIMATELY 10% of HL-A-identical unrelated combinations do not show significant stimulation in the MLC test.[1,2] Lebrun et al.[3] and Mempel et al.[2] showed that HL-A-identical parent–child combinations quite frequently can be MLC-identical. An analysis of available family data on heterozygous Four-locus-identical parent combinations shows that HL-A3,7 is by far the most frequently reported haplotype in such cases of HL-A- and MLC-identical parent–child combinations. These findings suggested to us that genetic linkage disequilibrium gives a strong association between the Four-locus determinant HL-A7 and a specific LD determinant that we shall call LD7a.

In this report we describe that HL-A3, 7-homozygous individuals are very frequently also homozygous for the LD determinant LD7a. We have used such homozygous cells as test cells to characterize the HL-A7-linked LD determinant in unrelated Danes.

The approach of typing for LD determinants by the use of LD-homozygous cells has also been used independently by Mempel et al.[4] and by van den Tweel et al.[5] We have further extended the test-cell panel to include well-defined LD-heterozygous test cells. This has been done by selecting cells carrying the SD antigens HL-A3, 7 and the LD determinant LD7a on one of their haplotypes. MLC testing between these haploidentical cells makes it possible to characterize the LD determinants on the other haplotypes.

From the Tissue Typing Laboratory and Blood Grouping Department, State University Hospital, Copenhagen, Denmark.

This study was supported by grants from the Danish State Research Council, the Research Foundation for Copnehagen, Greenland, and Faroe Islands, the Foundation for Research in Multiple Sclerosis, and by AB Gambro.

© 1973 by Grune & Stratton, Inc.

MATERIALS AND METHOD

The one-way MLC tests were performed as previously described.[6] All results obtained are given as stimulation ratios (SR) (c.p.m. in the combination $A + B_m$ divided by c.p.m. in the combination $A + A_m$).

Our normal material consists of 658 one-way MLC tests. The distribution of the log ratios are close to normal for each of the three groups: (1) A total of 479 unrelated HL-A-nonidentical combinations had a mean SR (using logarithms in the calculations) of 15.2 (4.1–58.6: 95% confidence limits). (2) Another 127 combinations were haploidentical family combinations with mean SR of 7.95 (2.09–30.2). (3) Fifty-two combinations were HL-A-identical sibling combinations, mean SR, 1.05 (0.54–2.07).[7] We observed no cases of overlapping between zero-haplotype and one-haplotype differences.

We have recently described an intermediate group of MLC responses with SR consistently between the zero-haplotype differences and the one-haplotype differences. This intermediate group has average SRs between 1.5 and 3.5. When tested repeatedly, the HL-A-haploidentical sibling combinations with LD identity belong to this group.[7,8]

Our data in this study are grouped according to the four different SR groups: (1) SR corresponding to HL-A-identical sibling combinations; (2) SR corresponding to the intermediate group;[7] (3) SR corresponding to haploidentical sibling or child–parent combinations; (4) SR for the two-haplotype-different combination.

For this study we selected test cells homozygous for the HL-A haplotype 3,7 obtained from family ST (Fig. 1). In this family the parents shared the haplotype HL-A3,7, and the HL-A3,7-homozygous cells did not stimulate any of the parents' cells. Furthermore, these cells did not stimulate those of the siblings when these carried the HL-A3,7 haplotype. The HL-A3,7-homozygous cells (A) must then also be homozygous for the LD determinant LD7a, and they have been used as test cells to identify the LD7a determinant.

We tested 34 normal individuals who all carried the HL-A7 determinant on at least one of their haplo-

Definition of the Homozygous Test Cells

Family ST

2,W15/3,7 Father — 2,W27/3,7 Mother

2,W15/3,7	3,7/3,7	3,7/2,W27	2,W15/2,W27
Sib. 1–3	Sib. 4*	Sib. 5–7	Sib. 8–10

Nonreactive Parent–Child Combinations

Parent		Child
2,W15/3,7	− ⇄ −	2,W15/3,7
2,W15/3,7	− ⇄ +	(3,7/3,7)m*
2,W27/3,7	− ⇄ −	2,W27/3,7
2,W27/3,7	− ⇄ +	(3,7/3,7)m*

*Sibling 4 is considered homozygous for the SD determinants HL-A3 and 7 and for the LD determinant LD7a. These test cells are called A.

Fig. 1. **→ +, denotes one-way stimulation; → −, denotes one-way nonreactivity. The HL-A-identical parent–child combinations are mutually nonreactive in MLC tests. The HL-A3,7-homozygous cells do not stimulate any of the parents' or siblings' cells, except those lacking HL-A3, 7 (sibs. 8–10), but respond normally to all family members.**

types. They represent 22 unrelated HL-A7-carrying haplotypes.

RESULTS

The first part of the study focused on the linkage between the Four antigen, HL-A7, and the LD determinant LD7a, compared to the linkage between the HL-A7 antigen and the different LA antigens.

Table 1 shows the parental HL-A genotypes in three Danish families. All six parents carry HL-A7 on one haplotype, but only one haplotype in each family is HL-A3,7, while the other is either 1,7 or 2,7. In each family the LD determinants linked to HL-A7 must be identical within the family because of the nonreactive parent–child combinations shown in the table. The LD7a-homozygous test cells (A) could not stimulate cells from any of these individuals, indicating that the six different HL-A7-carrying haplotypes in these three families all have the LD7a determinant. It is worth noting that this determinant was present also in the three haplotypes lacking HL-A3. Thus the association between HL-A7 and LD7a might be even stronger than that between HL-A3 and 7.

In the second part of this study we focused on the frequency of the LD7a de-

Table 1. MLC Nonreactivity Between Four-Locus-identical (HL-A7-identical) Parent–Child Combinations

Family	Paternal HL-A Genotypes	Maternal HL-A Genotypes	Nonreactive Combinations		
			Parent		Child
BY	28,W15/1,7	1,8/3,7	28,W15/1,7	− ⇄ −	28,W15/3,7
			1,8/3,7	− ⇄ +	1,7/3,7
			1,8/3,7	− ⇄ −	1,8/3,7
KR	9,12/3,7	11,5/2,7	11,5/2,7	− ⇄ −	11,5/3,7
RJ	10,W18/3,7	2,W5/2,7	2,W5/2,7	− ⇄ +	2,W5/3,7

All individuals included in this table did not respond on stimulation by the unrelated homozygous test cells HL-A3,7 (A) (see legend to Fig. 1).

Table 2. HL-A Genotypes and the LD Determinant LD7a in Unrelated Danes

Family	Person		HL-A Genotype	LD-Determinant Haplotype 1	LD-Determinant Haplotype 2	Numeration of LD7a Determinant
ST	P.ST.	(F)	2,W15/3,7	—	7a	1
	M.ST.	(M)	2,W27/3,7	—	7a	2
	A.ST.	(Ch)	3,7/3,7	7a	7a	*(A)
BY	P.BY.	(F)	2,W15/1,7	—	7a	3
	M.BY.	(M)	1,8/3,7	—	7a	4
	E.BY.	(Ch)	1,7/3,7	7a	7a	
	B.BY.	(Ch)	1,8/1,7	—	7a	
KR	P.KR.	(F)	9,12/3,7	—	7a	5
	M.KR.	(M)	11,5/2,7	—	7a	6
	L.KR.	(Ch)	11,5/3,7	—	7a	
RJ	P.RJ.	(F)	10,W18/3,7	—	7a	7
	M.RJ.	(M)	2,W5/2,7	—	7a	8
	MO.RJ.	(Ch)	2,W5/3,7	—	7a	
AN	P.AN.	(F)	28,W5/3,7	—	7a	9
	M.AN.	(M)	3,5/3,7	—	7a	10
	B.AN.	(Ch)	3,7/3,7	7a	7a	†(B)
FR	P.FR.	(F)	W25,W18/28,12	—	—	
	M.FR.	(M)	1,BC/3,7	—	7a	11
	M.FR.	(Ch)	10,W18/3,7	—	7a	
Unrelated	LCN.		3,7/3,7	7a	7a	12,13‡(C)
	DV.		10,W18/3,7	—	7a	14
	JJ.		2,W16/3,7	—	7a	15
	BJ.		2,7/3,7	—	7a	16

Test cells homozygous for the LD7a determinant; * A; † B; ‡ C.
F: father; M:mother; Ch: child.

terminant in unrelated Danish individuals carrying HL-A7. Sixteen other unrelated HL-A-genotyped normal persons with this antigen were selected and tested with the LD7a-homozygous test cells (A). This study revealed eight new HL-A3,7 haplotypes with this characteristic LD determinant represented in six individuals.

Our studies have so far included 41 individuals representing 22 haplotypes with the HL-A7 antigen. Sixteen (73%) of these haplotypes carry the LD7a determinant (Table 2), and thus this LD determinant seems to be the most frequent on HL-A7 haplotypes.

Table 3 shows some of the SR values obtained in these studies. Two LD7a-homozygous test cells (A and B) were used to define the HL-A3,7-linked LD determinant in the cell donors 1–5. Obviously the test cells A and B are identical with respect to SD as well as to LD determinants. Furthermore, none of the donors 1–5 could respond to these test cells.

The HL-A3,7/2,7 individual (BJ) was not LD7a-homozygous for the LD7a determinant, as her cells consistently stimulated the HL-A3,7-homozygous cells A and B. The HL-A3,7/10,W18 cells (HJ) did not stimulate the test cells and could thus be LD7a-homozygous or LD-7a/O on the LD locus. The other HL-A3,7-heterozygous cell donors did stimulate both test cells A and B.

Table 4 shows the assumed LD determinants in these seven individuals. Table 5 gives the results obtained in repeated MLC testings between four of the HL-A3,7-heterozygous individuals. Surprisingly, HJ (3,7/10,W18) did not stimulate HL-A3,-7/10,W18 (MF); 3,7/2,W16 (JJ); or 3,7/9,-W16 (CJ) cells significantly. The stimula-

Table 3. The HL-A7-linked MLC Determinant (LD7a) in Unrelated Danes

Responder Cells	Stimulating Cells							
	3,7/3,7$_m$		1m BJ	2m HJ	3m MF	4m	5m	
	A	B	3,7/2,7$_m$	3,7/10,W18$_m$	3,7/10,W18$_m$	3,7/2,W16$_m$	3,7/9,W16$_m$	−§/−§$_m$
3,7/3,7 A		0.8 0.9 1.0 1.0	7.5 9.7 11.5 13.5	1.2 1.3	4.7 4.7 5.0 5.5 8.0	5.8 8.6 9.3 11.5 18.8	7.1 7.5 14.3	N = 16* 5.6– *14.0*– 34.9
3,7/3,7 B	0.7 0.8 1.0 1.0		9.0 15.5	1.0 2.1	3.0 4.6 7.9	4.7 6.1 11.0	6.9	
1 BJ 3,7/2,7	0.8 1.6 2.8 4.1	2.3 3.1						
2 HJ 3,7/10,W18	1.1 1.9	0.8 1.4						
3 MF 3,7/10,W18	1.4 1.8 3.0 3.8	1.6 2.3 2.7						
4 3,7/2,W16	1.2 1.4 2.0 2.2	1.1 1.3 1.3						
5 3,7/9,W16	1.9 2.3 2.6	2.2						
−§/−§	N = 6* 3.8– *10.8*– 30.4	N = 6* 3.2– *10.5*– 34.5						

Characterization of the LD7a determinant by the homozygous test cells A and B.
*The SR obtained are given as mean value with 95% confidence limits.
N = number of independent, repeated testings.

Table 4. Evaluation of MLC Data From Table 3

	A 3,7/3,7$_m$	3,7/2,7$_m$	HJ 3,7/10,W18$_m$	MF 3,7/10,W18$_m$	3,7/2,W16$_m$	3,7/9,W16$_m$	§/§	MLC-Locus Genotypes	
3,7/3,7	0 h	1 h	0 h	1 h	1 h	1 h	2 h	X	X
3,7/3,7	0 h	1 h	0 h	1 h	1 h	1 h	2 h	X	X
3,7/2,7	0 h	1 h	0 h	1 h	1 h	1 h	2 h	X	W
3,7/10,W18 (HJ)	0 h							X	X/O
3,7/10,W18 (MF)	0 h							X	Y
3,7/2,W16	0 h							X	Z
3,7/9,W16	0 h							X	Q
§/§	2 h								

X, LD7a; W, LD7b; Y, LD-W18; Z, LD-W16a; Q, LD-W16b; O, Null-determinant.

0 h, 1 h, and 2 h: MLC responses compatible with zero, one, and two HL-A haplotype responses. See Materials and Method.

tion ratios obtained are compatible with those obtained when testing haploidentical siblings presumed to be identical on the major MLC locus,[7] and thus these intermediate stimulations could be due to differences at a minor MLC locus located within the HL-A chromosomal region.

The HL-A3,7/10,W18 of MF did not stimulate HL-A3,7/2,W16 (JJ) cells in repeated testings and stimulated CJ (3,7/9,-W16) only very weakly. In contrast, MF had a normal one-haplotype response to these HL-A3,7-haploidentical unrelated cells. From these studies we deduced the LD genotypes of these four individuals. As shown in the right part of Table 5, HJ (3,7/10,W18) could still be homozygous LD7a/LD7a or heterozygous LD7a/O. MF (3,7/10,W18) could be LD7a/LD-W18a, but if so the haplotypes 2,W16 and 9,W16 also must carry the LD-W18a determinant. However, the 2,W16 and the 9,W16 haplotypes must then carry extra and different LD determinants, LD-W16a and LD-W16b, in addition to their LD-W18a determinant, because of the mutual stimulation between JJ and CJ.

DISCUSSION AND CONCLUSIONS

These studies demonstrate that the Four antigen HL-A7, at least in the Danish population, is very frequently associated with a very specific and quite common MLC determinant, which we call LD7a. When this determinant is present in a single dose in unrelated individuals, they react mutually in MLC tests as haploidentical siblings. In another study we have shown that this LD7a determinant is characteristic for a majority of patients with multiple sclerosis.[9]

This study has primarily focused on the two different methods for typing of LD determinants. As is shown by us and independently by two other groups,[4,5] this can be done by means of LD-homozygous test cells. In addition, we have shown that it is also possible to use LD-heterozygous test cells when these carry one well-defined LD determinant. Furthermore, our study also demonstrates that the LD determinants of one HL-A haplotype may be composed of more than one specificity. We have described the inclusion of the LD-W18a determinant in two different HL-A haplotypes carrying the W16 antigen. We have also described an HL-A haplotype, 10,W18, which may not carry any LD determinant (HJ). This might reflect a high degree of complexity within the chromosomal region that determines the LD characteristics.[10]

Note added in proof: Our continuous work on the characterization of the LD7a determinant in the outbred Danish population has shown that the LD7a determinant is present in approximately 50% of normal individuals who carry HL-A7. In addition, LD7a is present in about 5 to 10% of normal individuals lacking HL-A7.

Table 5. Identical MLC Determinants Among Unrelated HL-A Different Normal Individuals

Responding Cells	Preliminary MLC Genotype (Table 4)		Stimulating Cells: HJ 3, 7/10, $W18_m$	MF 3, 7/10, $W18_m$	3, 7/2, $W16_m$	3, 7/9, $W16_m$	–§/–$§_m$	Deduced MLC Genotypes on Haplotype 1	2
HJ 3, 7/10, W18	X	O		4.4 4.9	7.6 9.3	10.1	9.0 11.7 14.4 20.1 22.7	LD7a	LD7a or null
MF 3, 7/10, W18	X	Y	1.4 2.3		*N* = 6* 3.8–6.3–11.8	5.6 10.1	4.9 7.3 7.4 10.1 12.3 19.9	LD7a	LD-W18a
3, 7/2, W16	X	Z	1.7 2.3	*N* = 6* 1.3–1.8–2.5		7.4 9.2 10.7 11.8	7.9 11.5 12.7 14.4 14.5 16.2	LD7a	LD-W18a + LD-W16a
3, 7/9, W16	X	Q	2.6	2.5 2.8 3.7	6.3 8.5 8.9 10.0			LD7a	LD-W18a + LD-W16b
–§/–§	§	§	*N* = 6* 3.2–9.7–28.9	*N* = 6* 5.6–16.1–46.3	*N* = 7* 5.2–12.2–28.4	*N* = 4* 4.0–8.5–17.7	*N* = 12* 3.7–15.0–60.8	§	§

The SR obtained are given as mean values with 95% confidence limits.

REFERENCES

1. van Rood JJ, Eijsvoogel VP: Lancet 1:698, 1970

2. Mempel W, Grosse-Wilde H, Albert E, Thierfelder S: Transplant Proc 5:401, 1973

3. Lebrun A, Sasportes M, Dausset J: Transplant Proc 5:363, 1973

4. Mempel W, Grosse-Wilde H, Albert E: Transplant Proc 5:1529, 1973

5. van den Tweel JG, Blussé van Oud Alblas A, Keuning JJ, et al: Transplant Proc 5:1535, 1973

6. Dupont B, Andersen V, Hansen GS, Svejgaard A: Transplantation 14:557, 1972

7. Dupont B, Good RA, Hansen GS, et al: Proc Natl Acad Sci (in press)

8. Yunis EJ, Amos DB: Proc Natl Acad Sci 68:3031, 1971

9. Jersild C, Dupont B, Hansen GS, et al: Transplant Proc 5:1791, 1973

10. Dupont B, Jersild C, Hansen GS, et al: Transplant Proc 5:1481, 1973

Linkage Disequilibrium Between HL-A7 and the MLC Specificity Pi

By E. D. Albert, W. Mempel, and H. Grosse-Wilde

AFTER the establishment of the fact that MLC is genetically determined by at least one locus clearly separated from but closely linked to the HL-A system, it became of interest to analyze MLC reactions between individuals of an unselected unrelated population. It has been known for several years that among unselected individuals a nonstimulation in MLC occurs only in a very low incidence, while 25% of the sibling combinations are mutually nonstimulatory. This information has been used to suggest the existence of one MLC locus with at least 20 different alleles of approximately equal gene frequencies.[1] The fact that 99% of the HL-A-identical siblings are MLC-nonstimulatory and that only 1% shows the recombinant behavior of stimulation suggests a rather close linkage between the MLC locus and the HL-A system. As is well known from the immunoglobulins,[2] the MNSs system,[3] and, most notably, from the HL-A system,[4] the alleles of two closely linked loci tend to show linkage disequilibrium for certain combinations of alleles. It can therefore be expected that there is some degree of linkage disequilibrium between certain HL-A antigens and MLC determinants. This expectation is in very good agreement with the finding that among unrelated individuals selected for HL-A identity there are as many as 10% nonstimulatory pairs as compared to about 0.1% nonstimulations in the random unrelated population.

From this one can conclude that selection for HL-A identity results in a selection for MLC identity by means of a linkage disequilibrium between the HL-A and the MLC system.

Furthermore, if one assumes that incompatibility for two MLC alleles generally results in a higher stimulation than incompatibility for one allele only (this has been shown for one- and two-haplotype different siblings[5]), one can predict that on the average the degree of MLC stimulation will increase with the number of HL-A incompatibilities and that this effect will be more pronounced if the incompatible HL-A antigens belong to the locus which is located in closer proximity to the MLC locus. These expectations are fully confirmed by our recently published data,[6] which show that incompatibilities at the second HL-A locus are correlated with a significantly higher stimulation ratio than are incompatibilities at the first HL-A locus, as it had been established previously in families showing crossing-over between HL-A and MLC.

If one assumes only one MLC locus closely linked to the second HL-A locus one would expect that among individuals identical for the antigens of the second HL-A locus the stimulation ratio should be the same as for individuals identical for the antigens of both loci. There is however a significantly higher stimulation ratio for the individuals who are identical only for the antigens of the second HL-A locus, suggesting that there is one additional MLC locus in closer proximity to the first HL-A locus responsible for a low-grade stimulation.[6] These data confirm earlier findings in crossing-over families by Eijsvoogel[7] and

From the Kinderpoliklinik der Universität München and Institut für Hämatologie, Abteilung Immunologie der GSF München.

Authors are members of Sonderforschungsbereich 37, München.

Supported in part by Deutsche Forschungsgemeinschaft, grant Al 92/7.

© 1973 by Grune & Stratton, Inc.

more recently by Thorsby[8] and by Revillard,[9] showing a slight but definite stimulation associated with the LA locus fragment of a recombinant chromosome.

From all this we conclude that the observed population data can be most economically explained by the existence of two MLC loci, one causing generally strong stimulation in close linkage to the second HL-A locus (therefore provisionally named LD-2) and another one somewhere in the proximity of the first HL-A locus (LD-1) producing definite but low-grade stimulation.

It is essential for this concept that there is a considerable linkage disequilibrium between the different alleles of these systems reflecting the close linkage and also possibly the action of selection, which could conceivably favor certain combinations of alleles of the major histocompatibility complex consisting of two HL-A and two MLC loci.

After the first MLC specificity has been defined[6] and after typing of unrelated individuals with the MLC-homozygous reference cells Pi and Fr,[10] we have attempted to estimate the gene frequency of Pi and the haplotype frequency as well as the linkage disequilibrium parameter (Delta) for the HL-A7-Pi haplotype.

Among 45 unrelated unselected individuals 6 were found to possess the Pi specificity of which 4 also were HL-A7 positive. This corresponds to a phenotype frequency of $f = 0.14$ and allows a gene frequency estimate $[g = 1 - (1 - f)^{1/2}]$ for Pi of approximately $g = 0.07$.

In an unrelated population of 67 persons who had been selected for the presence of HL-A7 (most of them had HL-A2-7 or 3-7) Pi was found 24 times (36%). From this one could conclude that probably 36% of all HL-A7 genes are coupled with the MLC determinant Pi. This percentage, however, must be corrected because non-HL-A7-bound Pi determinants might also be present in this population. The correction has to take into account that of the 24 Pi positive individuals some may not have the HL-A7-Pi haplotype ($= 2 \times 0.02 \times 67 = 2.7$) and others could be homozygous HL-A7-Pi/X-Pi ($= 2 \times 0.02 \times 0.32 \times 67 = 0.85$), so that the corrected figure would be $24 - (2.7 - 0.85) = 22.15$. So, only the corrected number of 22.15 out of 67 (=33%) persons are expected to have the HL-A7-Pi haplotype, and therefore only 33% of the HL-A7 genes are coupled with Pi. (It should be stressed that in these rough approximations the corrections are only given in order to elucidate the principles involved in these calculations.) Since the gene frequency of HL-A7 in the Munich population is $g_7 = 0.15$,[11] one can easily deduce the observed haplotype frequency for HL-A7-Pi from $0.15 \times 0.33 = 0.050$. The linkage disequilibrium parameter (Delta) is defined as the difference between the observed haplotype frequency and the haplotype frequency expected on the basis of the gene frequencies of the antigens involved: Delta $= hf_{7\text{-Pi}}(obs) - (g_7 \times g_{Pi})$. In this case it is Delta $= 0.050 - (0.15 \times 0.07) = 0.050 - 0.011 = 0.039$. This Delta value corresponds quite well to the values observed within the HL-A system as per example $\text{Delta}_{3\text{-}7} = 0.040$ in the Munich white population.[11]

It should be stressed that the above-discussed HL-A7-Pi haplotype is only one of a large number of possible HL-A-MLC haplotypes and that the linkage disequilibrium must be expected to vary considerably for the different haplotypes as is the case in the HL-A system.

Finally, it can be stated that the existence of linkage disequilibrium—be it a regular feature of closely linked loci or be it the reflection of selection processes or both—has been instrumental in the definition of MLC specificities.[6,10,12,13]

REFERENCES

1. Bach FH, Bach ML, Najarian J, Simmons R (eds): Transplantation. Philadelphia, Lea & Febiger, 1972, pp 40–61
2. Ceppellini R: Genetica delle Immunoglobuline. XII Ann. Meet. Assoziatione Genetica Italiana, Parma, A.G.I. 1967, 12, 3
3. Race RR, Sanger R: Blood Groups in Man. Oxford, Blackwell, 1968
4. Joint report of the Fourth International Histocompatibility Workshop. Histocompatibility Testing, 1970, Copenhagen, Munksgaard, 1970, pp 17–47
5. Bach ML, Solliday S, Stambuk M: Histocompatibility Testing, 1970, Copenhagen, Munksgaard, 1970, pp 17–47
6. Mempel W, Grosse-Wilde H, Albert E, et al: Transplant Proc 5:401, 1973
7. Eijsvoogel VP, du Bois MJGJ, Melief CJM, de Groot-Kooy ML, Koning C, van Rood JJ, van Leeuwen A, du Toit E, Schellekens P: Histocomp. Testing 1972.
8. Thorsby: Transplant Proc 5:1523, 1973
9. Revillard: Transplant Proc 5:1855, 1973
10. Mempel: Transplant Proc 5:1529, 1973
11. Albert ED, Scholz S, Rosenthal I, et al: Histocomp. Testing, 1972. Copenhagen, Munksgaard, 1972
12. Dupont et al: Transplant Proc 5:1543, 1973
13. van Rood et al: Transplant Proc 5:1335, 1973

The Histocompatibility Complex of Rhesus Monkeys: III. Evidence for a Major MLR Locus and Histocompatibility-linked Ir Genes

By H. Balner, M. E. Dorf, M. L. de Groot, and B. Benacerraf

IN several mammalian species a chromosomal region has been identified with a number of closely linked genetic systems which have a major influence on histocompatibility and control other immunological traits which are believed to be of great biological significance. In mice, this major histocompatibility complex (MHC) has been shown to include at least two systems coding for serologically defined transplantation antigens (SD loci), one or more systems governing lymphocyte-defined (LD) factors which determine reactivity in mixed lymphocyte cultures, and, finally, systems which control the capacity to respond immunologically to defined, synthetic antigens (Ir loci). This volume contains a number of articles providing up-to-date information regarding the SD, LD, and Ir loci of several species. The current paper summarizes the available data for rhesus monkeys. Since rhesus monkeys are phylogenetically close to man, and since they are still the only outbred species for which information regarding SD, LD, as well as Ir genes are available, this short review underlines the potential value of this species for fundamental and applied studies in immunobiology.

SEROLOGICALLY DEFINED SYSTEMS (SD)

Two closely linked genetic systems controlling the rhesus monkey's major histocompatibility antigens have been identified.[1-3] The methods used for their identification were similar to those employed in human tissue typing and have been described previously.[1,4] Analogous to HL-A, the chromosomal region containing the two SD loci was called RhL-A and the relevance of this region to histocompatibility was proved by intersib skin grafting experiments; grafts exchanged between sibs that had inherited the same parental haplotypes (chromosomal region coding for maximally two SD antigens) had significantly longer survival times than those exchanged between sibs differing for one or two RhL-A haplotypes. However, matching unrelated monkeys for the known SD antigens of RhL-A does not improve kidney graft survival, nor mitigate the graft-vs.-host reaction in irradiated, bone-marrow-treated animals.

At the time of writing, about 75% of the gene products of the two segregant series of RhL-A are serologically identified (ten antigens per series); however, the number of recognized antigens is steadily increasing. As in the human HL-A region, recombination frequency between the two known SD systems is about 1%. So far, there is no evidence for a third SD system within the RhL-A region, and "minor" histocompatibility systems outside RhL-A have not yet been identified.

SYSTEMS DETERMINING REACTIVITY IN MIXED LYMPHOCYTE CULTURES (MLR)

MLR in rhesus monkeys has been studied since 1970 and the techniques have been described.[5] In 1971, it was shown that lymphocytes from rhesus siblings do not stimulate each other in mixed cultures if they are genotypically identical for RhL-A

From the Primate Center TNO, Rijswijk, The Netherlands, and Harvard Medical School, Boston, Mass. (For reprints write Primate Center TNO.)

Supported in part by a contract from the Dutch government and contract 6243-22/6/001 of the Commission of the European Communities (E.E.G.), Luxembourg.

This publication is contribution No. 829 of the Euratom Biology Division.

© 1973 by Grune & Stratton, Inc.

but are stimulatory if they differ for one or two RhL-A haplotypes. This suggested that disparity for RhL-A caused MLC stimulation.[6] Subsequent family studies indicated that there is indeed a major MLR locus in the RhL-A region but that it is separate from the SD loci of RhL-A.[7] Results depicted in Table 1 suggest that, like in man (and unlike in the mouse), this major MLR system is probably located outside the SD region of the RhL-A complex (for detailed information see Ref. 5). Recombination frequency between this MLR locus and the SD region is approximately 1.5%, and there is preliminary evidence that the system is situated near the locus that controls the SD antigens of the first segregant series.[7]

As could be expected from work done in man[8,9] and in the mouse,[10,11] there is evidence for additional MLR loci also in rhesus monkeys. For instance, cells from three genotypically identical sibs (RhL-A, SD) did not stimulate each other in MLC (as expected if one major MLR locus is assumed). However, when tested with cells from a half-sib, two combinations showed stimulation, while a third did not. Similar results, also suggesting the existence of further MLR loci, have since been found on several occasions. The number and location of additional LD loci and their relative strengths are not yet known.

"Defining" the gene products of the major MLR locus, by serological or other methods, is obviously a next step. Preliminary results suggest that the polymorphism of this MLR locus is not as high as that of the SD loci and that there is a considerable degree of linkage disequilibrium between the LD and SD systems of the RhL-A

Table 1. Evidence for Recombination Between the Major MLR Locus and the Region Coding for the SD Antigens of RhL-A.

Stimulation Between Full Sibs Genotypically Identical for RhL-A

Parents	Sib	V	JJ	AV	BU	Genotypes
♂ 381, ♀ 584	V					bd —,—/6, 11*
	JJ	7.68				bc —,—/6, 14
	AV	9.46	1.91			bc —,—/6, 14
	BU	6.44	1.67	.59		bc —,—/6, 14
	CZ	8.08	*6.40*	*5.09*	*6.16*	bc —,—/6, 14

Parents	Sib	BJ	FU	Genotypes
♂ 381, ♀ 594	BJ			bd —,—/9, r18
	FU	*4.57*		bd —,—/9, r18
	YY	9.38	6.77	ad 10, r17/9, r18

Parent	Genotype
♂ 381	ab 10, r17/—,—
♀ 584	cd 6, 14/6, 11*
♀ 594	cd 6,—/9, r18

Absence of stimulation between full sibs differing for one RhL-A haplotype

Parents	Sib	AE	FL	Z	Genotypes
♂ 598, ♀ 589	AE				ad 6, 13/6, 13
	FL	*0.67*			bd r19, r17/6, 13
	Z	10.60	8.27		ac 6, 13/—, r17
	BP	9.37	7.62	8.64	bc r19, r17/—, r17

Parent	Genotype
♂ 598	ab 6, 13/r19, r17
♀ 589	cd —, (r17)/6, 13

Stimulation in bilateral MLC; mean values of triple tests given in cpm $\times 10^{-3}$, interesting results are italicized.
For details regarding assignment of parental haplotypes (see Ref. 5).

Table 2. Low MLC Reactivity Between Half-Sibs Differing for One Haplotype

Parents		G	GG	DV	AX	CK	Genotypes	
♂ 599 ♀ 581	G						bc_1	10, 13/9, 11*
	GG	0.88					bc_1	10, 13/9, 11*
	DV	1.43	1.64				bc_1	10, 13/9, 11*
♂ 599 ♀ 493	AX	*1.57*	*1.57*	*2.36*			bc_3	10, 13/9, 11*
	CK	*1.44*	*.96*	*1.79*	*.89*		bc_3	10, 13/9, 11*
	DM	*2.49*	*2.82*	*.80*	1.65	1.95	bc_3	10, 13/9, 11*

♂ 599	ab	R1, —/10, 13
♀ 581	c_1d_1	9,11*/R1,—
♀ 493	c_3d_3	9, 11*/10, —

Parents		FU	YY	CU	Genotypes	
♂ 381 ♀ 594	FU				bd_4	—, —/9, r18
	YY	6.77			ad_4	10, r17/9, r18
♂ 381 ♀ 324	CU	*1.68*	8.34		bc_6	—, —/9, r20
	EM	6.34	*1.57*	7.67	ac_6	10, r17/9, r20

♂ 381	ab	10,r17/—,—
♀ 594	c_4d_4	6,—/9,r18
♀ 324	c_6d_d	9,r20/10,—

Stimulation in bilateral MLC; mean values of triple tests given in cpm × 10^{-3}, interesting results are italicized.
For details regarding assignment of parental haplotypes see Ref. 5.
The maternal haplotypes are given subscripts to emphasize origin from different mothers.

region.[5] Table 2 shows examples of virtually negative MLCs between siblings sharing only one paternal RhL-A haplotype. Nonreactivity occurred most frequently if the other haplotype (from unrelated mothers) carried identical SD antigens, a finding which suggests linkage disequilibrium between the LD and SD systems. The availability of multiple half-sibs in our rhesus colony (offspring sired by the same father) obviously facilitates the identification of the most common LD determinants of RhL-A. An alternative method to define the gene products of the major MLR locus uses "typing cells" homozygous for LD or sera raised specifically against presumed LD determinants. Such sera, which are not lymphocytotoxic, have been raised in rhesus monkeys and been shown to inhibit MLR specifically.[7]

Further evidence for linkage disequilibrium between LD and SD parameters comes from the screening of unrelated individuals in bi- and unilateral MLR. Cells unmatched for SD antigens very rarely show low or negative MLR. If matched for three or four RhL-A antigens (SD), chances to share the same LD determinants improve considerably; bilateral MLR were low in 7%–8% of about 140 SD-identical combinations and some of these were negative in unilateral MLR.

Studies are in progress to test the relative importance of SD and LD matching for allograft survival in rhesus monkeys. Host-donor combinations have been selected as follows: SD-identical and MLR-positive (>90%), SD-identical and MLR-negative (<10%), SD-nonidentical with low MLR (very rare), and the usual control group of SD-nonidenticals with high MLR.

PRELIMINARY EVIDENCE FOR HISTOCOMPATIBILITY-LINKED SYSTEMS CONTROLLING THE IMMUNE RESPONSE TO SYNTHETIC ANTIGENS

Interest in the genetic control of the immune response was stimulated by the find-

Table 3. Humoral Response of Related Rhesus Monkeys to Three Synthetic Antigens*

Parents and Offspring	RhL-A Geno-type	(TG)AL	GA	DNP-GL
♂ 600		—	+	++
♀ 669		—	+	+
AC	ad	—	—	++
BI	ad	—	—	++
CR	ad	—	—	++
EL	bc	—	+	++
FS	bc	—	+	++
♀ 597		—	++	—
AB	bc	—	++	++
BF	bc	—	++	++
DW	ac	—	++	++
CG	ad	—	—	++
♀ 603		—		
T	bd	—		
DF	bd	—		
FO	bd	—		

		Tentative Ir genes (TG)AL	GA	GL
♂ 600	a	—	—	++
	b	—	+	++
♀ 597	c	—	++	—
	d	—	—	—

Parents and Offspring	RhL-A Geno-type	(TG)AL	GA	DNP-GL
♂ 599		+	+	++
♀ 581		—	++	—
G	bc	—	+	++
GG	bc	—	+	++
DV	bc	—	+	++
AG	ac	++	++	++
CF	ac	++	+	++
♀ 498		—	+	++
NN	ac	++	+	++
AQ	ac	+	++	++
ED	a/bd	—	++	++
♀ 590		+		
CV	bd	+		
EI	ad	+		

		Tentative Ir genes (TG)AL	GA	GL
♂ 599	a	++		++
	b	—		++

Parents and Offspring	RhL-A Geno-type	(TG)AL	GA	DNP-GL
♂ 381			++	+
♀ 584			++	+
V	bd		++	—
JJ	bc		++	+
AV	bc		++	+
BU	bc		++	+
CZ	a-bc		++	+
♀ 432			—	++
N	ad		++	++
FN	ad		++	++
CP	ac		++	++
♀ 324			—	++
CU	bc		++	—
EM	ac		++	++

		Tentative Ir genes (TG)AL	GA	GL
♂ 381	a		++	++
	b		++	—

Symbols in columns under abbreviations (TG)AL, GA and DNP-GL are arbitrary ratings of antibody levels against the three synthetic antigens (see text). Left—open spaces mean that immunizations had not been done. Symbols at the bottom of the table indicate that the data contained in the body of the table are compatible with the assignment of hypothetical Ir genes (responsible for specific humoral responses) on parental RhL-A haplotypes.

Parents are indicated with numerical symbols, offspring with letters. Offspring within a column share the same father (♂ at top). Paternal RhL-A haplotypes are indicated with a and b (same for each column), maternal haplotypes with c and d (different for each family).

Child ED is a paternal recombinant within the SD region of RhL-A (genotype a/bd), child CZ inherited the MLR determinant of paternal haplotype a and the SD determinants of haplotypes b and c (genotype a-bc).

ing that resistance of mice to various oncogenic viruses[12] and the response to synthetic antigens[13] are controlled by systems closely linked to the major histocompatibility system, H-2. The control of responses to synthetic antigens by so-called Ir genes has been studied mostly in inbred strains of mice and guinea pigs (reviewed in Ref. 14). More recently, attempts have been made to correlate human disease states with the occurrence of certain HL-A antigens[15] or with the inheritance of a particular HL-A haplotype in affected families.[16] The obvious importance of the subject led us to initiate studies of Ir genes also in the rhesus monkey.

In initial experiments,* we studied humoral responses to the synthetic polypeptide (TG)AL,† one of the antigens originally used to identify the Ir-1 locus of mice.[13] (TG)AL 100 μg/kg in saline was given subcutaneously, 3 times at weekly intervals. Antibody determinations were performed at Stanford University using the customary techniques.[17] After it was shown that unrelated animals could be high (++), medium (+) and low or nonresponders (−), members of several rhesus families were immunized. Table 3 summarizes results of part of those preliminary studies: all offspring of ♂ 600 were nonresponders but those of ♂ 599 included some responders and were informative. In the families with ♀ 581 and ♀ 498, the capacity to respond seemed to correlate with the inheritance of the paternal RhL-A haplotype *a*. Interestingly, the SD-recombinant child ED did not inherit the capacity to respond to (TG)AL. ED carries the first-series SD antigen of the paternal haplotype *a*, the second series antigen of haplotype *b*. The medium response of child CV, not carrying the paternal haplotype *a*, is probably due to inheritance of the maternal haplotype *d*.

The Ir studies were continued using antigens which had been employed primarily to demonstrate histocompatibility-linked Ir genes in guinea pigs.[14,18] Tested were humoral and cellular responses to synthetic amino acid copolymers containing glutamic acid as well as alanine, lysine or tyrosine, abbreviated as GA, GL, and GT, respectively. Pilot studies had shown that distinct humoral and cellular responses to these antigens were obtained only if complete Freund's adjuvant (CFA) was used. Deep intramuscular injections of 100 μg/g of GA and 50 μg/g of the dinitrophenyl conjugate of GL (plus CFA) were given on day 0, followed by intradermal skin tests with both substances on day 21 (in doses of 10 and 50 μg per antigen). Serum samples were taken on days 0, 21, and 28. In vitro reactivity of lymphocytes to the antigens was tested on day 21.

Table 3 summarizes results of the humoral response to GA and GL-DNP by members of several rhesus families (a detailed report is given elsewhere by Dorf et al.[19]). Antibody determinations were performed at Harvard University using a modified Farr test.[18] Titers obtained at 3 and/or 4 wk after initial immunization were considered and animals are rated as high (++), medium (+), and nonresponders (−). In several of the families, the data again suggest that the capacity to respond to an antigen is inherited with a particular RhL-A haplotype. On this basis, hypothetical Ir genes responsible for the capacity to respond to any one of the three antigens have been tentatively assigned to parental RhL-A haplotypes (bottom of Table 3).

It is clear that all results depicted in Table 3 have to be regarded as provisional. More elaborate family studies of the same type are in progress whereby the response to the copolymer GT is also being investigated.

Testing the in vivo and in vitro cellular

*Collaboration with H. O. McDevitt (Stanford), E. Mozes and M. Sela (Rehovot), and J. J. van Rood (Leiden).

†(TG)AL is a branched copolymer of polyalanine (A) and polylysine (L) with the addition of random sequences of tyrosine (T) and glutamic acid (G).

responses to the mentioned antigens has not been particularly successful, so far. Results of skin reactions were very difficult to score (the intradermal injections on day 21 are nevertheless maintained as booster doses). Results of in vitro proliferative responses of lymphocytes to the antigens were erratic and showed a poor correlation with the outcome of humoral responses. However, recent studies have shown that this technique can be improved (modifications of antigen dose, timing, etc.) and the modified test is maintained as a potentially valuable parameter in studying the genetic control of cellular reactivity.

SUMMARY

The rhesus monkey's major histocompatibility complex, RhL-A, is described. While mapping of genetic systems in this region has not reached the sophisticated stage attained for the analogous complex of mice, encouraging progress has been made. Adjacent to two closely linked highly polymorphic systems controlling the serologically defined antigens of RhL-A there is a system which exerts an important influence on reactivity in mixed lymphocyte cultures. This major MLR system is closely linked to but outside the region of the two systems controlling the serologically defined parameters. Identification (typing) of the gene products of this MLR is in progress. Furthermore, evidence has been obtained that immune-response genes may also be located in this chromosomal region. Preliminary results indicate that the humoral response to several synthetic antigens is genetically controlled by systems which are part of the major histocompatibility complex and thus represent the monkey's analogues of the murine Ir systems.

REFERENCES

1. Balner H, Gabb BW, Dersjant H, et al: Nature 230:177, 1971

2. Gabb BW, Piazza A, D'Amaro J, et al: Transplant Proc 4:11, 1972

3. Rogentine GN Jr, Merritt CB, Vaal LA, et al: Transplant Proc 4:21, 1972

4. Van Rood JJ, van Leeuwen A: J Clin Invest 42:1382, 1963

5. Balner H, Toth EK: Tissue Antigens 3:273, 1973

6. Appelman AWM, Balner H: Transplant Proc 4:17, 1972

7. Balner H, D'Amaro J, Toth EK, et al: Transplant Proc 5:323, 1973

8. Eijsvoogel VP, du Bois R, Melief CJM, et al: Transplant Proc 5:1301, 1973

9. Ward FE, Seigler HF: Transplant Proc 5:359, 1973

10. Bach FH, Widmer MB, Bach ML, et al: J Exp Med 136:1430, 1972

11. Festenstein H, Abbasi K, Sachs JA, Oliver RTD: Transplant Proc 4:219, 1972

12. Lilly F: Nat Cancer Inst Monogr 22:631, 1966

13. McDevitt HO, Benecerraf B: Adv Immunol 11:31, 1969

14. Benacerraf B, McDevitt HO: Science 175, 273, 1972

15. Marsh DG, Bias WB, Hsu SH, et al: Science 179:691, 1973

16. Levine BN, Stember RH, Fotino M: Science 178:1201, 1972

17. McDevitt HO, Sela M: J Exp Med 122:517, 1965

18. Bluestein HG, Green I, Benacerraf B: J Exp Med 134:458, 1971

19. Balner H, Dorf ME, de Groot ML, et al: Transplant Proc 5:1555, 1973

Phenotypic Expression of the Main Histocompatibility Complex (DL-A) in Randomly Selected Mongrel Dogs: I. Serologically Detectable (SD) DL-A Antigens and Mixed Leukocyte (MLC) Reactivity

By R. Bachvaroff, A. Ozaki, F.D. Cannon, N. Mollen, D.A. Blumenstock, J.H. Ayvazian, J.W. Ferrebee, and F.T. Rapaport*

IT is generally agreed that there exists in the canine species a major system of histocompatibility (MHC), for which the term DL-A has been proposed.[1] The studies of Mollen et al.[2] have provided evidence that serologically detectable (SD) leukocyte surface antigens transmitted as Mendelian autosomal dominants in the Cooperstown colony are a component of the canine MHC. Donor–recipient combinations selected on the basis of serologic and genetic[3] evidence of DL-A SD identity have resulted in the regularly reproducible survival of bone marrow allografts in supralethally irradiated recipients[4] that have also developed permanent tolerance to skin, kidney,[4] and lung[5] allografts obtained from the donor of marrow.

Studies of the segregation of the currently detectable DL-A SD alleles in 141 consecutive matings in the Cooperstown colony have shown that the DL-A SD products are transmitted en bloc from parent to offspring, with no instance of independent segregation.[3] A total of six different patterns of DL-A antigens was observed in this colony—an expression of the limited genetic pool encountered in the selectively bred lines of dogs raised in the Cooperstown colony.[6] In contrast, when the same DL-A antigens were used to study cell samples obtained from a population of 100 randomly selected unrelated mongrel dogs, 31 different patterns of DL-A SD antigens were observed and there were a number of statistically significant positive and negative associations between individual DL-A antigenic component(s) within this population of mongrel dogs.[3] This observation provided further support for the concept that the loci determining DL-A SD products were components of a complex immunogenetic system (MHC) governed by one principal region or complex, located on an autosomal pair of canine chromosomes.[3] These studies have recently been confirmed and extended by Vriesendorp et al.,[7] who have provided further evidence of the polymorphism of the SD components of the DL-A system and have shown further analogies between the DL-A SD loci and the corresponding analogues detected in other species.[8] Vriesendorp et al.[7] have also reported the existence of two principal DL-A SD loci, each of which determines a separate series of alleles.

Recent studies indicate that the SD loci of the mammalian MHC are not the only factors capable of conditioning allograft responses. The products of an additional locus(i), which has been shown to be located in close proximity to the second HL-A SD[9] and to the H-2K SD loci[10] in man and mouse, respectively, and which appear to determine the recognition phase of the allograft response, have been of particu-

Irma T. Hirschl Career Scientist Award.

From the Department of Surgery and Institute of Reconstructive Plastic Surgery, New York University Medical Center; the Research Service, Manhattan Veterans Administration Hospital, New York, N.Y.; and the Mary Imogene Bassett Hospital, Cooperstown, N.Y.

Supported by grants from the John A. Hartford Foundation, the Billy Rose Foundation, and the Irwin Strasburger Memorial Medical Foundation, and by NIH grant AM-02215 and U.S. Atomic Energy Commission Contract AT-(30-1)-2005.

©1973 by Grune & Stratton, Inc.

lar interest in this regard. Donor-recipient differences at this locus are detectable in vitro by the mixed leukocyte culture (MLC) technique, and the differences in the MHC which lead to lymphocyte activation in the MLC have been attributed to this locus(i), termed LD.[9] A number of different authors, and particularly Rudolph et al.,[11] Hartzman et al.,[12] Templeton and Thomas,[13] and Storb, Rudolph, and Thomas,[14] have adapted MLC techniques for canine studies. In general, skin and bone marrow allografts have been found to have a better chance to survive for longer periods of time in littermate dogs in which both DL-A SD and LD compatibility occurred.[14]

There has been a paucity of data, however, on the distribution of MLC reactivity between pairs of randomly selected unrelated mongrel dogs, with particular regard to a correlation of the results with the DL-A SD phenotypes of the animals under study. The present report describes the results of the 56 consecutive reciprocal MLC tests in such a canine population, whose DL-A SD phenotypes were determined simultaneously.

MATERIALS AND METHOD

A group of male unrelated mongrel dogs weighing 18–24 lb, maintained on a standard diet, underwent DL-A SD tests with a battery of lymphocytotoxic antisera recognizing 12 antigens by a standard technique.[4] The DL-A SD specificities (or sets of specificities) detectable under these conditions included b, c, d, e, f, g, h, k, l, m, n, and o.[6] Blood samples were drawn simultaneously for MLC tests by the technique of Hartzman et al.[12] so that the lymphocytes of each dog were tested in MLC against cells obtained from each of the other donors in the group. Each MLC test was performed in quadruplicate. The MLC reactions were expressed as the rate of ^{3}H thymidine incorporation by the responding cells, in counts per minute. Mild to moderate reactions involved those instances where the ^{3}H thymidine uptake rates exceeded the control value by a factor of at least 3 to 10 ×; strong reactivity required uptake values exceeding 10 ×. The assessment of major and minor DL-A SD phenotypic incompatibilities between cells acting as stimulatory cells (i.e., mytomycin-treated cells) and the responding cells was based upon the criteria of Dausset et al.[3]

EXPERIMENTAL RESULTS

As noted in Table 1, lymphocytes from each donor were nonreactive in the MLC test to at least one and occasionally more than one cell sample obtained from 7 other donors, with the exception of dog 881, whose cells reacted moderately or strongly against cells obtained from all other donors, and dog 882, whose cells behaved in similar fashion, but only reacted moderately to cells obtained from donor 883. It may be of particular interest that MLC nonreactivity occurred in as many as 8 out of 56 MLC

Table 1. Relationship Between DL-A Phenotypes and MLC* Reactivity in Randomly Selected Mongrel Dogs

Dog	Code Letter	DL-A Phenotype*	One-Way MLC Reactions with Cells Obtained from Donor Dog† Am	Bm	Cm	Dm	Em	Fm	Gm	Hm
877	A	bkf lgnoe	1,443‡	7,957	1,095	5,556	20,301	19,233	10,949	21,245
878	B	bkc lgne	19,105	2,970‡	10,693	4,521	22,144	15,553	18,652	10,505
879	C	kc gne	5,146	8,203	2,124‡	18,351	15,255	12,680	1,060	12,351
880	D	bkc n	21,715	13,078	4,227	1,701‡	26,298	15,437	3,885	37,062
881	E	c lgn	29,986	10,663	11,550	31,346	350‡	24,193	2,487	33,441
882	F	lge	31,663	21,488	1,640	17,716	22,024	362‡	1,813	42,951
883	G	bkc ne	11,163	2,108	1,222	6,590	2,708	18,151	490‡	399
884	H	kc lgne	9,146	12,879	29,374	3,102	30,876	1,762	7,922	2,309‡

*Phenotypes listed according to population studies in mongrel dogs. By Dausset et al, Journal of Experimental Medicine 134:1228, 1971.

†MLC Reactivity expressed as rate of incorporation of (^{3}H) Thymidine (counts/minute).

‡Autologous Control Counts

m, mitomycin-treated cells.

Table 2. Relationship Between DL-A Phenotypic Incompatibilities and MLC Reactivity in Randomly Selected Mongrel Dogs*

		One-Way MLC Reactions with Cells Obtained from Donors Bearing the DL-A Incompatibilities Listed															
		Am		Bm		Cm		Dm		Em		Fm		Gm		Hm	
Dog #	Code	cpm	DL-A Inc	cpm	DL-A Inc	cpm	DL-A Inc	cpm	DL-A Inc	cpm	DL-A Inc	cpm	DL-A Inc	cpm	DL-A Inc	cpm	DL-A Inc
877	A	1,443	—	7,957	c	1,095	c	5,556	c	20,301	c	19,233	none	10,949	c	21,245	c
878	B	19,105	f	2,970	—	10,693	none	4,521	none	22,144	none	15,553	none	18,652	none	10,505	none
879	C	5,146	b,f,l,o	8,203	b,l	2,124	—	18,351	b	15,255	l	12,680	l	1,060	b	12,351	l
880	D	21,715	f,l,g,o,e	13,078	l,g,e	4,227	g,e	1,701	—	26,298	l,g	15,437	l,g,e	3,885	e	37,062	l,g,e
881	E	29,986	b,k,f,o,e	10,663	b,k,e	11,550	k,e	31,346	b,k	350	—	24,193	e	2,487	b,k,e	33,441	k,e
882	F	31,663	b,k,f,n,o	21,488	b,k,c,n	1,640	k,c,n	17,716	b,k,c,n	22,024	c,e	362	—	1,813	b,k,c,n	42,951	k,c,n
883	G	11,163	f,l,g,o	2,108	none	1,222	none	6,590	none	2,708	l,g	18,151	l,g	490	—	399	l,g
884	H	9,146	b,f,o	12,879	b	29,374	none	3,102	b	30,876	none	1,762	none	7,922	b	2,309	—

*The same symbols are used in this table as outlined in Table 1.

Table 3. Summarized Correlation Between MLC Reactivity and DL-A Antigen Incompatibilities in Randomly Selected Dogs

Estimate of Compatibility based on DL-A Antigens detected in Mitomycin-treated Cell Samples, which were absent the Reacting Cells	MLC Reactions Observed in the Presence of Varying Degrees of DL-A Compatibility (Number of Individual Dog Combinations Tested)'		
	Nonreactivity*	Mild to Moderate Reactivity*	Strong Reactivity*
Major DL-A⁺ Incompatibilities	4	11	16
Minor DL-A⁺ Incompatibilities	3	6	3
No Incompatibility	2	7	4

*Mild to moderate reactivity was interpreted in those instances where the (^{3}H) Thymidine uptake values exceeded control values by a factor of at least 3 to 10 times; strong reactivity required uptake values exceeding 10 times.

⁺Dausset et al: J Exp Med, 134:1222, 1971

tests performed in matching each member of a group of eight mongrel dogs against the other seven animals.

Table 2 illustrates the relationship between DL-A SD phenotype incompatibilities (i.e., SD antigen(s) present in stimulatory cells but absent in responder cells) and the results of the MLC tests. There appeared to be a general lack of correlation between DL-A SD antigen(s) incompatibility and the intensity of the MLC reaction in most instances. For example, lymphocytes from dog 877 were stimulated with equal intensity by cells from donor 881, incompatible for DL-A SD antigen c, and by cells from DL-A SD-compatible donor 882.

When the overall results were pooled (Table 3) it was observed that when 31 donors whose cells contained major detectable DL-A SD incompatibilities (3 cases) with the responding cells there were strong (16 cases) or mild to moderate (11 cases) MLC reactions; of 12 donors whose cells contained minor DL-A SD incompatibilities (3 cases) with the responding cells, 9 cells induced strong (3 cases) or mild to moderate (6 cases) MLC reactions. Of the 13 MLC reactions performed with cells obtained from DL-A SD phenotypically compatible donors, there were 4 strong responses, 7 mild to moderate reactions, and 2 negative reactions.

Table 4. Mixed Leukocyte Culture Reactivity and DL-A Compatibility in Randomly Selected Mongrel Dogs

Number of individual dog combinations tested	56	
Number of concordant results	38	(67.9%)
Reactivity in the absence of detectable DL-A incompatibilities	11	(19.6%)
Nonreactivity in the face of detectable DL-A incompatibilities	7	(12.5%)

Further analysis of these data (Table 4) indicates that 38 of the 56 combinations tested gave MLC responses which were concordant with the DL-A SD states of donor-recipient compatibility (67.9%). In 11 cases (19.6%), MLC reactivity occurred in the absence of detectable DL-A SD incompatibilities and 7 dogs were (12.5%) nonreactive to cells obtained from DL-A SD-incompatible donors.

DISCUSSION

Any attempt to interpret the results of this study is clearly limited by the small number of mongrel dog combinations tested by the MLC technique and by the known shortcomings of the sera currently available for the detection of the SD antigens in the canine species.[6,7] In spite of these limitations, however, the relatively large percentage of MLC nonreactive donor-recipient pairs of mongrel dogs observed in this study (16%) suggests that the polymorphism of the LD locus(i) products may be more limited in the dog than it appears to be in man.[15–17]

The significant parallelism between lymphocyte reactivity and the presence or absence of serologically detectable DL-A SD incompatibilities in the stimulating cells used in the MLC tests extends to the canine species the concept of the existence of a linkage disequilibrium between the SD and LD loci of the major histocompatibility complex. A number of authors have reported similar findings in man.[18]

The results of this study further support the value of MLC testing as a marker for an additional component of the canine MHC, the LD locus(i).[9] Studies in dogs[14] and in man[17] have given evidence of the advantage of simultaneous MHC SD and LD identity for transplantation purposes. A number of other as yet unknown genetic determinants may also be of great importance.

ACKNOWLEDGMENT

The technical assistance of Miss E. Kunen is greatly appreciated.

REFERENCES

1. Rapaport FT, Hanaoka T, Shimada T, et al: J Exp Med 131:881, 1970

2. Mollen N, St John D, Cannon FD, et al: Transplantation 6:939, 1968

3. Dausset J, Rapaport FT, Cannon FD et al: J Exp Med 134:1222, 1971

4. Rapaport FT, Watanabe K, Cannon FD, et al: J Exp Med 136:1080, 1972

5. Blumenstock DA, Lempert N, Singer KM, et al: Transplantation, 10:241, 1970

6. Rapaport FT, Ozaki A, Cannon FD, et al: Transplant Proc 5:845, 1973

7. Vriesendorp HM, Rothengatter E, Bos E, et al: Transplantation 11:440, 1971

8. Ceppellini R: In Amos DB (ed): Progress in Immunology, New York, Academic Press, 1971, p 973

9. Bach FH: Transplantation Proc 5:23, 1973

10. Klein J: Transplant Proc, 5:11, 1973

11. Rudolph RH, Hered B, Epstein RB, et al: Transplantation 8:141, 1969

12. Hartzman RJ, Segall M, Bach ML, et al: Transplantation 11:268, 1970

13. Templeton JW, Thomas ED: Transplantation 11:429, 1971

14. Storb R, Rudolph RH, Thomas ED: J Clin Invest 50:1272, 1971

15. van Rood JJ, Eijsvoogel VP: Lancet 1:698, 1970

16. Bach FH, Day E, Bach ML, et al: Tissue Antigens 1:39, 1971

17. Koch CT, Eijsvoogel VP, Fredericks E, et al: Lancet 2:1334, 1971

18. Dausset J, Sasportes M, Lebrun A: Transplant Proc 5:1511, 1973

One-Way Nonstimulation in MLC Related to DL-A Homozygosity

By H. Grosse-Wilde, P. Baumann, B. Netzel, H. J. Kolb, W. Mempel, R. Wank, and E. D. Albert

RECENT reports of MLC data in man[1] and mice[2] have clearly established that the mixed lymphocyte culture is genetically determined by one or more loci closely linked to but separate from the loci coding for HL-A or H-2 antigens. In order to perform MLC experiments in situations not easily found in humans, the dog was selected as an outbred species for which two closely linked loci governing the expression of histocompatibility antigens have been defined.[3] Templeton and Thomas[4] have demonstrated that MLC reactions in dog families can be predicted by serological histocompatibility testing. After the definition of the first human MLC specificity in HL-A–MLC-homozygous individuals, it was our objective to use the opportunity presented by several litters of a closely bred beagle colony to identify DL-A-homozygous dogs. This paper gives evidence for the definition of two dog MLC specificities found in DL-A-homozygous animals.

MATERIALS AND METHOD

DL-A typing was performed using a microlymphocytotoxicity test as described elsewhere.[5] A battery of 180 cytotoxic antisera, kindly provided by Drs. Vriesendorp and van der Does from Holland and by Drs. Thomas and Storb from Seattle, was used to define the following DL specificities: DL1, 2, 3, 7, 10 of the first series and DL4, 5, 6, 8, 11, 12, 13, 14 of the second series.

From Institut für Hämatologie, Abteilung Immunologie der GSF München and Kinderpoliklinik der Universität München.

Authors are members of Sonderforschungsbereich 37, München.

Supported in part by Deutsche Forschungsgemeinschaft, grant Al 92/7.

© 1973 by Grune & Stratton, Inc.

MLC METHOD

An appropriate volume of heparinized blood (50 U/ml) was drawn by venipuncture. The blood was divided in two equal parts, one of which was x-irradiated with 2500 R. Buffy coat was produced by centrifugation at 250 g for 10 min. The supernatant cell-free plasma was pooled. The WBC layer and some of the adjacent erythrocytes were aspirated and diluted (approx. 1:5) with Waymouth medium MB 752/1 (Gibco) containing 1% glutamine (Flow Lab), 10,000 U/100 ml medium penicillin, 10,000 μg/100 ml medium streptomycin (Gibco) and 6.5 ml 4% $NaHCO_3$/100 ml medium. This cell suspension was layered on Ficoll Isopaque (specific density 1.077/20°C). After centrifugation at 1,000 g for 10 min, the interface was apirated and washed three times with culture medium. The remaining buffy-coat-poor blood was centrifuged once more at 1,000 g for 10 min, and the supernatant cell-free plasma was added to the original plasma pool.

The responding cells (RC) and the x-irradiated stimulating cells (SC) were adjusted with culture medium to a cell concentration of 3×10^6 lymphocytes/ml; 0.1 ml (3×10^5 lymphocytes) of the RC suspension and SC suspension were pipetted into each well of a microtiter plate (Greiner). Finally, 0.02 ml of the fresh pooled plasma was injected using a tuberculin syringe and a special adapted Hamilton dispenser. The culture plates were covered with a microtiter lid (Greiner) and kept at 38°C in an incubator with 5% CO_2 and humidified atmosphere for 5 days in a slightly inclined position (30°) to achieve a closer cell-to-cell contact. On the fifth day, 0.02 ml (2 μCi) of a thymidine (methyl ^{3}H) solution (Amersham, specific activity 5 Ci/mmol) was injected in each well; 16 hr later the culture plates were centrifuged at 500 g for 10 min, and the cell-free radioactive supernatant was discarded. The washing procedure included the addition of 0.1 ml 0.9% NaCl solution per well, rocking for 2 min on a microtiter mixer, centrifugation at 500 g for 10 min, and discarding the wash fluid. After washing, 0.1 ml of 0.25% trypsin in Hanks' solution was added per well. The plates were incubated for 3 min in a CO_2 incubator and then rocked on a mixer for 2 min. The resulting suspension of radioactive-labeled cells were harvested with a multiple-sample precipitator (Hiller) with distilled water on glass-fiber filter strips (Reeve Angle). The strips were dried on a heating plate for 10 min and then individually cut into plastic counting vials; 3 ml toluol plus PPO and POPOP were added and the vials were counted in a scintillation counter (Packard TriCarb Model 2450). The results are given as mean c.p.m. from triplicates.

RESULTS

Typing results in family 221 (Fig. 1) show that the parents (dogs 2567 and 2790) share the DL-A haplotype 2, 4, whereas they differ in the haplotypes 3, 12 and 2, 5. It can be seen from Fig. 1 that two pups (dogs 2215 and 2217) are homozygous for the DL-A2, 4 haplotype. Dog 2218 is serologically identical with his mother (DL-A2, 4/3, 12) and dog 2216 is identical with his father DL-A2, 4/2, 5).

In family 527 the parents (dogs 2541 and 2825) are DL-A-identical with the genotype DL-A2, 4/2, 5 (Fig. 2). Although they are not littermates, they both originate from a closely bred beagle colony. The typing results of the nine pups are consistent with the genotyping of the parents: there are five dogs (5270, 5272, 5273, 5275, 5276) that are homozygous for the DL-A haplotype 2,5. One dog (5271) is homozygous for DL-A2, 4, and three pups show the heterozygous combination DL-A2, 4/2, 5. Family 224 has the same father as family 527 (2541), whose genotype is DL-A2, 4/2, 5. The mother (2557) of family 224 was shown to possess the DL-A genotype 2, 4/3, 12. Thus also in this family the parents share one DL-A haplotype (DL-A2, 4), giving rise to two pups (2240 and 2243) who are homozygous for DL-A2, 4. Two pups are serologically identical with their mother (DL-A2, 4/3, 12) and one is identical with his father (DL-A2, 4/2, 5). The remaining three dogs (2242, 2244, 2246) present the combination DL-A2, 5/3, 12. One of these (dog 2242) was chosen as a control cell in the MLC experiment of litter 527.

MLC RESULTS

In litter 221 (Fig. 1) the DL-A-identical littermates 2215 and 2217 show as expected

Father (2567) DL-2-4/2-5

Mother (2790) DL-2-4/3-12

	Dog No.	DLA	Ax	Bx	Cx	Dx
A	2215	2-4 2-4	.459	.599	9.288	7.501
B	2217	2-4 2-4	.318	.466	14.198	13.487
C	2216	2-4 2-5	.426	.700	.378	11.113
D	2218	2-4 3-12	.533	.449	7.019	.378

MLC-Reactions (cpm) of Litter 221.

Index «x» means X-Irradiation with 2500 R.

Fig. 1. One-way and two-way nonstimulations involving DL2, 4 homozygotes in litter 221.

Father (2541) DL-2-4/2-5

Mother (2825) DL-2-4/2-5

	Dog No.	DLA	Ax	Bx	Cx	Dx	Ex	Fx	Gx	Hx	Ix	Kx
A	5270	2-5 2-5	.251	.157	.340	.156	.158	.843	.959	.653	3.984	3.440
B	5272	2-5 2-5	.277	.181	.263	.343	.364	1.697	3.579	1.094	6.442	7.549
C	5273	2-5 2-5	.368	.290	.340	.524	.474	3.069	3.444	1.018	7.393	7.098
D	5275	2-5 2-5	.365	.237	.495	.345	.321	5.375	5.372	1.841	6.522	10.253
E	5276	2-5 2-5	.227	.158	249	.363	.299	.943	2.282	.646	2.950	8.008
F	5271	2-4 2-4	1.697	2.504	1.474	4.100	3.004	.189	1.331	.755	5.077	5.676
G	5274	2-5 2-4	.153	.237	.320	.372	.372	.284	.221	.373	.473	7.826
H	5277	2-5 2-4	.155	.241	.302	.341	.207	.185	.435	.334	.363	3.306
I	5278	2-5 2-4	.516	.379	.440	.453	.333	.355	.360	.329	.597	9.620
K	2242	2-5 3-12	.444	.274	.352	.371	.380	2.102	2.828	2.262	7.008	.375

MLC-Reactions (cpm) of Litter 527.

Index «x» means X-Irradiation with 2500 R.

Fig. 2. One-way and two-way nonstimulations in litter 527 involving DL2, 4 and DL2, 5 homozygotes.

mutual nonstimulation. Dogs 2215 and 2216, who are homozygous for DL-A2, 4, are clearly stimulated by dogs 2215 (DL-A2, 4/2, 5) and 2218 (DL-A2, 4/3, 12), while in turn they are not stimulating the 2216 and 2218 as responders. This demonstrates a true one-way nonstimulation, which must be expected if both DL-A2, 4 haplotypes present in each of the homozygous dogs 2215 and 2217 carry identical MLC determinants. The last combination 2216 (DL-A2, 4/2, 5) versus 2218 (DL-A2, 4/3, 12) results in a two-way stimulation.

Figure 2 summarizes the MLC results of litter 527, which includes dog 2242 of litter 224 as a control. In the table the dogs are listed according to their DL-A genotypes: the first five pups (5270, 5272, 5273, 5275, 5276) are all DL-A-identical (DL-A2, 5/2, 5) and accordingly show mutual nonstimulation in all possible combinations. The second group of serologically identical dogs consists of dogs 5274, 5277, 5278 with the genotype DL-A2, 4/2, 5. Also this group presents mutual nonstimulation. As described above for litter 221, in this experiment lymphocytes from the five homozygous dogs (DL-A2, 5/2, 5) demonstrate clear one-way nonstimulations with all heterozygous partners possessing the DL-A2, 5 haplotype, including dog 2242, who originates from a different litter but has the same father and who inherited the DL-A2, 5 haplotype from this father. Likewise the DL-A2, 4/2, 4 homozygote (dog 5271) shows one-way nonstimulation with all three littermates, who carry the DL-A2, 4 haplotype in the heterozygous state.

As expected, strong stimulations in both directions were observed in the combinations of dog 5271 (DL-A2, 4/2, 4) with the five DL-A2, 5/2, 5 homozygotes (5270, 5272, 5273, 5275, 5276) and with dog 2242 (DL-A2, 5/3, 12).

In Fig. 3 the stimulation ratios of the above-described experiments are plotted on a logarithmic scale in order to visualize the relation between nonstimulation in both directions of DL-A-identical littermates and bidirectional stimulation in the one-haplotype-different situation on one side as compared to the observed one-way nonstimulation, which consists of a stimulation in one direction and a nonstimulation in the

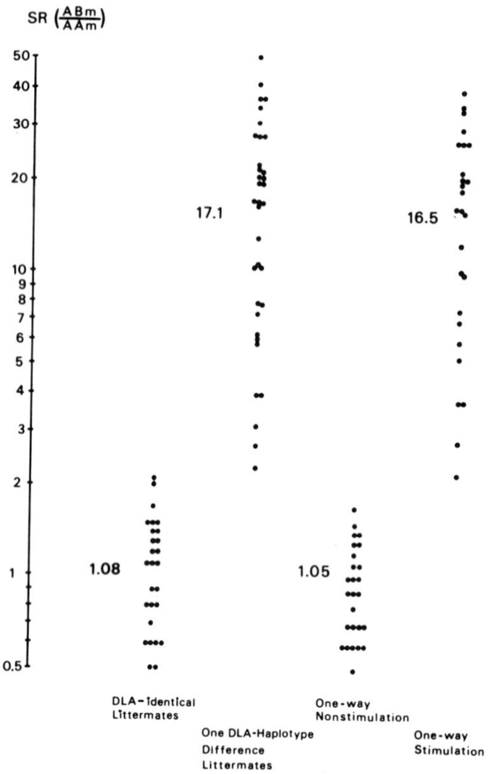

Fig. 3. Comparison of MLC stimulation ratios of DL-A-identical and one-allele-different combinations (first two columns) with the respective results in the homozygous versus heterozygous combination (last two columns).

opposite direction. The mean stimulation ratios are virtually identical (SR of 1.08 vs. 1.05 and SR of 17.1 vs. 16.5) in both stimulating and nonstimulating groups.

DISCUSSION

MLC testing has been accepted as an integral part of histocompatibility testing in man and mice. The establishment of two separate MLC loci has provided the challenge to attempt the definition of single MLC alleles, the first of which has recently been defined in individuals who could be shown by family analysis to be homozygous for the HL-A as well as for the MLC determinants.[6] Such cells are now serving as reference for MLC typing. In this presentation it could be shown that typing for MLC specificities can be applied also in the dog and that DL-A–MLC-homozygous dogs can be found quite frequently in closely bred colonies. Although final evidence for the separation between the DL-A and MLC loci has not been given as yet,[3] in view of the striking analogies in other species concerning the major histocompatibility complex it can quite reasonably be assumed that there is a separate MLC locus in dogs. The MLC data of a crossing-over between the DL-A loci[3] indicate that the MLC reactivity is determined on the chromosomal fragment that carries the second DL-A locus.

On the basis of the DL-A family analysis, it has been possible to find a number of DL-A homozygotes who could be shown to be homozygous also for MLC by one-way nonstimulation with heterozygotes and by mutual nonstimulation with other homozygotes. The one-way nonstimulation of these cells has become an important tool for the MLC typing of unrelated cells.

It is quite obvious from Fig. 3 that the observed one-way nonstimulations show a very clear difference between the nonstimulation in one direction and the stimulation in the other direction, which corresponds quantitatively very well to a one-allele difference between siblings. In the analogous situation in human MLC, there were a number of low-grade stimulations where one-way nonstimulations had to be expected according to the genetic analysis. This low-grade paradoxical reaction is not satisfactorily explained, and it seems quite remarkable that this disturbing reaction has never been observed in our dog experiments. It could be that the paradoxical stimulation is due to a blastogenic factor released by the mitomycin-treated cells, and it may be that either dog cells are unable to produce this factor or that the X-irradiation used for the inactivation of the stimulating cells does not allow the production or the release of blastogenic factor. On the other hand, it might be argued that in a closely bred colony there is a high degree of chance compatibility for minor loci that might otherwise produce this low-grade stimulation by a cumulative effect. This, however, seems unlikely because one would have to expect a low stimulation in a considerable number of DL-A- or HL-A-identical siblings, which clearly is not the case.

In conclusion, it can be stated that in dogs DL-A–MLC-homozygous cells are particularly good reference cells for the typing of MLC determinants. Selective breeding provides the opportunity to produce a larger number of different homozygotes for use in a MLC typing cell panel.

REFERENCES

1. Eijsvoogel VP, du Bois MJGJ, Melief CJM, et al: Histocompatibility Testing, 1972. Copenhagen, Munksgaard, (in press)

2. Bach ML, Widmer MB, Bach FH, et al: Transplant Proc 5:369,1973

3. Vriesendorp HM, Westbroek DL, D'Amaro J, et al: Tissue Antigens 3:145, 1973

4. Templeton JW, Thomas ED: Transplantation 11:429, 1971

5. Albert ED, Storb R, Erickson VM et al: Tissue Antigens (in press)

6. Mempel W, Grosse-Wilde H, Albert ED, et al: Transplant Proc 5:401, 1973

The Ag-B Locus of Rats: A Major Histocompatibility Complex?

By Joy Palm and Darcy B. Wilson

THE H-2 histocompatibility genes of the ninth linkage group in the mouse were thought for many years to reflect a highly polymorphic multiple allelic locus; although no function could be assigned to the products of this locus nor to those of the comparable major histocompatibility locus in man (HL-A), they could be detected and defined serologically and were recognized as the principal antigens associated with the homograft reaction. Subsequently, as a result of genetic analyses of the fine structure of the H-2 region, the relatively simple system of allelic genes at a single locus was revealed to be a cluster of separable, functionally distinct genes (subloci), which, though usually inherited as a complex, exhibit low levels of recombination.[1] These findings have led to the use of the term major histocompatibility complex (MHC) to describe a chromosomal region of closely linked genes whose products are intimately involved with the cell surface (Tla, H-2D, H-2K) and exert a controlling influence on lymphocyte function (Ir-1, Ir-IgG, and Ir-IgA). More recently, a strong case has been made[2-5] for further complexity of the MHC region, both in man and in the mouse, from data suggesting the existence of genes specifying two operationally distinct immunogenic systems: one, serologically defined (SD) antigens that elicit the production of antibodies upon immunization and are specified in the mouse by two subloci, D and K; two, lymphocyte-defined (LD) antigens, not yet identified serologically, that are capable of stimulating proliferative activity of allogeneic lymphocytes in mixed lymphocyte interactions (MLI).

The concept that the chromosomal fine structure controlling major histocompatibility complexes (MHC) in mammalian species may be composed of a large number of independent genes with functionally dissimilar gene products presents a multiple challenge to immunogeneticists working with species in which the existence of even two subloci for serologic determinants remains to be determined. The rat is a case in point. Is the organization of two (or more) subloci with an integrated genetic control by separate genes of immune response, lymphocyte determinants, and various serum proteins (e.g., Ss-Slp[6]) a prototype for all mammalian species? Or may a simpler situation exist in which: (1) the serologically complex SD antigens are determined by a single locus of alternative alleles, (2) there is no basis for distinguishing between SD and LD antigens, and (3) non-SD loci (e.g., those for immune response), while possibly chromosomally associated, may not be incorporated within a typical gene complex.

Distinguishing between these alternatives in additional species will be essential to an understanding of the ways in which these genes may interact to influence the development and effectiveness of immunocompetence, including that which dictates a predisposition to certain malignant and autoimmune diseases or leads to rejections of transplanted tissues and organs. Of particular interest in the field of lymphocyte function, for example, is recently accumulated evidence that indicates that killer-cell activity generated in mixed lymphocyte interaction and involving acti-

From the Wistar Institute of Anatomy and Biology, Philadelphia, Pa., and the Department of Pathology, University of Pennsylvania, Philadelphia, Pa.

Supported by NIH grants CA-10097, AI-09275, and AI-10961.

©1973 by Grune & Stratton, Inc.

vation of allogeneic lymphocytes by LD antigens seems to be directed to SD specificities on target cells.[5] One interpretation placed on these findings is that two lineages of lymphocytes may participate in the generation of effector cells during the course of an immune response.

The purpose of this communication is to describe briefly the current status of immunogenetic research in rats and to indicate some of the differences between rats and mice that may serve to elucidate the genetic and molecular basis for the phenotypic and functional properties associated with a major histocompatibility locus.

THE MAJOR HISTOCOMPATIBILITY LOCUS OF RATS

Variously designated as R-1, Ag-B, and RtH-1,[7-9] a locus has been defined in rats on the basis of antigenic products which exhibit a readily detectable serological complexity, multiple alleles, and an overriding immunogenicity in tissue transplantation. These antigens also play a singular role in eliciting graft-vs-host (GvH) reactions with nonsensitized lymphocytes[10] and serve as stimuli for allogeneic lymphocytes in mixed lymphocyte interactions (MLI).[11] Genetic control of all of these features is inherited as a unit for which no evidence of an intragenic recombination potential has yet been obtained. An additional similarity to the H-2 and HL-A regions of mouse and man is the association of the Ag-B locus with genes controlling immune responsiveness to antigens of limited diversity such as (T-G)-A–L,[12] or to some enzymes.[13] These characteristics indicate a functional and immunological homology of the Ag-B chromosomal region with the MHCs of mouse and man and may also reflect a genetic homology with respect to an integrated gene complex. One might anticipate that closely related rodent species will be more alike than different, and in fact many gene homologies between rat and mouse linkage groups are becoming apparent.[14]

However, the evolution of integrated gene complexes,[15] such as H-2 appears to be, undoubtedly involves a variety of chromosomal rearrangements including interactions with the centromere, translocations, inversions, gene duplications, and/or recombinations that may vary from species to species. These serve to create the variability that makes individuals more or less fit for their environments and upon which in turn the processes of natural selection may operate. Detecting genetic homologies of complex loci among different species depends upon both the individual variability (polymorphism) that is maintained in the population and, perhaps more importantly, the access of the investigator to that variability.

The rat and mouse differ in a number of immunobiologic and genetic parameters, and the question of genetic homology, particularly as it relates to chromosomal fine structure and multiple genes, is unresolved. A consideration of the ancestry of currently available rat strains, the number of Ag-B alleles distinguishing these, the lack of detected recombination, the paucity of other genetic markers on the relevant chromosome, as well as the data accumulating from various kinds of immunobiological experiments, raises the possibility that an MHC as complex as that proposed for the mouse may not be typical of rats.

POLYMORPHISM AT Ag-B (H-1) LOCUS

The limited number of serologically distinct Ag-B alleles that have been defined in domesticated stocks following many years of random breeding do not encourage the belief that Ag-B intralocus recombinations of selective advantage are an important factor in rats, at least under domestic conditions. At a recent Transplantation Society Congress, for example, 10 serologically distinct Ag-B (H-1) allelic products were described.[16,17] Among the 52 inbred rat strains typed, 47 were found to fall into only five groups with respect to the allele each possessed. Most of these strains, though admittedly of common ancestry from the now defunct commercial rat colony of the Wistar Institute, had been separated from their common source for upwards of 30 or more years during which time most were maintained as random breeding colonies.

Of the 10 alleles mentioned above, 7 have appeared in inbred strains known to have Wistar ancestry although only 4 can be traced directly to the Wistar colony.[18] Thc 3 additional non-Wistar alleles occurred in single strains, at least 1 of which, BN, is known to be derived from feral stock. A related observation is that of the currently available random-bred, genetically heterogeneous stocks that have been serotyped, each has exhibited not more than two segregating Ag-B (H-1) alleles.[16] Apparently, this is the minimum number required in order to maintain the maternal–fetal histoincompatibility required for optimum reproduction of segregating populations differing at non-Ag-B H loci.[19] These facts suggest a stability of inheritance of the SD genes in the periods between separation from the common source and the initiation of the inbreeding process, or that recombination does not exert an overwhelming selective advantage under animal colony conditions. To date, evidence of genetic recombination has been sought in two ways: by testing for the occurrence of new Ag-B alleles with respect to SD regroupings, and for the separation of SD and MLC determinants. Neither approach has as yet been fruitful, but the number of animals tested is insufficient to exclude the possibility of recombination frequencies of the magnitude associated with the H-2 or HL-A subloci.

It is unclear whether the limited heterogeneity of alleles in so many rat strains is a result of their common ancestry or whether this is a characteristic of the species. Numerous studies have indicated that the clone(s) of lymphocytes reactive to the antigenic products of a chosen Ag-B allele is quite large. Various estimates have indicated that as many as 3 to 12% of the circulating lymphocytes of one individual respond in the GvH reaction and in the MLI to the major alloantigens of a second individual.[21,22] Assuming functional unipotentiality of these responding cells and that the total repertoire of circulating T cells in the rat is reactive to H antigens, this would place upper and lower limits on the number of reactive allelic products at the Ag-B locus capable of stimulating lymphocytes in the MLI at 8 and 30. This important question probably can be resolved with studies of wild rats currently in progress.

The study of wild rats will be important also for additional confirmation of what appears to be a major, and possibly MHC significant, dissimilarity between the relevant chromosomes of rat and mouse with respect to both antigenic and nonantigenic markers. In mice, two multiple-allelic loci occur within the ninth linkage group in very close proximity (as judged by recombination) to H-2. Each may have contributed to the observed complexity of the mouse MHC and neither has been found to occur in rats. These are the Tla (thymus-leukemia antigen) locus and the T (brachyury) locus with its associated group of unstable, highly mutable t alleles. The importance of the t alleles, of which two types, lethal and viable, exist, resides in the capacity of most of the lethal mutants to suppress recombination.[15] These genes occur at high frequency in wild mice[15] and their appearance may have been one factor for the evolutionary development of clustering and unitary inheritance of the various genes now attributed to the H-2 complex.[23] An additional feature of the H-2 locus, its proximity to the centromere, may be similarly relevant. Information on centromere location with respect to the rat Ag-B locus is unknown.

Despite extensive scrutiny by several investigators of both wild and domesticated stocks, evidence for a T-t-like locus in rats has not been found.[24] Studies of radiation-induced mutants also have failed to provide evidence for tail abnormalities.[25] Castle and King studied one tail mutation, "stub," which is now lost. It was more similar to the mouse stub mutation than to the mouse brachyury, though it did present some of the pleiotropic features of the latter.[25] If the apparent absence of t-like mutations in the rats is real, it is possible that the close "complex gene" type of organization of the various functionally distinct rat counterparts to genes of the H-2 region may not occur. A case in point may be the recent demonstration that in the rat the gene for susceptibility to experimental allergic encephalomyelitis, EAE, though on the Ag-B chromosome (provisionally designated linkage group VI, LG-VI) apparently is separated by some 9–15 map units from Ag-B.[26] Establishing the relationship of this locus to those determining other immune responses will be important, particularly if they also prove to map outside the SD-defined locus. In this regard, comparative studies of segregating populations and congenic lines (of which a number are available[8,9]) may be especially informative.

THE MIXED LYMPHOCYTE INTERACTION IN RATS

The conditions necessary for the mixed lymphocyte interaction (MLI) with rat cells appear to differ somewhat from those prevailing with mouse cells, in that Ag-B incompatibility of donor lymphocyte and target cell is apparently required. In contrast, positive responses have been reported in mice with both H-2 and non-H-2 incompatible strain combinations. An important multiple allelic non-H-2 locus for the MLI in mice, the M locus, has been described by Festenstein (these Proceedings). This locus is not linked to H-2, H-7, or Ly-1, and the antigenic products do not seem to affect skin graft survival, or elicit a GvH reaction.

In rats little, if any, response occurs with peripheral blood or thoracic duct lymphocytes from strain combinations which though compatible at the Ag-B locus, are sufficiently incompatible at other H loci that skin grafts exchanged between such individuals are rejected promptly and GvH reactions can be recorded.[27] The data in Tables 1 and 2 illustrate this point. Table 1 shows that only strains differing with respect to the major Ag-B locus display proliferative responses in vitro. Table 2 shows the results of MLI responses following interaction of cells from two congenic rat strains with their parental prototypes. BN.B2 rats are BN strain animals which possess the WF Ag-B^2 chromosomal region, and BN.B4 animals possess the DA Ag-B^4 chromosomal region.[8] This table shows that (1) differences with respect to the Ag-B locus alone are sufficient to induce proliferative activity in the MLI and (2) cells from donors similar only with respect to the Ag-B chromosomal region are nonreactive. These data have been supplemented by tests of 8 additional strains with similar results. Therefore, at this time, studies with the rat provide no basis for distinguishing between LD and SD determinants; a continuing search for Ag-B serologically identical, MLC-positive strains, as well as for recombination alleles, is being made in order to

Table 1. MLI of Ag-B-compatible Inbred Rat Strains

Responding Cells	Ag-B Allele	Stimulating Cells*				
		Fischer	Lewis	BH	DA	ACI
Fischer 344	B^1	120	131	147	4083	7900
Lewis	B^1	101	135	100	5721	7041
BH	B^1	117	175	99	4144	4344
DA	B^4	6133	5200	8700	127	98
ACI	B^4	5212	6970	9713	128	142

*Stimulating cells were mitomycin treated.

Table 2. MLI of Ag-B-incompatible Inbred Rat Strains

Responding Cells	Ag-B Allele	Stimulating Cells*				
		BN	DA	BN.B2	BN.B4	WF
BN	B^3	187	10104	7144	6109	
DA	B^4	11404	151		149	
BN.B2	B^2	7198		170		147
BN.B4	B^4	6001	181		171	
WF	B^2		4012	184		174

*Stimulating cells were mitomycin trated.

detect the possible occurrence of the LD phenomenon in rats and to determine its biochemical and genetic basis.

SUMMARY

As a result of recent explosive interest in the immunogenetics of histocompatibility systems, a detailed genetic analysis of the H-2 region of mice has indicated an unexpectedly complex fine structure. This raises the important question of whether this complexity in the mouse is a prototype for the major histocompatibility loci of other vertebrate species, and whether such associations, per se, are necessary for effective immunocompetence of the individual. Evidence favoring such genetic homology of the major H locus in the mouse and rat is the association of the gene(s) determining serologically detectable antigens which activate lymphocytes in the MCI and GvH reactions, with the genes controlling immune responsiveness. Contrary evidence for homology of a gene complex includes the lack of recorded intralocus recombination and the apparent lack of the associated loci, Tla, T-t, which may have been important for the maintenance of this complex in the mouse.

REFERENCES

1. Klein J, Shreffler D: Transplant Rev 6:3, 1971
2. Amos DB, Bach FH: J Exp Med 128:623, 1968
3. Yunis EJ, Amos DB: Proc Nat Acad Sci 68:3031, 1971
4. Eijsvogel VP, Van Rood JJ, duToit ED, et al: Eur J Immunol 2:413, 1972
5. Bach FH: Transplant Proc 5:23, 1973
6. Shreffler DC, Passmore HC: In Lengerova A, Vojtišková (eds): Proceedings of a Symposium on Immunogenetics of the H-2 System. Basel, Karger, 1971.
7. Bogden AE, Aptekman PM: Ann N Y Acad Sci 97:43, 1962
8. Palm J: Transplantation 11:175, 1971
9. Štark O, Křen V, Frenzl B, and Křenová D: Folia Biol 14:425, 1968
10. Elkins WL, Palm J: Ann N Y Acad Sci 129:573, 1966
11. Wilson DB: Prog Immunol 1:1045, 1971
12. Gunther E, Rüde E, Štark O: Eur J Immunol 2:151, 1972
13. Wurzburg U: Eur J Immunol 1:496, 1971
14. Gasser, DL, Silvers WK, Reynolds HM, Black G, Palm J: Biochem Genet (in press)
15. Dunn LC, Bennett D, Beasley AB: Genetics 47:285, 1962
16. Štark O, Křen V, Gunther E: Transplant Proc 3:165, 1971
17. Palm J: Transplant Proc 3:169, 1971
18. Palm J, Black G: Transplantation 11:184, 1971
19. Palm J: Transplant Proc 2:162, 1970
20. Nisbet NW, Simonsen M, Zaleski M: J Exp Med 129:459, 1969
21. Wilson DB, Blyth JL, Nowell PC: J Exp Med 128:1157, 1968
22. Ford WL, Atkins RC: Advan Exp Biol Med 29:255, 1973
23. Klein J: Transplant Proc 5:11, 1973
24. Dunn LC, Gluecksohn-Schoenheimer S, Curtis MR, et al J Hered 33:65, 1942
25. Taylor BA: Genetics 60:559, 1968
26. Gasser DG, Newlin C, Palm J, and Gonatis NC: Science 181:872, 1973
27. Wilson DB: J Exp Med 126:625, 1967

Evidence of a Third HL-A Locus

By B. G. Solheim and E. Thorsby

IN previous reports[1,2] we have described an antiserum from a multiparous woman, SA-AJ, which might detect an antigen belonging to a third segregant HL-A series. Subsequent studies[3] disclosed a very close association between antigen AJ and four specificities of the second HL-A series; i.e., HL-A5, W15, W22, and HL-A27. More recently, Svejgaard et al.[4] reported additional sera, SA-532, RH-UPS, and RH-315, which seemed to detect determinants mutually exclusive to AJ and which also showed strong associations with some second-series specificities. Taken together, the results indicated that the specificities AJ, 532, UPS, and 315 might either be determined by alleles at a closely linked third HL-A locus or be public (supertypic) specificities of some HL-A antigens belonging to the second segregant series.

To study this further, we performed blocking experiments with $F(ab')_2$ fragments from different HL-A antisera detecting second or AJ-series specificities. Furthermore, aggregation and capping at the cell surface of the corresponding antigens were induced by means of intact IgG anti-HL-A antibodies + anti-human IgG. A preliminary report of our studies has appeared,[5] and a full report appears elsewhere;[6] only a short summary will be given here.

RESULTS AND COMMENTS

Previously HL-A-typed lymphocytes were first incubated at 15°C for 2 hr with $F(ab')_2$ fragments from a particular HL-A antiserum. After washing, the cells were retyped using different HL-A antisera and a modified NIH technique involving incubation at 15° C for 3 hr in the presence of 5 mM NaN_3 to avoid extensive aggregation by $F(ab')_2$ fragments of HL-A antigens at the cell surface. The method is essentially identical to that reported by Richiardi et al.[7] The results of our experiments show that $F(ab')_2$ fragments of antisera detecting antigens of the AJ series will only inhibit the cytotoxic effect of intact Ig from the same serum and not the cytotoxic effect of antisera recognizing first- and second-series specificities. Thus, the AJ, 532, and UPS antigenic determinants are separate from those determining antigens of the first and second series [$F(ab')_2$-anti-315 was not tested].

To investigate whether the antigens of the AJ series were situated on other molecules than those carrying first- and second-series specificities, aggregation/redistribution of HL-A specificities at the cell surface was induced, following the method of Bernoco et al.[8] Previously HL-A-typed lymphocytes were first incubated with a given antiserum for 2 hr at 20°C. The cells were washed and reincubated for 30 min at 4°C with rabbit anti-human IgG. New washing was performed and the cells then incubated for 30 min at 37°C to induce aggregation and typed either with the modified NIH technique or the KN technique[9] in the presence of 5 mM NaN_3.

To test the suitability of the method, cells were first incubated with antisera assumed to detect public specificities of the first or second HL-A series; (2+W28), (5+W5), and (5+17+W21+SL). It could be shown that preincubation of cells with, for example, anti(2+W28) inhibited cytotoxicity both with anti-HL-A2 and anti-W28 sera (second line, Table 1). Thus it could be confirmed that the specificity (2+W28) most

From the Tissue Typing Laboratory, Rikshospitalet University Hospital, Oslo, Norway.

Financial support from Anders Jahre's Fund for the Promotion of Science.

© 1973 by Grune & Stratton, Inc.

Table 1. Separate Aggregation at the Cell Surface of Antigens belonging to the First, Second, and AJ Series of Specificities

Pretreatment	Typing*
None	3, W28, W10(UPS), W5
anti-(2+W28)	3, , W10(UPS), W5
anti-UPS	3, W28, W10 , W5
anti-W10	3, W28, (UPS), W5
None	3, 11, 5(SL), W5(315)
anti-315	3, 11, 5(SL), W5
anti-SL(5+17+W21+SL)	3, 11, , W5(315)

*Population studies[4] have revealed a very close association between W5 and 315, and W10 and UPS.

probably is public or common to HL-A2 and W28.

Different cells were then preincubated either with antisera detecting first- or second-series specificities, or with antisera recognizing specificities of the AJ series. Two of our experiments are depicted in Table 1. The results show that specificities belonging to the first, second, or AJ series must all be parts of different molecules. AJ, 532, UPS, and 315, therefore, most probably are antigens determined by alleles at a third HL-A locus.

To confirm independent aggregation/redistribution at the cell surface of second- and AJ-series specificities, immunofluorescence studies were carried out. Lymphocytes (HL-A2, W19, 8, 27, 532) were first incubated with anti-HL-A27 (or anti-532) for 2 hr at 20°C, followed by treatment with rhodamine-labeled anti-F(ab′)$_2$ antibodies for 30 min at 4°C. After washing, the cells were incubated for 30 min at 37°C, then incubated with anti-532 (or anti-HL-A27) for 30 min at 4°C, followed by incubation for 30 min at 4°C in the presence of FITC-labeled anti-IgG. The cells were then processed for fluorescence microscopy.

We observed fluorescence on essentially all cells. The red fluorescence was aggregated in spots or caps, while the green fluorescence was diffusely distributed in the cell membrane in addition to being superimposed on the aggregated rhodamine-labeled complexes.

CONCLUSION

Our studies demonstrate that at least three series of serologically detectable HL-A antigens seem to exist, each determined by separate but closely linked loci (SD1, SD2, and SD3). Studies of families with a recombinant child[4,10] show that the probable third HL-A locus is more closely linked to the second than to the first HL-A locus. However, since we have not found families demonstrating unambiguous recombination between the SD2 and SD3 loci, we do not know whether the third locus is situated between the first and second HL-A loci or on the other side of the second locus.

ACKNOWLEDGMENTS

We are grateful to Dr. Staub-Nielsen, Copenhagen, Dr. Sandberg, Gothenburg, Dr. Kissmeyer-Nielsen, Århus, Dr. Spärck, Copenhagen, Dr. Sachs, London, Dr. Mayr, Basel, and Dr. van der Putte, Leuven, for providing us with some of the antisera used in these studies.

REFERENCES

1. Thorsby E, Sandberg L, Lindholm A, et al: Scand J Haemat 7:195, 1970
2. Sandberg L, Thorsby E, Kissmeyer-Nielsen F, et al: in: Histocompatibility Testing, 1970 Copenhagen Munksgaard 1970, p 165
3. Thorsby E, Lindholm A, Sandberg L, et al: Vox Sang 21:69, 1971
4. Svejgaard A, Staub-Nielsen L, Ryder L, et al: In Histocompatibility Testing, 1972 Copenhagen, Munksgaard, 1973, p 465
5. Solheim BG, Bratlie A, Thorsby E: Scand J Immunol 2:457, 1973
6. Solheim BG, Bratlie A, Sandberg L, et al: Tissue Antigens (in press)
7. Richiardi P, Carbonara AO, Mattiuz PL, et al: In Histocompatibility Testing, 1972 Copenhagen, Munksgaard, 1973, p 455
8. Bernoco D, Cullen S, Scudeller G, et al: In Histocompatibility Testing, 1972. Copenhagen, Munksgaard, 1972, p 527
9. Kissmeyer-Nielsen F, Kjerbye E: In Histocompatibility Testing, 1967, Copenhagen, Munksgaard, 1967, p 381
10. Solheim BG, Thorsby E: Unpublished data

Genetic Analysis and Biological Properties of Products of the Third SD (AJ) Locus of the HL-A Region

By W. R. Mayr, D. Bernoco, M. De Marchi, and R. Ceppellini

THE concept of a major histocompatibility complex (MHC) composed of a number of linked genes related in origin and in function[1] has arisen in the last decade from the observations collected in many mammalian species, particularly man and mouse. It is useful for convenience of communication, at least on a temporary basis, to distinguish MHC components on the basis of current modes of detection, chiefly into SD (serum-defined) and LD (lymphocyte-defined) genes, as suggested by Bach.[2] The biological meaning of this distinction is not yet clear and may be only marginal. Moreover, SD is mainly based on the standard complement-dependent lymphocytolysis (CdL), while other methods, also making use of alloantisera, as indirect immunofluorescence (IIF),[3] inhibition of lymphocyte activation (ILA),[4] and lymphocyte–antibody lytic interaction (LALI),[5] are likely to detect MHC products that are missed by standard CdL. On the other hand, typical SD products play a role as targets of cell-mediated lysis (CML),[6,7] and their participation in MLC, at least in regard to the level of ^{3}H-thymidine incorporation, cannot be excluded.[8]

These reservations do not disavow the fact that products of SD-1 (LA) and SD-2 (Four) loci, in comparison to other polymorphisms of MHC (e.g., MLC, Ir) are better immunogens for the induction of humoral antibodies and are more easily recognized with standard serological CdL techniques.

The history of the partition of HL-A antigens between two different but closely linked loci is germane to a discussion of the existence of a third SD locus. In 1965, Dausset et al.,[9] on the basis of correlations at the population level, hypothesized that "all the [HL-A] antigens belonged to one complex system." In 1967, Ceppellini et al.[10] confirmed this hypothesis and also introduced the concept of two segregant series of mutually exclusive alleles, not independent and therefore controlled by two linked loci. This was definitely validated by the finding of crossing over between the two loci.[11] This model was reached by applying the tools of formal genetics, i.e., fit of gene frequencies with the Hardy-Weinberg law in populations and segregation analysis in families. The picture was not obscured by misinterpretation of cross reactions because it was soon realized[9,10] that HL-A antigens, later reported to be polypeptides controlled by one cistron, are likely to cross-react either because they share some but not all determinants in different areas of the molecule or because they are characterized by different but structurally similar determinants that may fit with the same antibody population. These two classical sources of cross-reactivity each have a genetic basis because they reflect relatedness in evolution of the mutant alleles.[12] Another condition, operationally difficult to distinguish from the first two, again due to genetics, is cross-reactivity at the supramolecular level due to nonrandom association of alleles at different loci, which are usually closely linked and control chemically related products. An extreme case of such a situation is observed for the IgG subclasses (constant part) of man, as al-

---

From the Basel Institute for Immunology, Basel, Switzerland, and Istituto de Genetica Medica dell'Università, Torino, Italy.

The work done in Torino has been supported in part by NIH grant AI 08896 and in part by CNR contract, Centro di Studio per l'Immunogenetica e l'Istocompatibilità.

© 1973 by Grune & Stratton, Inc.

ready discussed in detail by Ceppellini and co-workers,[10,13] where Gm^b factor would allow the splitting of Gm^a positive (homozygous) sera into a European variety (Gm^b negative) and an African variety (Gm^b positive). On the other hand, Gm^b could be interpreted as a cross-reaction bridging Gm^a (African) with Gm^f (European), while Gm^a would also be a cross-reaction bridging Gm^b (African) with Gm^g (European), and so on in a circuitous but formally correct way of interpreting. The source of these confusing interrelations is the strong linkage disequilibrium, peculiar for different ethnic groups, between alleles at the two closely linked and phenogenetically related cistrons $\gamma 1$ and $\gamma 3$.[13] The intricacies of the Gm system, however, were easily resolved by the study of myelomatous proteins at the molecular level,[14] reflected at the cellular level by exclusion of gene expression.[15]

It is to the credit of Sandberg and co-workers[16] to have presented in 1970 very good evidence for the existence of a specificity, SA-AJ, that fulfilled a number of criteria for belonging to the HL-A system but fitted into neither SD-1 nor SD-2 segregant series, thus likely representing the first product of a third locus (SD-3) of the HL-A region characterized by a strong positive association with two SD-2 antigens, A5 and W27. Two years later, however, the same group of workers,[17] while presenting additional data in support of SD-3, discussed complicated alternatives under the influence of theories postulating an endless heterogeneity of HL-A antigens.[18,19] The dilemma was justified by the lack of the only discriminative evidence at the genetic level, i.e., separation of SD-3 antigens from members of the other two loci by crossing over with a relatively high frequency. In fact, even crossing over, if very rare, in the absence of molecular evidence cannot allow a distinction between the alternatives of two mutational sites located in the same cistron or in two adjacent cistrons. In the meantime, however, Richiardi et al.[20] and Bernoco et al.[21] had worked out two new tools facilitating the molecular analysis at the cell surface of the products of HL-A genes. By applying these techniques, the dilemma was solved in favor of SD-3.[22,23] Co-capping experiments, which are equivalent to an artificial and selective exclusion of gene expression at the cell surface, showed that SD-3 antigens were physically independent from the other HL-A antigens present on the cell, hence corresponding to different polypeptides.

In the present paper, the evidence forwarded by the Scandinavian authors for the existence of SD-3 is fully confirmed and extended. Moreover, the possible relevance of SD-3 antigens for MLC and CML is analyzed. Finally, the distribution of these products in different tissues and some peculiarities of their functional behavior are reported.

MATERIALS, METHOD, AND DEFINITIONS

Panels of lymphocytes and antisera. HL-A specificities are indicated according to the joint report of 1972.[19] The terms monospecific, supertypic (public), subtypic (private), cross-reacting, and corresponding symbols are used as described by Richiardi et al.[20] The three loci of the HL-A region whose products are currently recognized by serology are here indicated as SD (serum-defined): SD-1 = LA, SD-2 = Four, SD-3 = AJ.

The lymphocytes used in the experiments came from a panel of 700 donors typed for all HL-A specificities described at the Histocompatibility Workshop of 1972[19] and for four alleles of the SD-3 locus. Some of them were genotyped through family analysis. When possible they were selected for being full-house, i.e., with all the HL-A antigens identified.

The alloantisera employed were obtained from volunteers immunized by planned blood transfusion in Torino and Parma[24] or from multiparous women screened in Tübingen and Wien. The HL-A specificity of the sera had already been studied and classified as far as complement-dependent lysis (CdL) is concerned by means of population and family analysis and, for some of them, by absorption/elution techniques. All antigens have been defined using the CdL technique described below.

Antigens and antibodies of SD-3. While waiting for the decisions of the nomenclature committee, for minimizing confusion, they are indicated by the letter T (third) followed by numbers corresponding to the

Table 5. Independent Resistance to Lysis of Different HL-A and Non-HL-A Antigens at the Cell Surface

1st Anti-HL-A Coat + Anti-human Ig	SD-1 (LA)						SD-2 (Four)								SD-3 (AJ)				Non-HL-A	
	A 1	A 2	A 11	W 23	W 24	W 26	A 7	A 8	A 12	A 13	W 5	W 15	W 18	W 27	T 2	T 4	T 5	T 6	Le^a	A_1Se
(1) autol. serum				+	+			+	+							+				
anti-A12				+	+			+	−							+				
anti-T4				+	+			+	+							−				
(2) autol. serum			+			+				+				+	+					
anti-A7*			+			+				+				−	+					
anti-T2			+			+				+				+	−					
(3) autol. serum		+			+		+				+					+				+
anti-W5		+			+		+				−					+				+
anti-T4		+			+		+				+					−				+
(4) autol. serum		+					+					+				+				
anti-W15		+					+					−				+				
anti-T4		+					+					+				−				
(5) autol. serum	+	+						+					+				+	+	+	
anti-A8	+	+						−					+				+	+	+	
anti-W18	+	+						+					−				+	+	+	
anti-T5	+	+						+					+				−	+	+	
anti-T6	+	+						+					+				+	−	+	

Column heading printed over all antigen columns: Typing after Strip.

Lysostrip (as described under Method and in reference 26): after a first treatment with an anti-HL-A serum, followed by anti-human Ig and incubation at 37°C for 15 min, lymphocytes become resistant to lysis upon addition of new antiserum and C′ for those specificities carried by the same physical units that were stripped during first treatment.

HL-A typing after strip is according to NIH technique, but incubation (3 hr) is carefully maintained at 16°C. Antisera were previously absorbed for removing cold pancytotoxins: + strong positive; − definitely negative reactions.

Correct phenotype of cells results from controls, where autologous serum has been used for the strip.

Note lack of co-resistance to lysis, i.e., physical independence between all products of different HL-A genes. Also $Lewis^a$ and A_1Se reactivities are not affected. Anti-human Ig alone (controls) does not strip any surface antigen.

*Anti-A7 (ShBS) contains a A7 × W27 cross-reacting antibody CdL-negative against antigen W27 (see reference 5).

Table 6. SD-3 as Target for CML and LALI; Family Amrhein

Stimulators and Haplotypes		MLC* ^3H c.p.m.	CML† Target Ch-2	LALI‡ T1	T2	T3
Father	*ab*	78,908	83%	>1000	>1000	0
Mother	*cd*	1,805	—	0	0	300
Ch-1	*ac*	36,474	42%	>1000	0	0
Ch-2	*bd*	27,976	100%	0	>1000	300
Ch-6	*bc*	22,836	102%	0	>1000	0
Ch-7	*ad*	46,761	49%	>1000	0	300

Haplotypes

a: A11; W15; T1 b: W32; W10; T2

c: A3; A7; T− d: W32; W10; T3

*MLC: unidirectional; responder is always the mother.

†CML: effector is always the mother activated in MLC by the various stimulators. Target is always Ch-2 (homozygous at SD-1 and SD-2). Total release $^{51}CrCl$, 8,403 c.p.m.; spontaneous release, 2,141 c.p.m. When Ch-2 is the stimulator, experimental release is 5,118 c.p.m. = 48%. This last figure has been taken as 100% (specific lysis) and damage of the same Ch-2 target after MLC activation by others (cross-lysis) has been expressed as percentage of specific lysis (see reference 43).

‡LALI: with three anti-SD-3 antisera, expressed as serum dilution still giving significant ^{51}Cr release over controls (see reference 5).

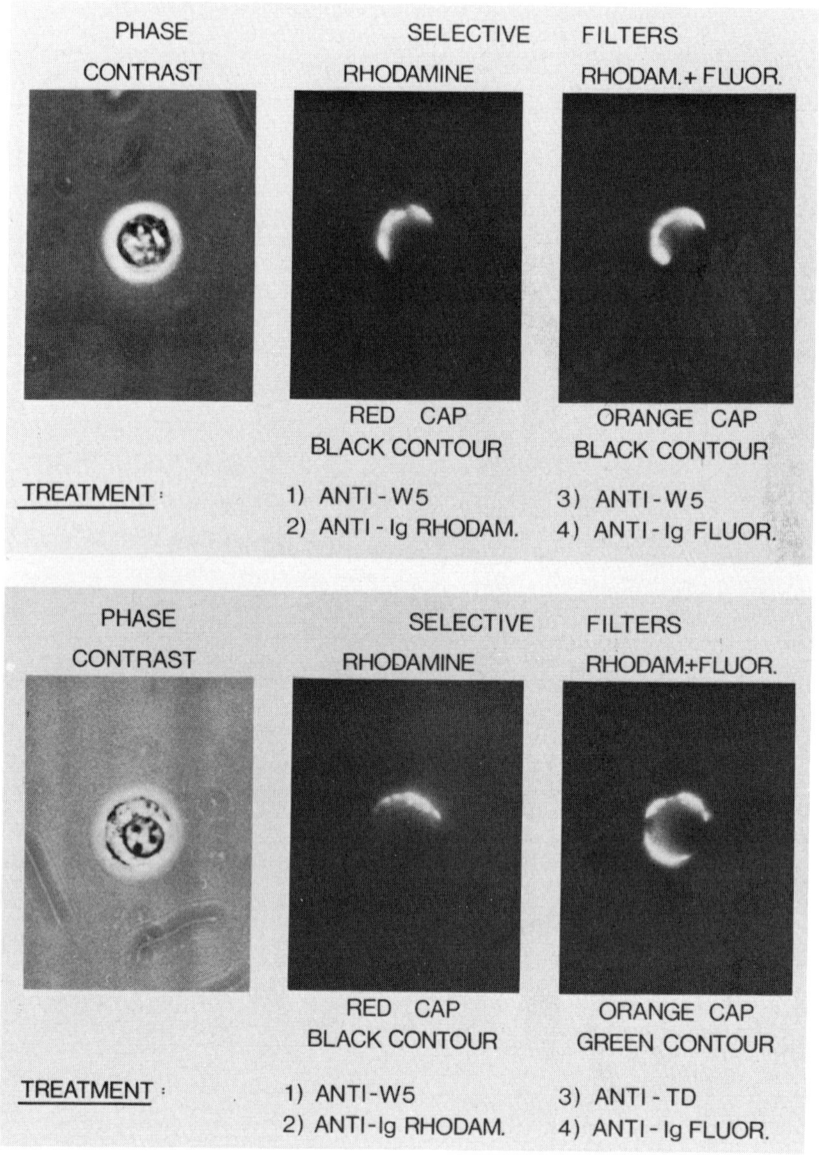

Fig. 1. Fluorostrip showing independent capping of the physical units carrying W5 and T4 (TD) determinants of the SD-2 and SD-3 loci, respectively. These two antigens have been selected because they have been mixed up even by "George,"[19] due to a high Δ. Technique as described by Bernoco et al.[21] Sequence on top shows that strip with anti-W5 (1) followed an anti-human Ig (2) has sequestered into a cap all W5 molecules as shown by the cell contour remaining black after steps (3) and (4). Sequence at the bottom shows that same strip does not prevent contour staining when anti-T4 (TD) is used in step (3). The lymphocytes from donor 3 of Table 5 were full-house at SD-1 and SD-2.

areas of the same structure or if they are carried by different physical units.

(b) Fluorostrip. For deciding between the two alternatives, the fluorostrip was carried out according to the technique described by Bernoco et al.[21] As shown in Fig. 1, anti-W5 does not strip T4 and vice versa.

(c) Lysostrip. Lysostrip was done in all possible combinations, with special atten-

tion to those SD-2 and SD-3 antigens known to be often associated in the same haplotype (Table 5). In no case was there co-capping between the antigens of these two loci, nor between SD-1 and SD-3. Anti-IgG per se is not able to cap any HL-A antigen. Anti-HL-A sera for the three loci did not interfere with the reactivity of other polymorphic antigens, as A_1Se and Lewis[a] expressed at the lymphocyte surface,[31,32] whether synthesized by the lymphocyte itself or absorbed from the serum.

By contrast, a rabbit anti-human $\beta 2$ microglobulin serum of high specificity induced resistance to CdL upon addition of Ab + C′ for all antigens of the three HL-A loci, even on cells that had not previously been exposed to anti-HL-A coating. This suggests that $\beta 2$ microglobulin may in some way be associated with HL-A antigens. Other alternatives, however, cannot be ruled out. This important finding will be presented in detail elsewhere.[33]

SD-3 and Cell-mediated Immunity

(a) MLC. A family was found where the two parents carried a haplotype that had the same SD-1 (W32) and SD-2 (W10) but was different for SD-3 (T2 in the father, T3 in the mother). Of 10 children (only some combinations are reported in Table 6), those apparently homozygous for SD-1 and SD-2 and two more that differed from the mother (the responder) only for SD-3 gave a lower activation, thus suggesting that the so-called SD antigens may participate in controlling at least the magnitude of ^{3}H-thymidine incorporation, once the LD differences have derepressed the responder lymphocytes.

(b) LALI. As shown in Table 6, SD-3 antigens are excellent targets for lymphocytotoxicity due to interaction between humoral antibodies and normal lymphocytes. Note that the three anti-T sera tested had CdL titers between 1:2 and 1:16.

(c) CML. As shown in Table 6, the fact that cross-lysis by child 6 and by the father was very high in comparison to specific lysis due to child 2 suggests that either SD-3 or other components of MHC, or, less likely, non-HL-A differences, are excellent targets for CML. Thus the assumption that SD-2 antigens have in this respect a privileged role is incorrect.[34]

SD-3 Antigens at the Cell Surface

(a) Expression on different cell lineages. Quantitative studies by using radiolabeled anti-IgG are in progress. For the moment, the data based on the number of cells that are necessary for absorbing out the same number of cytotoxic units, as well as the impression given by immunofluorescence (indirect method), suggest that the amount of antigens expressed on lymphocytes and platelets is approximately the same for SD-3 as for SD-1 and SD-2.

SD-3 antigens are also expressed on all lymphocyte lineages, because with appropriate dilutions of antisera, all cells are killed by CdL and all cells fluoresce by IIF. Pure B lymphocyte preparations, obtained from two patients with typical chronic lymphocytic leukemia, also exhibited a normal expression of their SD-3 antigens.

(b) Desensitization and spontaneous resistance. Desensitization in the first hour seems to develop at a higher rate for the majority of SD-3 antigens tested than for SD-1 and SD-2 antigens (Fig. 2a). At later times, the speed of desensitization becomes the same for all HL-A antigens. The quicker initial rate is probably related to spontaneous resistance, which is very rarely observed for SD-1 and SD-2 antigens but in our experience is rather common with SD-3 antigens (Fig. 2b). This interesting phenomenon is not due to extrinsic characteristics of the antisera tested (e.g., addition of NaN_3 as antibacterial preservative) because: (*i*) it has also been observed with antibodies absorbed and eluted from platelets of appropriate phenotype; (*ii*) mixing of anti-SD-3 sera with anti-SD-1 or anti-SD-2

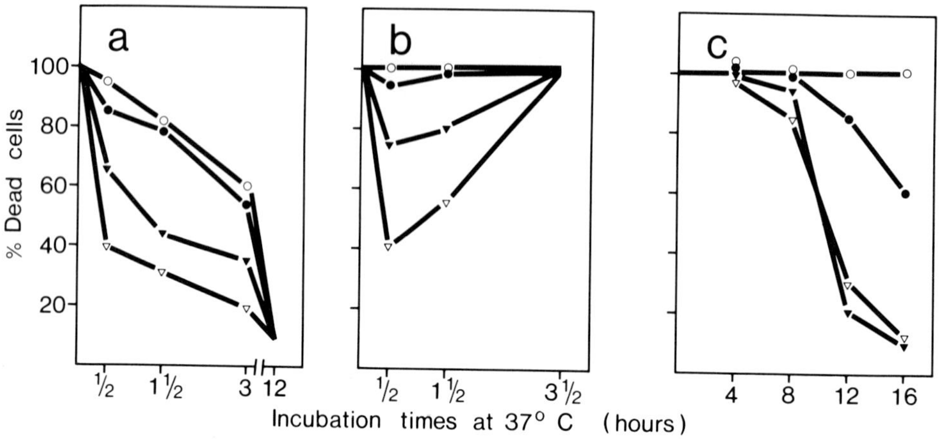

Fig. 2. Desensitization (a), spontaneous resistance (b), and exhaustion (c) for different HL-A antigens. Legend: Same donor's cells used in the three experiments, HL-A2,3,12,W5,T2,T4. Note, however, that different time scales have been used. ○ = anti-A2, ● = anti-A12, ▽ = anti-T2, ▼ = anti-T4. (a) Desensitization: cells sensitized with 4U of Ab, 3 hr at 4°C; washed; incubated at 37°C in RAS for the times indicated (up to 12 hr); washed at 4°C; C′ alone (4U) added; incubated 3 hr at 16°C. (b) Spontaneous Resistance: cells sensitized with 4U of Ab, 3 hr at 4°C; washed; incubated at 37°C in RAS for the times indicated; washed at 4°C; 4U of same Ab + 4U of C′ added; incubated 3 hr at 16°C. (c) Exhaustion: cells, nonsensitized by Ab, incubated at 37°C in RAS with 100 μg cycloheximide; washed at 4°C; 8U of Ab + 8U of C′ added; incubated 3 hr at 16°C.

does not induce spontaneous resistance for SD-1 or SD-2 antigens.

(c) Recovery and exhaustion. As extensively discussed by Cullen et al.,[26] after strip the rate of recovery (within the limits of the methods used) seems to be the same for products of the three SD loci. In all cases, recovery was completely blocked by cycloheximide at the dose used (0.1 mg/ml). NaN_3 interfered with recovery in a differential way because at 24 hr expression of SD-1 antigen was normal and SD-2 antigen was only partially repressed, but by marked contrast the SD-3 antigen (T4) had completely disappeared from the cell surface (Fig. 2b in reference 26). This was the first hint that some biological properties of products of the various loci of the HL-A region might be different.

This has been definitely and very clearly confirmed by exhaustion, where cycloheximide is added to lymphocyte suspensions, cultured in autologous serum and previously exposed neither to strip by anti-HL-A nor to any other treatment (e.g., enzymatic digestion). Figure 2c depicts a typical experiment: at 16 hr after the addition of the drug, in excess of lytic reagents (8 Ab U + 8 C′ U), HL-A2 induces 100% killing, HL-A12 induces about 50% killing, while T2 and T4 seem to have disappeared. This experiment has been repeated on a number of different cells. In all cases after 16 to 24 hr SD-3 antigens could not be recognized anymore by CdL, SD-2 antigens expression was significantly but not completely reduced, and SD-1 antigens were almost unaffected. This differential behavior seems to be common to all antigens of a given locus, although minor variations for alleles of the same locus have been observed.

CONCLUSIONS

The data here presented support the previous findings of the Scandinavian authors[16,17] and establish on a definite basis the existence in the HL-A region of a third locus, which controls surface components recognized by CdL (hence the SD-3 denomination) and resembling for many characteristics the other already known HL-A antigens. This fact has important implications in many different directions. Here only the major points will be briefly considered.

Formal Genetics

For the geneticist the finding is not unexpected because a number of chromosomal regions are known in higher organisms composed of genes with the following characteristics: (*a*) some of them are derived one from the other by gene doubling and then differential, though related, evolution;[1] (*b*) hence they are often also related in function; (*c*) they are kept together (or even brought together from different parts of the genome) because they interact functionally, possibly at the level of the chromosome itself, and represent an epistatic block of genetic information, according to Fisher's theory.[35] As already discussed, the IgG region is a typical example of such a situation, but the MHC already shows many features fitting with the model: (*a*) cross-reactions between products of HL-A SD-1 and SD-2[37] and of H-2D and H-2K,[38] in agreement with a common origin of the pairs of genes by duplication; (*b*) the striking homology of MHC in many species, which is firm evidence of a strong selective force that keeps together through evolution a number of related genes; (*c*) the high linkage disequilibrium between alleles of relatively distant genes (as HL-A1 and HL-A8), which also suggests a selective advantage of some haplotypic combinations.

In this respect the Δ between SD-2 and SD-3 are particularly high. This suggests that the recombination frequency between these two genes is smaller than between SD-1/SD-2 or SD-1/SD-3. This is confirmed by family data (Table 3), although it is not yet known whether SD-3 is located between SD-1 and SD-2 or between SD-2 and the major LD.[39] In fact, the report of Löw[36] needs to be confirmed. This may be an important point because the region between SD-2 and the major LD seems to be critical for disease association.[40]

The high Δ between W5 and T4 may be a good reason for maintaining the view that disease association is due to linkage between SD loci and some other genes, possibly equivalent to murine Ir, as strongly suggested by the findings of Levine et al.[41] in the case of ragweed hay fever. Very high associations between specific antigens and diseases, as W27 and ankylosing spondylitis[42] support, however, the alternative view of a direct physiological connection between given antigens, as components of the cell surface and susceptibility to disease.

Phenogenetics

This last remark opens up the question of the functions of SD-3 antigens in comparison to the products of other MHC loci. Obviously there is no answer at the moment, but the respective role of alleles at the three SD loci, in respect to susceptibility to disease, to immune response, to cell membrane function, to graft rejection in vivo, and to MLC and CML in vitro must be reevaluated by taking into consideration also SD-3. For example, at variance with other reports,[34] Trinchieri et al.[43] found that both SD-1 and SD-2 antigens were competent targets for CML, although association with SD-2 gave a higher crosslysis (60% versus 48%). In view of the data presented here (Table 6), it is likely that the association measured was often with SD-2 + SD-3, due to the high linkage disequilibrium between some alleles of these two loci. Thus probably all antigens recognized by CdL are also recognized by CML.

On the basis of the present evidence, limited however to different lymphocyte lineages and to platelets, SD-3 products do not seem to be differentiation antigens[40] anymore than the other HL-A.

Biological Characteristics

Strict similarity between products of the three SD loci by no means should be taken for granted for their various biological characteristics. Actually, the data presented here and in the joint paper[26] suggest that the behavior at the cell surface of antigens of the three loci in regard to interaction with antibody and complement (spontaneous resistance) and to susceptibility to cycloheximide and NaN_3 (exhaustion) is quite different.

Further studies with adequate biochemical methods are in progress, and for the moment only some possibilities can be anticipated. Our feeling is that the two phenomena observed are not unrelated. The easiest exhaustion by drugs of SD-3 antigens can be explained by a smaller pool of preformed molecules that are parking below the outer layer of the cell surface, ready to replace the molecules removed by microaggregation, shedding, or proteolytic treatment.[44] This would also justify the easiest induction of spontaneous resistance by alloantibody against SD-3 antigens.

Other alternatives, as different turnover or molecular size or affinity for the lipid layer, must also be considered. The important point is that drugs may differentially control the expression at the cell surface of the products of the various genetic units of the HL-A region, with obvious implications for new approaches to the problems of graft rejection, immune surveillance, and HL-A-associated diseases.

SUMMARY

The existence of a third locus (SD-3, AJ) in the HL-A region, closely linked to SD-2 (Four), controlling antigens easily recognized by complement-dependent lymphocytolysis, has been confirmed through genetic and molecular evidence. Six alleles (besides the blank) have been identified. Their distribution in different cell lineages and their relevance for MLC, CML, and LALI have been studied. Cycloheximide and other drugs inhibit the expression of SD-3 antigens at the cell surface more easily than expression of SD-1 and SD-2. SD-3 antigens also frequently undergo spontaneous resistance to lysis upon addition of Ab + C′. These findings suggest that some biological properties (e.g., pool of preformed molecules, turnover, affinity for the lipid layer) may differ for products of the various HL-A loci.

ACKNOWLEDGMENTS

We gratefully acknowledge the generous gifts of sera from Drs. H. V. Bashir, C. P. Engelfriet, H. Festenstein, I. van de Putte, G. Rizzo, L. Sandberg, and A. Svejgaard. We express our gratitude to the blood donors of Hoffmann-La Roche, Basel, and particularly to the families Amrhein and Holzgang for their collaboration. We thank Mrs. Marietta Bernoco, Mrs. Dorothea Mayr, and Miss Claretta Finà for their expert technical assistance.

REFERENCES

1. Ceppellini R: Progress in Immunology. New York, Academic, 1971, p. 973

2. Bach FH: in McDevitt H, Landy M (eds): Genetic Control of the Immune Response. New York, Academic, 1972, p. 105

3. van Leeuwen A, van Rood JJ: Transplant Proc 5:1539, 1973

4. Ceppellini R, Bonnard GD, Coppo F, et al: Transplant Proc 3:63, 1971

5. Trinchieri G, De Marchi M, Mayr WR, et al: Transplant Proc 5:1631, 1973

6. Ceppellini R: in McDevitt H, Landy M (eds): Genetic Control of the Immune Response. New York, Academic, 1972, p. 256

7. Eijsvoogel VP, du Bois R, Melief CJM, et al: Transplant Proc 5:1301, 1973

8. Thorsby E: Research in Immunochemistry and Immunobiology, vol 5 (in press)

9. Dausset J, Ivanyi P, Ivanyi D: Histocompatibility Testing 1965. Copenhagen, Munksgaard, 1965, p. 51

10. Ceppellini R, Curtoni ES, Mattiuz PL, et al: Histocompatibility Testing 1967. Copenhagen, Munksgaard, 1967, p 149

11. Kissmeyer-Nielsen F, Svejgaard A, Ahrons S, Staub Nielsen L: Nature (Lond) 224:75, 1969

12. Bodmer W, Bodmer J, Adler S, et al: Ann NY Acad Sci 129:473, 1966

13. Ceppellini R: Genetica delle Immunoglobuline, Atti Ass Genet It 12:1, 1966

14. Kunkel HG, Allen JC, Grey HM: Cold Spring Harbor Symposia on Quantitative Biology. 29:443, 1964

15. Pernis B, Chiappino G, Kelus AS, Gell PGH: J Exp Med 122:853, 1965

16. Sandberg L, Thorsby E, Kissmeyer-Nielsen F, Lindholm A: Histocompatibility Testing 1970. Copenhagen, Munksgaard, 1970, p. 165

17. Svejgaard A, Staub Nielsen L, Ryder LP, et al: Histocompatibility Testing 1972. Copenhagen, Munksgaard, 1973, p 465

18. Thorsby E, Lindholm A, Sandberg L, Staub Nielsen L: Vox Sang (Basel) 21:69, 1971

19. Joint Report of the Fifth International Histocompatibility Workshop: Histocompatibility Testing 1972. Copenhagen, Munksgaard, 1973, p 619

20. Richiardi P, Carbonara AO, Mattiuz PL, Ceppellini R: Histocompatibility Testing 1972. Copenhagen, Munksgaard, 1973, p 455

21. Bernoco D, Cullen SE, Scudeller G, et al: Histocompatibility Testing 1972. Copenhagen, Munksgaard, 1973, p 527

22. Svejgaard A, Staub Nielsen L, Ryder LP, et al: Histocompatibility Testing 1972. Copenhagen, Munksgaard, 1973, p 472

23. Solheim BG, Bratlie A, Sandberg L, et al: Tissue Antigens (in press)

24. Curtoni ES, Scudeller G, Mattiuz PL, et al: Tissue Antigens 2:415, 1972

25. Bøyum A: Scand J Clin Lab Invest 21(suppl):97, 1968

26. Cullen SE, Bernoco D, Carbonara AO, et al: Transplant Proc 5:1835, 1973

27. Naito S, Mickey MR, Hirata A, Terasaki PI: Tissue Antigens 1:219, 1971

28. Bernoco D, Mattiuz PL, Miggiano VC, Ceppellini R: Giornale Batteriologia, Virologia Ed Immunologia 64:272, 1971

29. Piazza A, Mattiuz PL, Richiardi P: Tissue Antigens 2:156, 1972

30. Mattiuz PL, Ihde D, Piazza A, et al: Histocompatibility Testing 1970. Copenhagen, Munksgaard, 1970, p 193

31. Jeannet M, Bodmer JG, Bodmer WF, Schapira M: Histocompatibility Testing 1972. Copenhagen, Munksgaard, 1973, p 493

32. Mayr WR, Bernoco D, Rovis L, Ceppellini R: in preparation

33. Poulik MD, Bernoco D, Ceppellini R: in preparation

34. Eijsvoogel VP, du Bois MJGJ, Melief CJM, et al: Histocompatibility Testing 1972. Copenhagen, Munksgaard, 1973, p 501

35. Fisher RA: Genetic Theory of Natural Selection (2 ed). New York, Dover, 1958

36. Löw B: quoted as personal communication in reference 17

37. Belvedere MC, Curtoni SE, Mattiuz PL: Tissue Antigens (in press)

38. Shreffler DC, David CS, Passmore HC, Klein J: Transplant Proc 3:176, 1971

39. Yunis EJ, Amos DB: Proc Natl Acad Sci USA 68:3031, 1971

40. Bodmer WF: Nature 237:139, 1972

41. Levine BB, Stember RH, Fotino M: Science 178:1201, 1972

42. Schlosstein L, Terasaki PI, Bluestone R, Pearson CM: N Engl J Med 288:704, 1973

43. Trinchieri G, Bernoco D, Curtoni SE, et al: Histocompatibility Testing 1972. Copenhagen, Munksgaard, 1973, p 509

44. Cone RE, Marchalonis JJ, Rolley RT: J Exp Med 134:1373, 1971

45. Rizzo G: personal communication

46. Morton NE: Am J Hum Genet 9:55, 1957

Possible Relationships Among HL-A Histocompatibility Components

By Miriam Segall and Fritz H. Bach

THE separation of loci of the major histocompatibility complex (MHC) into two types, genetically and functionally distinct, is a dichotomy that has been documented by many researchers in the last few years. One type of locus controls antigens that on immunization appear to provoke the formation of cytotoxic and/or agglutinating antibody; these antigens have been called serologically defined (SD) antigens, and the loci controlling them, SD loci. The products of the other type of locus lead to activation in the in vitro mixed leukocyte culture (MLC) test; these loci are called lymphocyte-defined (LD) loci. The LD–SD terminology is a heuristic one; although LD differences may in the future be detected by serologic tests and SD differences by lymphocyte responses, it is still necessary to make a distinction on the basis of the functional dichotomy described above. Genetically, loci of both SD and LD types are found closely linked in the MHC in both man and mouse, and it is with these MHC loci that we will be concerned in this article.

The distinction between SD and LD has been very clearly drawn in mouse studies and in family studies in man. SD differences alone either do not lead to MLC activation or do so only weakly; LD differences can lead to MLC activation even in the absence of SD differences. However, several investigators have shown a correlation of SD-antigen identity with low (and in a few cases no) stimulation in MLC in unrelated human subjects. In an attempt to harmonize these apparently contradictory results, we have suggested that there may be linkage disequilibrium between SD and LD alleles in the human population, resulting in a genetic and consequent phenotypic association of certain LD and SD alleles on the same chromosome. We here present results of further studies designed to illuminate the relationship between SD antigens and MLC reactivity in the unrelated human population.

MATERIALS AND METHOD

HL-A Typing. Cells were typed by Dr. D. Bernard Amos, using a microcytotoxicity technique,[1] or by Dr. Flemming Kissmeyer-Nielsen using microcytotoxicity and complement-fixation techniques.[2] Only cells with four identified antigens for the SD1 (LA) and SD2 (Four) loci were used.

Freezing. All cells were frozen by the procedure we have discussed in detail elsewhere[3] and stored in liquid nitrogen until used.

MLC. The MLC technique used was the micromethod in tissue culture plates that we have previously described,[4] with some modifications to accommodate the apparently greater sensitivity of the frozen cells to centrifugation and pH changes after inactivation for use as stimulating cells.[3] Stimulating cells in these experiments were inactivated with 4,000 R X-irradiation.

Analysis of Results. Each experiment was done three times; such a set of three repeat experiments constitutes a series. In order to make comparisons between repeat experiments and between series, we adopted the approach discussed previously[5] of using stimulation by pools of stimulating cells to provide a standard for each responder. Thus each responder in every experiment was tested with three non-overlapping pools of 20 cells each, i.e., three separate standard stimulating cells were used. For each individual stimulator–responder combination in a given experiment, a stimulation value was calculated by dividing the c.p.m. in that combination by the average of the

---

From the Departments of Genetics, Medical Genetics, and Surgery, University of Wisconsin, Madison, Wis.

Supported by NIH grants AI08439, AI06525, and GM-15422; NF-MOD grant CRBS 246; and ONR grant N00014-67-A-0128-003.

M.S. is a NIH Trainee from NIGMS (grant GM-00398), Madison, Wisc.

This is Paper No. 1697 from the Laboratory of Genetics, University of Wisconsin, Madison, Wisc.

© 1973 by Grune & Stratton, Inc.

stimulation (in c.p.m.) of that responder by the three pools. The stimulation values for the three experiments of a series were averaged for each combination to give a mean stimulation value.

Definition of Low Stimulation. When the experiments were designed, the following analysis was planned: Given the SD-identical cells A and B, the combination AB_x could be compared to the combinations AC_x, AD_x, etc., testing whether A responds less to B_x than to other stimulators (analysis I, or analysis of SD-identicals as responders). The groups of SD-identical and -nonidentical combinations were tested to see whether the mean stimulation values in the former were significantly lower than in the latter, using the one-tailed Wilcoxon unpaired rank test (Mann–Whitney U test). In the example given above, the group $AB_x + BA_x$ was tested against the group of all four-specificity-different combinations involving responders A and B.

As we soon discovered, this analysis is subject to two important potential distortions. (1) A statistically significant difference can be obtained if one or both of the stimulators A_x and B_x provoke a low response in all responders tested. (2) A difference may be obscured if some of the non-SD-identical stimulators provoke a low response in all responders tested, or if one or both of the SD-identical cells provoke a high response in all responders tested. The situations mentioned may be biologically important, but in the present context they would only serve to confuse the interpretation of comparisons between SD-identical and -nonidentical cells.

To avoid such confusion, we have also analyzed the SD-identical cells as stimulators against a series of different responders (analysis II, or analysis of SD-identicals as stimulators). In this case the mean stimulation values of the combinations BA_x, CA_x, DA_x, etc., are used. Again using the Wilcoxon test, the group $AB_x + BA_x$ is compared to the group of all four-specificity-different combinations involving stimulators A_x and B_x. In this analysis, in some cases there are not enough combinations in a given group to attain significant p values in the Wilcoxon test; these groups are indicated in Table 1. Analyses of groups of combinations differing only by SD1 specificities were performed in the same way.

RESULTS

SD-identical Unrelated Individuals. The HL-A SD phenotypes of the donors tested are listed in Table 1. Also indicated is whether or not low stimulation was seen between the members of the pair or group. The p values give the probability that the degree of difference between the group of typing identicals and the group of combinations differing by all four SD specificities

Table 1. Stimulation by Cells Identical for SD1 and SD2 or for SD2

SD Phenotype	Analysis I* p value	Analysis II p value	SD Phenotype	Analysis I p Value	Analysis II p Value
2,Li,12,W16 (2)	N.S.	N.S.	2,Li,12,W16 (2)	N.S.	N.S.
			2,W26,12,W16		
2,3,W5,W16 (2)	0.025	0.053**			
1,11,5,8 (2)	0.018	0.033	1,11,5,8 (2)	<0.0005	<0.0005
			1,Li,5,8		
			2,3,5,8		
2,9,12,BB (2)	N.S.	N.S.			
1,2,8,W15 (3)	0.021	0.007			
1,3,7,8 (2)	0.025	0.053**	1,3,7,8 (2)	$\ll 0.0001$	$\ll 0.0001$
			1,2,7,8		
			2,3,7,8		
			3,11,7,8		
2,9,7,W15 (2)	N.S.	N.S.	2,9,7,W15 (2)	0.03	N.S.
			1,3,7,W15		
			3,28,7,W15		

*Analysis I: Comparison of the SD- (or SD2-) identical individuals as responders to each other and as responders to a group of individuals differing by four SD specificities. Analysis II: Comparison of the SD- (or SD2-) identical individuals as stimulators of each other and as stimulators of a group of individuals differing by four SD specificities.

Wilcoxon unsigned rank test, one-tailed, for difference between the two groups. Numbers in parentheses indicate the number of individuals of that phenotype tested.

**There were not enough values in the two groups in this comparison to reach a significant level of difference in the Wilcoxon test.

is due to chance. Analysis as responders (I) or as stimulators (II) gives the same results.

Donors Differing by LA (SD1) Specificities Only. Combinations where the cells differed from one another by one or two SD1 (LA), or one or two SD2 (Four), specificities were also tested as responders and stimulators. The results are summarized in Table 1. When SD-identical combinations showed low stimulation values, cells having the same SD2 antigens but different SD1 antigens were also low stimulators with these SD-identical cells and among themselves. When SD-identical combinations did not have low stimulation values, neither did combinations of cells differing for SD1 specificities only. The stimulation values in the SD-identical combinations were not included for these calculations.

The results with the group having SD2 specificities HL-A7, W15 and differing by SD1 specificities are somewhat ambiguous. The SD-identicals (2, 9, 7, W15) are not low stimulators or responders to one another. The members of the entire group having HL-A7, W15 in common show significantly low responses to one another compared to their responses to other stimulators (analysis I). However, these cells are not low stimulators of one another compared to their stimulation of other responders (analysis II). The significant difference seen in analysis I appears to be a result of generally low stimulation of all responders (regardless of those responders' SD phenotypes) by the cells of the group identical for HL-A7, W15. As discussed above under Method, although this generally low stimulation may be of biological interest, these SD2-identicals do not appear to be low stimulators among themselves.

The low stimulation values are seen in all combinations of the group having SD1 differences only. In all combinations tested where low stimulation values were seen, the combinations differing by one or two SD1 specificities were not distinguishable from the SD-identical combinations. The numbers in any one group are, however, small, and it is possible that a larger series will reveal statistically significant differences.

Use of Pools as a Standard Stimulator. Variation in the number of c.p.m. incorporated in a particular combination in repeat experiments is a familiar phenomenon. When large experiments are repeated this seems to be due primarily to an apparent variation in general responsiveness; a particular responder may give much higher c.p.m. with all stimulators in one experiment of a series than in another. The expression of stimulation as a fraction of pool mean (here called stimulation value) permitted the distinction between high and low stimulation when the stimulation of several different responders by a single stimulating cell was compared. Within a series of experiments the pools as standard stimulator substantially achieved their purpose in eliminating the variation due to differences in overall response (measured in c.p.m.) of different responding cells.[3] (Segall, unpublished data).

DISCUSSION

The correlation between LD antigens, as detected by MLC, and SD antigens, as detected by serotyping, and between graft prognosis and either of these methods of histocompatibility assessment, is presently a matter of intense investigation and, on occasion, equally intense dispute. It has become clear over the last year or two that MLC activation is not primarily a response to SD antigens but is controlled by loci closely linked to the SD antigens in both mouse[6,7] and man.[8] Unrelated SD-identical human subjects do, however, show low MLC stimulation[5,9] and sometimes non-stimulation.[10,11]

In studying a genetic problem of this magnitude and complexity, an obvious starting point is to look for possible correlations between HL-A SD antigens, as identified by typing, and MLC reactivity. The immediate clinical importance of any such correlation lies in the fact that although in the nonimmunized recipient MLC may be a better indicator of graft prognosis than SD disparity,[12–14] the MLC test as presently performed takes too long to be predictively applicable to cadaver transplantation. If it could be shown that certain incompatibilities for SD antigens are associated with relatively low MLC stimulation, retrospective analysis of transplant data may indeed indicate that transplantation across these incompatibilities involves less risk than transplantation across other incompatibilities. Typing could then be used in these situations for its implied statements about LD compatibility as measured by MLC. The data given in Table 1 indicate that apparent identity of SD antigens in unrelated individuals is not always associated with low MLC stimulation.

We have previously suggested[5] that low stimulation among SD-identical unrelateds may be most reasonably explained by a linkage disequilibrium, certain LD alleles being present on the same chromosome with certain SD alleles more often than expected from the frequencies of these alleles in the population. The situation with respect to the HL-A1,2,8,12 donors analyzed previously[5] may be very special. The occurrence together on the same chromosome (called a haplotype) of the antigens 1,8 or 2,12 is more frequent in white populations than expected from the frequencies of the individual antigens. Since the SD antigens of the SD1 and SD2 loci exhibit linkage disequilibrium in these haplotypes, disequilibrium involving other alleles in the region would not be surprising. The results presented here, however, suggest that the genetic situation is more complicated.

The data summarized in Table 1, concerning stimulation by SD1-different cells, indicate that in those cases where there is low stimulation between SD-identical unrelateds there is a similarly low level of stimulation between individuals differing from those SD-identicals and among themselves only for one or two LA (SD1) specificities. Hence the entire haplotype is not important for the phenomenon of low stimulation. The critical factor seems to be an association between certain SD2 and certain LD alleles. This is not surprising in view of the demonstration by Yunis and Amos,[8] confirmed by Eijsvoogel, van Rood, and others,[15] that a genetic region extremely important in control of MLC reactivity lies near the SD2 locus on the side away from SD1. These findings are also consistent with the data of Mempel et al.[16] Other combinations do not show low stimulation among either SD-identical or SD1-different cells.

The number of combinations tested in these experiments is not large, and any generalizations about mechanisms of MLC activation drawn from these data are unquestionably speculative. However, certain ideas about MLC and its relationship to SD antigens are suggested by our results. Of particular interest is the finding that, in our material, whereas combinations identical for HL-A8 and W15 or for HL-A8 and HL-A7 show reciprocal low stimulation, a group of combinations identical for W15 and HL-A7 (including a pair of typing identicals) does not.

The situation may thus be more complex than a simple linkage disequilibrium between Four and LD alleles. For example, in combinations with identity for SD2 (Four series) antigens the presence of HL-A8, or of the LD allele(s) associated with it, may lead to low stimulation in MLC through interaction of some kind, at either the genotypic or phenotypic level. A simple damping effect of HL-A8 or its associated LD allele(s) is probably ruled out by the fact that combinations identical for their two SD1 antigens and for HL-A8, and differing only by the second SD2 antigen, do not appear to be low stimulators.

In this context, another possibly significant observation is that in combinations where the only antigen carried by the stimulator cell but not by the responder is

HL-A8, stimulation may be low, and the same may be true of HL-A5 and W5, or of any two of these antigens. The combinations showing unequivocally low stimulation with identity for SD2 are phenotypes with one or two of these antigens. A detailed analysis of the various SD2 differences examined in these experiments is now being made.

All these results may suggest why a correlation between matching for SD2 antigens and kidney graft success in nonimmunized recipients has not been demonstrated. Matching for SD2 may indeed be effective in nonimmunized recipients when it involves a concurrent matching for linked LD alleles (either directly because of LD identity or indirectly because of interaction effects). In order to demonstrate an effect of matching for SD2 in the general population, it may be necessary to select those identities and incompatibilities which have been shown to be associated with low MLC stimulation in normal unrelateds.

We have mentioned the appearance of HL-A8 in many low-stimulating combinations and the possible low stimulation across HL-A8, HL-A5, and W5 differences. HL-A8 in kidney transplant recipients, and HL-A5 and/or portions of the complex of antigens cross-reactive with HL-A5 in various groups of patients, have been associated with heightened responsiveness of individuals carrying them, as measured by rejection of grafts or incidence of allergic or presumed autoimmune states.[17] Such behavior, of high responsiveness and low stimulation, is what would be expected from a universal donor type such as O in the ABO system. Some unpublished preliminary data suggest that there may also be individuals who are high stimulators with all responders. While no clear-cut phenomenon of universal donor or universal recipient should be expected to emerge in the tissue transplant field, the possibility that certain histocompatibility types will have tendencies in these directions should be borne in mind.

These investigations give some clues concerning the population genetics of the major histocompatibility complex in man, and perhaps some suggestions for practical testing for organ transplantation. However, they involve relatively few donors and more extensive research is certainly necessary. Also, especially in this complicated area, one must remember that things may be as they seem but not for the reasons ascribed.

ACKNOWLEDGMENT

We thank the officers and members of Local 171, Wisconsin State Employees' Union, A.F.S.C.M.E., for their help in obtaining the panel of blood donors tested in these experiments. We are most grateful to Barbara Stephan, Claudia Kan, and Genia Gordon for excellent technical assistance, and particularly for their cheerfulness and competence in the late stages of long experiments.

REFERENCES

1. Amos DB, Bashir H, Boyle W, et al: Transplantation 7:220, 1969

2. Kissmeyer-Nielsen F, and Thorsby E: Transplant Rev 4:1, 1970

3. Segall M, Bach ML, Proc Int Conf Cryopreservation Normal Neoplastic Cells (in press)

4. Hartzman RJ, Segall M, Bach ML: Transplantation 11:268, 1971

5. Segall M, Omodei-Zorini C, Bach FH, et al: Transplant Proc 5:383, 1973

6. Bach FH, Widmer MB, Segall M, et al: Science 176:1430, 1972

7. Bach FH, Widmer MB, Bach ML, et al: J Exp Med 136:1024, 1972

8. Yunis EJ, Amos DB, Proc Nat Acad Sci 68:3031, 1971

9 . Sorensen SF, Staub-Nielsen L: Acta Pathol Microbiol Scand 78B:719, 1970

10. van Rood JJ, Eijsvoogel VP: Lancet 1:698, 1970

11. Bach FH, Day E, Bach ML, et al: Tissue Antigens 1:39, 1971

12. Hamburger J, Crosnier J, Descamps B, Rowinska D: Transplant Proc 3:260, 1971

13. van Rood JJ, Koch CT, van Hooff JP, et al: Transplant Proc 5:391, 1973
14. Cochrun KC, Perkins HA, Payne RO, et al: Transplant Proc 5:391, 1973
15. Eijsvoogel VP, van Rood JJ, du Toit ED, et al: Eur J Immunol 2:413, 1972
16. Mempel W, Grosse-Wilde H, Albert E, et al: Transplant Proc 5:401, 1973
17. Morris PJ: In Contemporary Topics in Immunobiology, Vol 3, 1973

Standard Stimulating Cells and Mixed Leukocyte Cultures in Man

By David Osoba and Judy Falk

EXPERIMENTS with one-way mixed leukocyte cultures (MLC) fall into two categories. The technique can be used to investigate the genetic and cellular basis of responsiveness and stimulation in the mixed leukocyte reaction itself; it can also be used in clinical medicine either in matching donor–recipient pairs for organ and tissue transplantation or as a diagnostic test in the investigation of patients with suspected immunological deficiencies. As a diagnostic test, the procedure gives results that may clearly indicate lack of responsiveness or stimulation in certain kinds of immunological deficiency diseases. However, in situations where the deviation from normal may be more subtle the test is less reliable because of the difficulty of defining the upper and lower limits of a "normal response."

To be a sensitive assay for screening a population of individuals, any given test should fulfill at least two criteria. First, it must be quantifiable, and second, the result in each test should be directly dependent upon a change in only one variable while all other variables remain constant. Culture conditions for the MLC can be obtained that will fulfill the first criterion, i.e., quantification of the response. The second criterion is not usually fulfilled because when responding cells from different individuals are mixed with stimulating cells from different individuals in a series of tests, variables in both the responding cells and the stimulating cells are introduced each time the test is performed.

At least two sources of variables are present in each of the two cell populations in any particular MLC. There are genetic differences, determined by lymphocyte-defined (LD) loci and by serologically defined (SD) loci, between the two cell populations, and these differences vary for each mixture of responding and stimulating cells. Also, there may be quantitative and qualitative differences between individuals in the kinds of cells (including T cells, B cells and macrophages) that are necessary for a reaction to take place. These cellular differences between responding and stimulating individuals may also be subject to variation from time to time, depending upon physiological events in each donor.

Theoretically, it would be advantageous to reduce the number of variables present in either the responding cells or the stimulating cells. Since in most experiments the object of the investigator is to assess the response of the responding cells, it is clear that the variables in the stimulating-cell population must be controlled. This might be achieved by the use of a standard stimulating-cell preparation, thereby removing the variability produced by using different stimulating cells in each experiment. Under these conditions, the genetic and cellular variables affecting the test would be provided only by the responding-cell population.

Our studies have been designed toward developing a practical stimulating-cell preparation that would be constant from experiment to experiment. Such a preparation should allow a meaningful comparison

From the Tissue Typing Laboratory, Toronto Western Hospital, and the Department of Medicine, Ontario Cancer Institute, University of Toronto, Toronto, Ontario.

Supported by the Ontario Cancer Treatment and Research Foundation (Project 271) and the Medical Research Council of Canada (grant MA-1609).

Dr. Osoba is an Associate of the Medical Research Council of Canada.

© 1973 by Grune & Stratton, Inc.

of the responsiveness of cells from two populations of donors.

RESULTS

Only the most critical aspects of the methodology and a summary of the results will be presented here, since the details of the methods used and the results obtained are reported elsewhere.[1]

We attempted to obtain a standard stimulating-cell population by pooling cells from three individuals who had been selected on the basis of SD specificities. The SD specificities represented in this kind of cell pool included specificities from the major cross-reacting groups of HL-A specificities determined by both the first and the second loci. All selected pools were made to be as similar as possible to each other with respect to these specificities.

Peripheral blood cells were separated in a one-step Ficoll Hypaque method to obtain purified mononuclear cells. Mixtures of 5×10^5 responding cells and 5×10^5 irradiated (2500 rads) stimulating cells were incubated for varying periods of time. The responses were assayed in quintuplicate culture tubes by the uptake of tritiated thymidine added 18 hr before the cells were harvested.

In initial experiments with selected pools, the peak of tritiated thymidine incorporation was always on the sixth day of culture. When the number of cells of one population (either responding or stimulating) was kept constant and the number of cells of the other population was varied the dose–response curves were linear and extrapolated through 0. The log-log transformations of these data gave slopes not significantly different from 1 in both situations. Thus, we were satisfied that our method allowed the assay to be used quantitatively.

Since the primary objective of these experiments was to determine if responding cells from different individuals would give similar responses to selected pools of stimulating cells, the next step was to assess the responses of cells from a large number of normal individuals and to calculate the variance of these responses. To determine if the responses to stimulating cells from selected donors had a smaller variance than did the responses to stimulating cells from random donors, we compared the responses against these two kinds of stimulating pools of cells. As a further test of the validity of our idea of pooling cells to give a standard stimulating-cell population, the responses in both the above groups were compared with the responses against single-donor stimulating cells, i.e., a "classical" one-way MLC.

In all, cells from 30 normal responders were tested against selected pools, 40 against random pools and 30 against single donors of stimulating cells. To calculate the variance for each of these groups of responders, it was first necessary to determine whether the responses in each group were normally or log-normally distributed. Depending upon the nature of the frequency distribution, the variance would then be calculated either on the basis of each actual response or on the basis of the log of each response. We found that the frequency distribution of the responses in each group fit a log-normal distribution more closely than a normal distribution. Thus, the calculation of the mean of all responses for each group and the test for homogeneity of variance (F-distribution) were based on the log of the response by the cells of each individual in all three groups of experiments.

The geometric means of all the responses (on day 6 of culture) in each group were not significantly different from each other; for the 30 responses against selected pools of stimulating cells the mean was 88,200 c.p.m. (95% confidence limits = 80,700–96,500 c.p.m.), for the 40 responses against random pools of stimulating cells the mean was 97,800 c.p.m. (95% confidence limits = 82,600–115,900 c.p.m.), and for the 30 responses against single-donor stimulating cells the mean was 71,000 c.p.m. (95% confidence limits = 50,900–99,100 c.p.m.).

The variance of the logs of the responses against selected pools (0.0567) was less than either the variance of the responses against random pools (0.2734) or the variance of the responses against single-donor stimulating cells (0.7682). A comparison of the homogeneity of variance of the logs of the responses against each of the three kinds of stimulating cells showed a significantly greater homogeneity of variance for the responses against selected pools than for the responses against either random pools or single-donor stimulating cells ($p = < 0.01$ in both comparisons). Thus, it can be concluded that selecting three individuals on the basis of SD specificities as donors for a pool of stimulating cells gave results with the smallest variance in the responses by the responding cells.

Finally, we noted an inverse correlation between the magnitude of the variance and the number of different SD specificities we were able to detect in each of the three kinds of stimulating cells. When the variance was smallest (selected pools) the number of different SD specificities we detected was 9.7 per pool, whereas when the variance was greatest (single-donor) the number of specificities was 2.8. The number of specificities per random pool of stimulating cells was intermediate, i.e., 6.6.

DISCUSSION

The results of these experiments indicate that a standard stimulating-cell preparation can be achieved by selecting three donors for the stimulating-cell pool. This selection, based upon SD specificities, seems to be adequate in controlling the variables in the stimulating-cell preparation in that the responses by cells from healthy individuals always peak on the same day and the variance of the responses by the population of responders is small. Thus, under our conditions, a normal response can be defined in terms of c.p.m. of tritiated thymidine incorporated on day 6 and the upper and lower limits of this response can be set to give a range for the normal response. Presumably, if values are obtained that fall outside these limits, such values should be suspected of being abnormal. Therefore, this approach can be used to test cells from individuals who belong to a particular disease population in an attempt to determine deviations from the normal range of responsiveness. The method we have developed is practical. Whether or not it is useful in particular clinical situations remains to be determined.

If cells from patients with a particular disease are found to give abnormal responses, the next step would be to determine whether this abnormality has a genetic basis, e.g., association with closely linked loci in the major histocompatibility system, or whether there is an association with abnormalities in the cell populations that participate in the MLC. It is possible that changes in cell populations produced by disease either may remain constant with time or may vary with the clinical course of the disease. It is also possible that changes in the cell populations from time to time may result from physiological events in healthy as well as ill donors of responding cells.

An intriguing question that cannot be answered on the basis of these experiments alone is why a stimulating pool of cells selected on the basis of SD specificities gives results in which the responses have a smaller variance than if the pool of stimulating cells is obtained at random or from single donors. Current work in mouse[2] and man[3–5] suggests that responsiveness in the MLC is determined primarily by differences between the responding and stimulating cells not at the SD loci, but at the closely linked LD loci in the major histocompatibility complex. In the mouse a locus that segregates independently of H-2, the M locus, also determines the capacity of cells to act as stimulators.[6] Apparently, SD loci play a role in determining the gene products that serve as targets for the cytotoxic effector cells generated in the MLC,[7,8] although the results of some experiments in mice seem to provide an exception to this idea.[9]

One possibility that may explain our results is that there is a linkage disequilibrium between certain LD alleles and certain SD alleles, and that we have selected for particular LD alleles by selecting for the representation of certain SD alleles in the selected pools of stimulating cells. The description at this meeting of nonreactivity in MLCs by unrelated individuals sharing an SD specificity could be interpreted to mean that such individuals also share a common LD allele. This gives reason to suspect the existence of previously undetected linkages between SD loci of the second series and LD loci. An alternative interpretation is also possible. By analogy with the effects of the alleles of the M locus in mice,[6] there might well be a variation in the strength of stimulation determined by the alleles of the LD loci in man.

Even if a linkage disequilibrium between certain SD and LD alleles does exist, this does not necessarily imply that it plays a role in our results. There seems little doubt that LD differences act as a trigger to initiate the reaction, but it is still possible that differences between responding and stimulating cells for SD alleles are of importance in controlling the subsequent events, e.g., the magnitude of the response in the MLC. The inverse correlation between the variance of the response and the number of detectable SD differences in the three kinds of stimulating-cell preparations we have used in our experiments is consistent with such a possibility.

Whether or not a linkage disequilibrium between certain SD and LD alleles exists by no means excludes another possibility—both LD and SD alleles control the magnitude of the response in the MLC, but they act at different levels or stages of the response.

REFERENCES

1. Osoba D, Falk J: Cell Immunol (in press)
2. Bach FH, Widmer MB, Bach ML, et al: J Exp Med 136:1430, 1972
3. Yunis EJ, Amos DB: Proc Nat Acad Sci 68:3031, 1971
4. Eijsvoogel VP, Koning L, de Groot-Kooy ML, et al: Transplant Proc 4:199, 1972
5. Eijsvoogel VP, van Rood JJ, du Toit ED, et al: Eur J Immunol 2:413, 1972
6. Festenstein H, Abbasi K, Sachs JA, et al: Transplant Proc 4:219, 1972
7. Eijsvoogel VP, du Bois MJGJ, Melief CJM, et al: in Dausset J, Colombani J (eds): Histocompatibility Testing, 1972. Copenhagen, Munksgaard (in press)
8. Alter BJ, Schendel DJ, Bach ML, et al: J Exp Med 137:1303, 1973
9. Widmer MD, Alter BJ, Bach FH, et al: Nature New Biol 242:239, 1973

Mixed Leukocyte Culture Reactions With Man–Mouse Hybrid Cells

By K. Kano, H. Yoshida, and F. Milgrom

IT has strongly been suggested by data obtained in human family studies that activation in mixed leukocyte culture (MLC) reactions is due to disparity in cell membrane structures controlled by a locus (loci) separate from but closely linked to the HL-A locus.[1,2] The question whether serologically detectable HL-A antigens themselves can stimulate allogenic leukocytes in MLC still remained to be answered.[3]

Our previous studies[4,5] showed that some clones of man–mouse hybrid cells carry human histocompatibility antigens including HL-A antigens in addition to murine antigens while others retain murine antigens only. This is most probably due to the fact that preferential loss of human chromosomes takes place during long-term cultivation of the hybrid cells in the selective GHAT medium.[6]

In the present study, leukocytes of a donor NB, whose genotype was HL-A1, 12/3, 7, were fused with cultures of a murine cell line IT by the aid of inactivated Sendai virus.[4] Original hybrid culture 309 was obtained from colonies of heterokaryon cells. It was tested by means of mixed agglutination tests[7] for expected as well as other HL-A specificities using at least three HL-A typing sera for each specificity. The culture 309 gave positive results with antisera to HL-A1,3,7, and 12 antigens but not with antisera to other HL-A antigens. Clone 1 from 309 culture was also included in the present study. On this clone no HL-A antigens were demonstrated. The hybrid cells had been propagated in our laboratory for over one year prior to the present study.

Cultures of these hybrid cells and both parent cells were examined for their ability to stimulate allogenic leukocyte in one-way test performed according to the procedure of Bach and Voynow.[8] All stimulator cells were x-irradiated.[9] The degree of stimulation was measured by ^{3}H thymidine uptake and recorded as counts per minute (c.p.m.) in triplicate sets of tubes incubated for 1, 2, 3, 4, 5, 6, and 7 days.[8] Representative results of these experiments obtained on the 6th day of MLC, when the maximum c.p.m. values were noted in all combinations, are summarized in Table 1.

In this experiment, leukocytes KK with phenotype HL-A 2, 9, 7, and W22 were used. The control culture consisted of the responder leukocytes NB and x-irradiated autologous leukocytes NBx. The murine parent ITx cells gave c.p.m. value very similar to that of the control culture. MLC with NBx + KK gave an expected high c.p.m. value. Similar c.p.m. value was noted when (NB + IT)x was studied for stimulation of KK. The responder cells incubated with the hybrid cells gave virtually negative results, and there was no significant difference between c.p.m. in the experiment with the original culture which contained HL-A antigens and c.p.m. in the experiment with clone 1 which had no demonstrable HL-A antigens. Very similar results were obtained with other original hybrids and their clones, i.e., the number of c.p.m. was independent from presence or absence of the HL-A antigens. In addition to KK, leukocytes of other donors were used and results of studies were very similar to those obtained with KK.

From these results, it may be concluded

From the Department of Microbiology, School of Medicine, State University of New York at Buffalo, Buffalo, N.Y.

Supported by USPHS research grant AM-17317 from the National Institute of Arthritis, Metabolism, and Digestive Diseases.

© 1973 by Grune & Stratton, Inc.

Table 1.

	Stimulator Cells (x-irradiated)	HL-A Antigens Detected	Responder Cells	Mean c.p.m. on Sixth Day
Parents	NB	1,3,7,12	KK	52,903
	NB	1,3,7,12	NB	377
	IT	none	KK	320
	NB + IT mixture	1,3,7,12	KK	37,560
Hybrids	309, original	1,3,7,12	KK	1,204
	309 clone 1	none	KK	1,476

that the presence of serologically detectable HL-A antigens on the cells does not suffice for induction of a significant stimulation of allogenic leukocytes in MLC. The apparent loss of stimulating activity of the hybrid cells which retained HL-A antigens might have been due to unique makeup of the hybrid cell membrane. It appears possible that stimulating structures may be sterically blocked by the murine antigens on surface of the hybrid cells in such a way that their intimate contact with the responder cells is prevented. Another possibility is that expression of the stimulating structures may require cooperation of genes other than those on HL-A chromosomes and that chromosome(s) carrying these genes were deleted from the hybrid cells by the time when they were studied.

REFERENCES

1. Yunis EJ, Amos DB: Proc Nat Acad Sci 68:3031, 1971
2. Eijsvoogel VP, van Rood JJ, du Toit ED, et al: Eur J Immunol, 2:413, 1972
3. Bach FH: Transplant Proc 5:23, 1973
4. Kano K, Baranska W, Knowles BB, Koprowski H, Milgrom F: J Immunol 103:1050, 1969
5. Kano K, Knowles BB, Koprowski H, Milgrom F: Eur J Immunol, 2:198, 1972
6. Weiss MC, Green H: Proc Nat Acad Sci 58:1104, 1967
7. Milgrom F, Kano K, Witebsky E: JAMA 192: 845, 1965
8. Bach FH, Voynow NK: Science 153:545, 1966
9. Kasakura S, Lowenstein L: in Amos DB, van Rood JJ (eds): Histocompatibility Testing, 1965. Copenhagen, Munksgaard, 1966, pp 211–213.

On the Mechanism of Self-tolerance in Embryo-Fusion Chimeras

By Tommaso Meo, T. Matsunaga, and A. M. Rijnbeek

IN higher organisms endowed with a cellular system differentiated to recognize foreignness, the extent of individuality is learned and defined through a developmental process rather than established by the genotype.[1-3] Thus far, the only genetic contribution to the array of prohibited immune responses appears to be limited to particular alleles at immune-response loci that confer unresponsiveness to certain chemically defined immunogens.[4]

The direct demonstration that tolerance to autologous tissues is an epigenetic phenomenon was given by Triplett,[5] who showed that hypophyseal explants from tree-frog embryos were rejected when returned as dermal implants to the original donors at a metamorphic stage. These findings are complementary to those of Billingham et al.,[6] who described in dizygotic cattle twins the phenomenon of acquired allogeneic tolerance as a result of an *inborn hemopoietic chimerism.*

Subsequent work by Medawar's group on perinatally induced allogeneic unresponsiveness suggested that self-tolerance is due to an acquired central failure of the immune system (reviewed in reference 7). More recently, the concept of enhancement facilitation developed in tumor immunology has been extended by several authors[8-10] to account for the state of transplantation tolerance produced in *radiation-induced or neonatally induced chimeras.* It has been suggested that this type of tolerance is in fact accomplished by an active immune response leading to the production of humoral blocking factors (antibodies or antigen–antibody complexes) that specifically abrogate the cytotoxic activity of sensitized lymphocytes to the tolerated graft.

Contrasting evidence has also been presented by other investigators on the mechanism of tolerance in *embryo-fusion chimeras.* This type of chimerism differs from the aforementioned ones not only in the way in which it develops but also because of the more extensive and different morphogenetic consequences. However, in all probability this situation, although genetically anomalous, is the closest to the natural mechanism for the attainment of autologous tolerance. In these individuals, originating from the early fusion of two dizygotic embryos and characterized by an inborn chimerism expressed in virtually every tissue, the coexistence of coeval histoincompatible cell lineages precedes the acquisition of the immunologic discrimination between self and donor.

Mouse embryo-fusion chimeras have been demonstrated to be fully tolerant to skin grafts of either parental or F_1 hybrid genotype.[11,12] Ceppellini and his associates[13] examined a case of a tetragametic human chimera, conceivably equivalent to the tetraparental mouse, whose tissues in many body areas consisted of two populations of different sex. HL-A typing of peripheral lymphocytes disclosed a tetrallelic phenotype. The lymphocytes of this individual showed specific unreactivity in unidirectional MLR test with the cells of either of two siblings whose HL-A type differed by one haplotype from each of the two populations of the chimera. Selective elimination of either by means of differential killing with anti-HL-A sera did not abolish the unresponsiveness in the other population. The

From the Basel Institute for Immunology, Basel, Switzerland.

©1973 by Grune & Stratton, Inc.

two populations, used separately as responders, displayed a normal activation against unrelated stimulators but no activation against the sibs or against one another, and the chimera's serum showed no blocking effect on the reactivity of his own or his siblings' lymphocytes.

The specific unresponsiveness of the tetragametic individual coincides with that displayed in other cases of zygotic anomalies. Bach and Amos[14] and Van der Hart and Van Loghem[15] observed cases of mutually unreactive lymphocyte cultures between HL-A-incompatible dizygotic twins due to a presumptive, or in other instances ascertained, inborn hemopoietic chimerism. A similar specific unresponsiveness in MLR has also been demonstrated by Wilson and Nowell in rats inoculated at birth with lymphoid cells.[16]

The evidence from the tetragametic individual indicated a mechanism of tolerance of a central type due to functional deletion of self-reactive forbidden clones.

Different conclusions were reached by Wegmann et al.,[17] who found that lymph node cells of allophenic mice are able to destroy in vitro fibroblasts of parental strains and that preincubation of the target cells with serum of the allophenic mouse, but not of F_1 hybrids, specifically abrogated the cytotoxic activity of the lymphocytes. Furthermore, Phillips et al.[18] reported that in MLR the serum of allophenic mice specifically inhibited the capacity of the lymphocytes of parental genotype to stimulate genetically unrelated strains, although the capacity to respond was unaffected. It was suggested that the noncytotoxic blocking factors in the serum are directed against determinants of the H-2 complex.

Moreover, the observation that unstimulated cultures of chimeric lymphocytes displayed a spontaneous blastogenesis significantly higher than either parental or F_1 lymphocytes was taken as evidence for a state of reciprocally induced allogeneic reactivity between the two populations in the absence of tetraparental mouse serum. The apparent inconsistency of the latter observations with the findings of Ceppellini and his associates led us to undertake a search for conciliatory experimental evidence.

Eight C3H/HeJ ↔ C57BL/6J allophenic mice exhibiting chimerism in the coat color and serum Ig allotypes were selected and studied individually in unidirectional MLR. Our findings (detailed in a separate paper in preparation) can be summarized as follows:

(1) Splenic or lymph node lymphocytes from allophenic mice were totally unreactive to cells of either parental genotypes or heterozygous F_1, but were fully responsive against cells of genetically unrelated strains. The unresponsiveness was established in time-course studies on both spleen and lymph node cells.

(2) Lymphocytes from allophenic mice displayed normal capacity to stimulate cells of unrelated strains, but they induced differential degrees of activation in the cells of two parental genotypes. The phenomenon appears to be a reflection of the variable ratios of the two lymphocyte populations, as demonstrated in three cases where the ratio was determined in advance by means of selective cytotoxicity with anti-H-2 sera. The specificity of the stimulatory capacities of allophenic cells was confirmed by their failure to activate F_1 hybrid lymphocytes.

(3) Individual sera failed to show any specific effect in MLR cultures, neither parental cells nor cells from the chimeras being affected in their capacity to stimulate or to respond to genetically unrelated donors.

Since this work was initiated, a second report by Phillips et al.[19] appeared suggesting that chimeric lymphocytes produce specific factors in vitro, not clearly related to the blocking activity previously described,[18] that inhibit the MLR between parental cells. This interpretation is not in accordance with the findings of Ceppellini et al.[13] demonstrating intrinsic unresponsiveness in either population of the chimeric individual, which remains unaffected by the selective removal of the other by means of anti-HL-A antisera. The objection may be raised that such inhibitory factors are aspecifically taken up and released by ancillary cells of either genotype and therefore elude a selective elimination by either antiserum. However, this hypothesis is inconsistent with our further results.

(4) Cells of each parental type were mixed in bidirectional cultures with tetraparental cells with the aim of showing blocking factors released in culture. Should such factors be responsible for the mutual tolerance in the allophenic, they should also act upon nontolerant parental cells, turning off their responsiveness to either allogeneic population in the chimera. Not only was a marked stimulation obtained, but cultures containing increasing ratios of allophenic to parental cells exhibited higher proliferation, thus indicating that the tolerant cells acted as stimulators rather than as suppressor cells.

To conclude, no evidence was obtained in this series of experiments indicating a peripheral mechanism for tolerance in embryo-fusion chimeras, but the results can be explained in terms of and lend some additional support to the forbidden-clone hypothesis. We suggest that some inconsistencies with the results of Phillips et al. could be explained by the particular parental strain combination used in their first work.[18] It is possible that the high spontaneous incidence of reticulum cell sarcoma and the known immunologic abnormalities in the SJL strain[20] are reflected in the allophenic situation. The inconsistent finding of blocking factors in the serum of chimeras of a different genotypic composition (Phillips, reference 19 and personal communication) is in accordance with the above suggestion. Experiments are underway to test this possibility.

Our findings also prompt some observations relevant to the immunogenetics of MLR. First of all, the unresponsiveness of allophenic cells against the cells of corresponding F_1 implies that no hybrid determinants responsible for MLR stimulation are formed in heterozygous (C3H/HeJ × C57BL/6J) F_1. Furthermore, the demonstration that an MLR response toward specific genotypes can be deleted without apparent impairment of the reciprocal capacity to stimulate them raises some questions on the nature and the cellular expression of MLR determinants. Klein[21] has suggested that the determinants responsible for allogeneic stimulation might exhibit the sort of restriction shown by Zoshke and Bach[22] for MLR responsiveness. If Klein's observation is correct, it is tempting to question whether both recognition and stimulatory determinants toward a certain genotype are restricted to the same subpopulation of cells.

Thorsby's preliminary findings, discussed at this meeting, indicate that the use of the hot-pulse technique in unidirectional MLR, by destroying the population responding to a given donor also specifically removes the capacity of this population to stimulate, in a second MLR, the original donor cells. These results, if confirmed, would imply that in the allophenic mouse tolerant clones of lymphocytes do exist in which only the stimulatory capacity is retained. Using chimera cells as stimulators against the parental lymphocytes might ultimately represent a way to reveal their presence.

REFERENCES

1. Burnet FM: The Clonal Selection Theory of Acquired Immunity. Cambridge University Press, 1959
2. Jerne NK: Eur J Immunol 1:1, 1971
3. Cohn M: Cell Immunol 5:1, 1972
4. Benacerraf B, McDevitt HD: Science 175:273, 1972

5. Triplett EL: J Immunol 89:505, 1962
6. Billingham RE, Lampkin GH, Medawar PB, Williams HL: Heredity 6:201, 1952
7. Brent L: in Nisbet NW, Elves MW (eds): Immunological Tolerance to Tissue Antigens. Oswestry, England, Orthopaedic Hospital, 1971, pp 49–66
8. Voisin GA, Kinsky RG, Jansen FK: Nature 210:138, 1966
9. Hellström I, Hellström KE, Storb R, Thomas ED: Proc Natl Acad Sci USA 56:65, 1970
10. Allison AC: Lancet 2:1401, 1971
11. Mintz B, Silvers WR: Science 158:1484, 1967
12. Mintz B: Transplantation 9:523, 1970
13. Ceppellini R: in Amos B (ed): Progress in Immunology. New York, Academic, 1971, pp 973–1025
14. Bach FH, Amos DB: Science 156:1506, 1967
15. Van der Hart M, Van Loghem JJ: Vox Sang 12:161, 1967
16. Wilson DB, Nowell PC: J Exp Med 131:391, 1970
17. Wegmann TG, Hellström I, Hellström KE: Proc Natl Acad Sci USA 68:1644, 1971
18. Phillips SM, Martin WJ, Shaw AR, Wegmann TG: Nature 234:146, 1971
19. Phillips SM, Wegmann TG: J Exp Med 137:291, 1973
20. Wanebo HJ, Gallmeier WM, Boyse EA, Old LJ: Science 154:901, 1966
21. Klein J, Park JM: J Exp Med 137:1213, 1973
22. Zoschke DC, Bach FH: Science 172:1350, 1971

Cellular Reactivities Associated With Theta-Antigen Disparity

By A. B. Peck, F. H. Bach, and E. A. Boyse

THE development of cytotoxic lymphocytes in mixed leukocyte culture (MLC) with subsequent testing in cell-mediated lympholysis (CML) apparently requires (1) activation of responding leukocytes by alloantigens, possibly lymphocyte-defined (LD) differences, of the major histocompatibility complex (MHC) and (2) the presence on target cells of serologically defined (SD) MHC alloantigens, or antigens of loci closely linked to the loci determining the SD antigens, also present during the MLC activation phase.[1-3] For most species, MLC activation is governed by the MHC. In mouse, however, MLC activation can also be induced by genetic differences at loci segregating independently of the MHC as has been clearly demonstrated for the M locus in H-2-identical strains.[4] To date, though, non-MHC antigens appear ineffective as target antigens on normal cells.[5]

Theta (θ) antigen, an antigenic marker on thymus-dependent lymphocytes of the mouse, also appears capable of inducing MLC activation in a serum-free culture system using theta-congenic-resistant partners of strain A/Jax. The question to which the present report is addressed therefore is whether or not θ-antigen differences which induce MLC activation will also result in cell destruction in CML.

From the Laboratory of Genetics, University of Wisconsin, Madison, Wisc., and Memorial Sloan-Kettering Cancer Center, New York, N.Y.

Supported in part by NIH grants GM-15422, AI-08439, and AI-06525; ONR N00014-67-A-0128-0003; NF-MOD grant CRBS 246; and NCI CA 08748.

A.B.P. is a Research Fellow of the Wisconsin Heart Association.

This is Paper No. 1689 from the Laboratory of Genetics, University of Wisconsin, Madison, Wisc.

© 1973 by Grune & Stratton, Inc.

MATERIALS AND METHOD

Strains of mice used in this study are A/Jax, A/Thy-1.1 (formerly A/θ-AKR) and C57BL/10ScSn. MLC was performed in a serum-free culture medium according to the procedures described elsewhere.[6] MLC consisted of 0.5×10^6 responding spleen cells cultured with 0.5×10^6 x-irradiated stimulating spleen cells in microtiter plates. At 120 hr of culture 2.0 μCi tritiated thymidine (^{3}H-TdR) were added to each well for 12 hr. Cells were filtered through glass-fiber filters using an automatic multiple sample harvester, and total ^{3}H-TdR incorporation was determined in a scintillation spectrometer. Data are expressed as c.p.m. of the mean of triplicate cultures.

CML was performed by a modification of the technique described by Alter et al.[2] Effector cells were produced in MLC, 0.05 cc of fresh serum-free medium being added to each reaction well at 120 hr of incubation. Following a total incubation of 144–156 hr, the cells were collected from the wells, pooled, centrifuged, and washed once in serum-free medium. Target cell cultures containing 2.5×10^6 pooled cervical, axillary, brachial, and inguinal lymph node cells in 1 cc serum-free medium supplemented with 5% fetal calf serum were established 60–70 hr prior to CML, incubated 6 hr, then PHA stimulated. At time of assay the cells were pooled, centrifuged, resuspended in 0.5 cc supernatant, and labeled for 1 hr with 200 μCi $Na_2{}^{51}CrO_4$. The labeled cells were washed three times in serum-free medium. Cell destruction was performed in round-bottom microtiter plates—each well containing 1×10^6 effector plus 1×10^4 target cells. Cell killing was allowed to proceed 3 hr, after which the plates were centrifuged, the supernatant collected, and the quantity of released ^{51}Cr determined.

RESULTS

Table 1 shows results of reciprocal MLC between strains A/Jax and A/Thy-1.1, congenic-resistant partners possessing different prototypes of θ antigen,[7] as well as the responses of the θ-congenic partners against C57BL/10, a strain possessing H-2 and non-H-2 genetic differences. Moderate activation was evident for both A/Jax responding against A/Thy-1.1 and A/Thy-1.1 responding against A/Jax. Strong reactivity

Table 1. MLC Activation Induced by Theta Antigen in Theta-Congenic Mice

Responding Strain	Stimulating Strain	Genetic Difference	Mean c.p.m. (ratio) ± SD
A/Jax	A/Jax	none	439 ± 173 —
	A/Thy-1.1	θ antigen	3921 ± 1331 (8.9)
	C57BL/10	MHC, non-MHC	14079 ± 2614 (32.1)
A/Thy-1.1	A/Thy-1.1	none	3503 ± 548 —
	A/Jax	θ antigen	9282 ± 1026 (2.6)
	C57BL/10	MHC, non-MHC	19229 ± 4032 (5.5)

was demonstrated by both strains against C57BL/10.

Results of CML in which the A/Jax or A/Thy-1.1 strains were tested for their capacity to cause cell destruction of various target cells following sensitization against one another or C57BL/10 are shown in Table 2. No destruction of target cells was observed when the target antigen was θ. Target cell destruction in the CML assay did occur however when A/Jax and A/Thy-1.1 sensitized against C57BL/10 were reacted against C57BL/10 antigens, demonstrating that cytotoxic cells can be generated in this system given the necessary genetic differences.

DISCUSSION

MLC activation in mouse results from genetic differences associated with any one of at least three antigenic systems: MHC alloantigens, θ antigen, and M-locus (or minor histocompatibility loci) products. Since one apparent requirement in the production of effector lymphocytes capable of target cell destruction in CML is an activation or proliferation phase, each of these antigenic systems could play a role in CML since they all lead to a positive MLC response. Extensive genetic studies of mouse MLC–CML by Alter et al.[2] and Widmer et al.[8] have demonstrated that H-2K and H-2D alloantigens, or products of loci closely linked to those alleles determining SD alloantigens, in addition to the LD difference of C57BL/6By–B6.C–H(z1), serve as effective target antigens for cell destruction following MLC activation by these same antigens. In contrast, neither M-locus products, as shown by Festenstein,[4] nor θ antigen, as shown in the present report, serve as effective target antigens following MLC activation.

Unlike M-locus products, θ antigen is serologically detectable and easily demonstrated on cell surfaces of thymus-dependent lymphocytes. Nevertheless, it must be cautioned that θ antigen may be a differentiation antigen and that under the present assay conditions the lymph node cells used as targets may lose θ during the PHA-stimulation phase or ^{51}Cr-labeling procedures. Thus in vitro cell differentiation

Table 2. Lack of Cytotoxicity Between Theta-Congenic-Resistant Strains A/Jax and A/Thy-1.1

Responding Strain	MLC Stimulating Strain	Target-Cell Strain	% Specific ^{51}Cr release Mean ± SD
A/Thy-1.1	A/Thy-1.1	A/Thy-1.1	−4.05 ± 3.13
		A/Jax	−13.34 ± 9.29
		C57BL/10	−12.12 ± 8.72
	A/Jax	A/Jax	−17.72 ± 6.37
		A/Thy-1.1	−6.43 ± 2.91
		C57BL/10	−19.23 ± 6.86
	C57BL/10	C57BL/10	39.85 ± 13.09
		A/Thy-1.1	0.94 ± 2.47
		A/Jax	−8.76 ± 6.27
A/Jax	A/Jax	A/Jax	−6.02 ± 4.76
		A/Thy-1.1	−3.87 ± 2.63
		C57BL/10	−3.66 ± 3.24
	A/Thy-1.1	A/Thy-1.1	−5.10 ± 3.18
		A/Jax	−6.83 ± 4.63
		C57BL/10	−7.54 ± 3.92
	C57BL/10	C57BL/10	35.40 ± 2.83
		A/Thy-1.1	−1.30 ± 5.11
		A/Jax	−7.87 ± 2.97

could result in θ-negative target cells which then would be totally ineffective as targets for CML.

Assuming that lack of target cell destruction results not from the loss of θ antigen but the lack of production of effector cells during the activation phase, the findings remain compatible with the hypothesis that two or more cell populations are involved in MLC–CML.[2,3] One population, the MLC-reactive cells, recognizes foreign antigens and subsequently proliferates. The second population, the effector cells in CML, might be a later stage of the first, arising through differentiation, or may possibly be distinct from the first but requiring a type of T–T cell interaction. Based on this hypothesis, θ antigen affects only the first population—that is, inducing cell proliferation but not inducing killer lymphocytes. Thus, θ antigen may be a useful system in distinguishing between a one-cell and a two-cell hypothesis for MLC–CML.

SUMMARY

Theta antigen was shown to be capable of inducing MLC activation in a serum-free culture medium utilizing the congenic-resistant strains A/Jax and A/Thy-1.1, but proved ineffective in producing effector cells capable of killing ^{51}Cr-labeled, PHA-stimulated lymph node cells serving as target cells for θ antigen.

REFERENCES

1. Eijsvoogel VP, du Bois R, Melief CJM, et al: Transplant Proc 5:1301, 1973
2. Alter BJ, Schendel DJ, Bach ML, et al: 137: 1303, 1973
3. Schendel DJ, Bach FH: Transplant Proc 5:1651, 1973
4. Festenstein H, Abbasi K, Sachs JA, et al: Transplant Proc 4:219, 1973
5. Festenstein H: Transplant Proc (in press)
6. Peck AB, Bach FH: J Immunol Meth (in press)
7. John M, Carswell E, Boyse EA, Alexander G: Nature New Biol 238:57, 1972
8. Widmer MB, Alter BJ, Bach FH, et al: Nature New Biol 242:239, 1973

The T-Cell Receptor: Does It Stimulate Allogeneic Lymphocytes in MLC?

By H. Hirschberg, A. Kaakinen, and E. Thorsby

STUDIES in mice have shown that Ir-l-locus disparity is associated with strong MLC stimulation (Bach et al., *Science* 176:1024, 1972; Meo et al., *Transpl Proc* 5:377, 1973). This could indicate that T-cell receptor structures may function as an allogeneic stimulus in MLC.

We have studied this question in human MLC tests in our laboratory. Our experiments were based on the observations that living cells are necessary to cause stimulation in MLC and that it is possible to eliminate specifically a responding population of lymphocytes with a hot pulse of tritiated thymidine. The cells that are eliminated are presumed to be those that carry specific receptors for the initial stimulating cells, and we assume that this particular population of lymphocytes is therefore no longer capable of acting as a stimulant in MLC after ^{3}H-thymidine treatment.

In our experiments, one-way hot-pulse MLC combinations were established for a duration of approximately 80 hr. The protocol used has been described previously (Hirschberg and Thorsby, *J Imm Met* 1973, in press). These cultures were then washed to remove the excess of isotope and subsequently treated with mitomycin C. Let us designate these treated cultures as $(ABm)^{3H}m$. We then used these treated cultures as stimulating cells in combination with responding cells from B (the initial stimulating-cell donor) and with responding cells from third-party individual C. The lymphocytes from individual C were rendered incapable of responding to B by first treating them in a hot-pulse MLC: $(CBm)^{3H}$. This ensured that the responding cells from C only responded to stimulation by A when confronted with the combination $(ABm)^{3H}m$. Controls consisted of B or $(CBm)^{3H}$ responder cells in combination with mitomycin-treated 3-day MLC combinations, i.e., (ABm)m, which were not exposed to ^{3}H thymidine.

The results of a typical experiment from a series of eight are shown in Table 1. The experiments indicate that elimination of the specific population of cells proliferating in response to a particular allogeneic cell donor (A anti-B) significantly reduces the ability of the remaining A cells to stimulate responding cells from the same individual used as stimulator in the initial hot-pulse MLC (B). This can be seen from the table by comparing the control response B(ABm)m to the response of the test culture $B(ABm)^{3H}m$. A reduction of between 30 and 70% was observed in seven of eight of our experiments. This reduction seemed to be specific, since the ability of the ^{3}H-thymidine- and mitomycin-treated cells to stimulate lymphocytes from other donors was comparable to controls in all of our experiments. In the table, a comparison between the controls $(CBm)^{3H}(ABm)m$ and $(CBm)^{3H}(ABm)^{3H}m$ showed no significant differences. Control experiments also suggest that mitomycin-treated MLC cultures, (ABm)m, do not stimulate significantly better than normal mitomycin-treated cells, Am, in specific combinations, although exceptions have been observed. Other experiments also indicate that ^{3}H-thymidine treatment of cells prior to mytomycin treatment does not significantly alter their ability to stimulate: $B(Am)^{3H}$ vs. BAm.

Our experiments are at present limited, and the conclusions drawn from them must, by necessity, be of a tentative nature.

From the Tissue Typing Laboratory, Rikshospitalet, Oslo, Norway.
©1973 by Grune & Stratton, Inc.

Table 1. Functional Elimination of Cells From A With Receptors for Allogeneic Structures on B Also Reduces the Ability of A Cells to Stimulate B Cells in MLC Tests, While the Stimulation of Third-Party C Cells Is Not Reduced

Stimulating Cells	Responding Cells	
	B	$(CBm)^{3}H$
Bm	293 ± 37	705 ± 89
(ABm)m	6745 ± 428	4422 ± 289
$(ABm)^{3H}$m	1835 ± 375	4017 ± 317
Am	8923 ± 735	5115 ± 815

Results are expressed as mean c.p.m. in triplicates ± SE.

Nevertheless, our studies could indicate that structures on the T-cell receptor are able to stimulate directly allogeneic lymphocytes or potentiate the stimulatory effect of the other histocompatibility antigens on lymphocytes. It must be emphasized, however, that in none of our experiments was it possible to completely eliminate the specific stimulating ability of the treated cells. Thus structures on the T-cell receptor are at least not the only stimulatory agents causing an MLC response. This is also borne out by the positive MLC response obtained using parental responding cells in combination with mitomycin-treated F_1 hybrid stimulating cells. In addition, both endothelium and epithelium cells stimulate well in MLC tests, and such cell types would be expected to lack receptors toward non-self.

Which Antigens on Skin Cells Cause Allogeneic Stimulation of Lymphocytes In Vitro?

By H. Hirschberg, B. Rankin, and E. Thorsby

ALLOGENEIC epidermal cells can cause stimulation of human lymphocytes (Levis and Miller, *Lancet* 11:357, 1972). In experiments performed in our laboratory, we have confirmed these observations. Human skin cell suspensions were obtained by trypsinization and filtration through sterile cotton gauze. These cells gave clear-cut stimulation of allogeneic lymphocytes after 7 days of culture, with maximum response at a skin–lymphocyte ratio of 1:2.

In some preliminary studies, cells proliferating in response to allogeneic lymphocytes were eliminated by ^{3}H-thymidine hot-pulse treatment (Hirschberg and Thorsby, *J Imm Met* 1973, in press). After this treatment, the response toward mitomycin-treated lymphocytes from the donor was eliminated, while the response toward skin cells from the same donor was only slightly altered (see Fig. 1). On the other hand, when the responding lymphocytes were first confronted with skin cells in the initial hot-pulse MLC, the secondary stimulation response to the skin cells was not eliminated but the response to mitomycin-treated lymphocytes from the skin donor was greatly reduced.

Although more experiments are needed to confirm this apparent specificity, our studies indicate that epidermal cells possess antigenic structures, in addition to possible MLC-locus products, that are able to stimulate allogeneic lymphocytes to proliferation in vitro. Whether these are also determined by the MHS chromosomal region needs further study.

From the Tissue Typing Laboratory, Rikshospitalet, Oslo, Norway.

©1973 by Grune & Stratton, Inc.

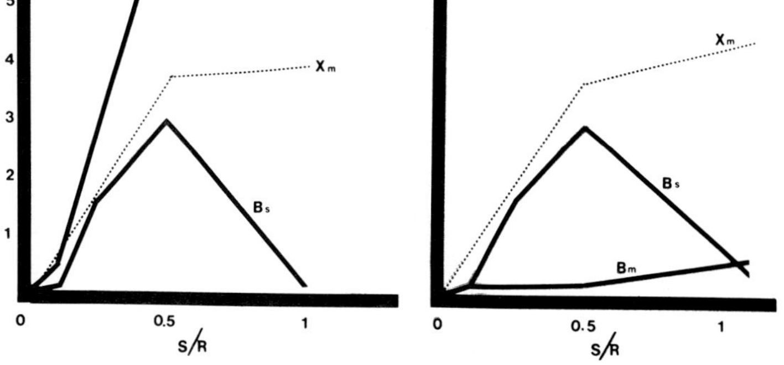

Fig. 1. The left part shows the response in cpm when responding lymphocytes from A are stimulated with mitomycin-treated lymphocytes from B (Bm) and X (Xm) and with skin cells from B (Bs). On the right part is given the secondary stimulation response when the responding cells of A toward mitomycin-treated lymphocytes from B (Bm) were first functionally eliminated in a hot-pulse MLC, e.g., (ABm)$^{^3H}$. The abscissa shows the ratio between the number of stimulating and responding cells.

Part II

The Destruction Phase—CML

Formation of Cytotoxic Lymphocytes in Mixed Leukocyte Culture Systems: Introduction

By J.-C. Cerottini, H. R. MacDonald, and K. T. Brunner

FOLLOWING the work of Häyry and Defendi,[1] compelling evidence has been obtained that cytotoxic lymphocytes (CL) may be generated in mixed leukocyte culture (MLC) systems. As measured by a ^{51}Cr assay system, CL activity was found to be directed against surface antigens carried by target cells syngeneic to the stimulating cells, whereas target cells syngeneic to the responding cells were unaffected.[2-3] As CL have also been found during the development of allograft responses and graft-vs.-host reactions (as reviewed by Cerottini and Brunner[4]) and appear to be involved in the effector phase of allograft immunity, at least in some model systems,[5] the demonstration of CL appearance in MLC systems has suggested the possibility of investigating in vitro the cellular events required for the generation of effector cells participating in transplantation rejection.

As emphasized in this symposium, considerable effort has been exerted in many laboratories to dissect the genetic factors involved in CL formation in vitro. This approach has been very useful in providing evidence for the dissociation between cell proliferation and CL formation in some MLC combinations.[6-8] Based on these findings, it has been suggested that the antigenic determinants recognized by CL were determined by genes identical with or closely linked to those controlling the serologically defined (SD) histocompatibility antigens, whereas cell proliferation depended on lymphocyte-defined (LD) antigenic differences determined by other genes in the major histocompatibility complex. Furthermore, data have recently been obtained suggesting that CL formation in MLC may require both SD and LD differences between responding and stimulating cells.[9]

It should be realized, however, that there exist several general shortcomings in the present assessment of CL. The main one is the lack of assays able to detect individual CL. (Although the virus plaque assay described by Bloom et al.[10] appears to detect sensitized T cells, including presumably CL, it is not yet established whether all CL and/or CL alone are enumerated in this system.) In the assay based on ^{51}Cr release from labeled target cells in the presence of sensitized lymphoid cell populations, it has been shown in some systems that there is a relationship between target-cell lysis and effector-cell concentration. Although the existence of such a relationship has proved to be very useful for estimating the relative frequency of CL in defined systems using the same target cells (see below), its general use may be restricted by the variation in susceptibility to lysis of different target-cell types. Another limitation of the ^{51}Cr assay method relates to the relatively high number of target cells needed in individual tests. With the specific activity of ^{51}Cr currently available, 10^4 to 10^5 labeled target cells per individual test are usually required to obtain a measurable reaction. Even taking into account the fact that several target cells can be killed by one CL, it appears that detectable lysis, i.e., killing of about 5% of the target cells, requires the presence of several hundred CL in the lymphoid cell population tested. It is thus evident that the lack of detectable cytotoxicity in a given test cannot be used as evidence of the absence of CL directed against the relevant target cells. These points deserve consideration when attempts are made to define the

From the Department of Immunology, Swiss Institute for Experimental Cancer Research, rue du Bugnon 21, CH-1011 Lausanne, Switzerland.

© 1973 by Grune & Stratton, Inc.

specificity of CL activity by assaying the effector cells on target cells with different genotypes.

In spite of these problems, a large body of quantitative information regarding CL formation in vitro has been obtained recently in well-defined MLC systems in the mouse. In the present introduction, we will briefly summarize the present stage of knowledge regarding the cellular requirements for CL generation and activity, the physical properties of CL during the course of culture, and the effect of repeated antigenic stimulation of MLC populations kept in vitro for prolonged periods of time.

RELATIVE QUANTITATION OF CL

Under well-defined conditions, it has been possible to obtain an empirical estimation of the relative frequency of CL present in MLC populations. This estimation has been based on the finding that there exists a linear relationship between the number of target cells lysed and the logarithm of the number of lymphoid cells added.[11–12] A detailed analysis of the conditions necessary for the demonstration of such a relationship can be found elsewhere.[13] In addition, dose–response curves obtained with different lymphoid cell populations have been found to be parallel both within and between experiments, provided the same target cells are used in the assay. It is thus possible to estimate the relative frequency of CL in different populations by comparing the number of lymphoid cells required to achieve a fixed value of cytotoxicity within a given incubation time. Examples of the practical use of this method have been published recently.[14–16]

This quantitative approach should be useful for defining the optimal culture conditions required for CL formation in MLC. According to the available data, the most effective culture system, at least for mouse lymphocytes, appears to be that described by Marbrook[17] as modified by Wagner and Feldmann.[2] However, recent studies in our laboratory indicate that cell populations containing a relatively high CL frequency can be obtained in mouse MLC performed in regular tubes, provided critical ingredients are added to the culture medium.[18] In particular it was found that the relative frequency of CL increased tenfold to thirtyfold after addition of 2-mercaptoethanol to the culture medium. Under these conditions, CL could be detected as early as 2 days after the onset of MLC and reached peak levels by day 4 or 5. This early appearance of CL, also noticed by Wagner and Feldmann,[2] is in contrast with the results reported by Häyry et al.,[3] who, although they used similar mouse strain combinations and the same target cells as in our experiments, found that cytotoxicity appeared relatively late in MLC and did not reach high values until the eighth culture day.

The same quantitative method has been used to investigate CL generation in MLC using spleen cells from immune mice as responding cells. Comparative studies of populations obtained at the peak of the response demonstrated a fivefold increase in the relative frequency of CL in secondary MLC as compared to primary MLC, although the kinetics of CL appearance was similar in both instances.[18]

CELLULAR REQUIREMENTS FOR CL GENERATION AND ACTIVITY

In the mouse, conclusive evidence has been obtained that CL formed in vitro are thymus-derived (T) cells, as is the case in allograft responses (see review[4]). Also in agreement with the findings made with in vivo sensitized cell populations, it is evident that the cytotoxic activity of MLC-generated CL is due to the direct contact of the effector cells with the relevant target cells, rather than to the release of soluble factors, and is independent of the presence of other cell types such as B cells or macrophages.[3,15,19] In addition, it has been found that removal of B cells from the responding cell population before the onset of MLC had no effect on the relative frequency of CL obtained at the peak of response, suggesting no B–T cell cooperation during the induction phase.[3,15] On the other hand, cooperation between two T-cell subsets has recently been suggested by Wagner.[20]

The results of comparative studies of CL generation in MLC containing stimulating cells of different types again emphasize the usefulness of CL quantitation. Under optimal conditions, B cells were found to stimulate as well as if not better than T cells, whereas the relative frequency of CL was tenfold and fortyfold lower in cultures containing macrophages and fibroblasts, respectively, as the source of stimulating cells.[21] Further investigation is needed to extend these findings to species other than the mouse.

PHYSICAL CHARACTERISTICS OF CL

Cell separation by zonal velocity sedimentation, as described by Miller and Phillips,[22] has been used to characterize the size of CL generated in MLC.[16] The results demonstrated that the effector cells collected on day 4 were a relatively heterogenous, rapidly sedimenting population. The maximum enrichment was obtained in the fractions containing very large cells. A relatively large number of CL were also present in less rapidly sedimenting cell populations, whereas the small lymphocyte region was virtually devoid of cytotoxic activity. Similar experiments performed on lymphoid cells obtained from secondary MLC gave identical results.[18] In contrast, the majority of CL present in day-15 MLC were found in the small lymphocyte region.[23] Moreover, when CL-enriched blast cells were isolated from MLC populations at the peak of response and subsequently cultured on syngeneic fibroblast monolayers for 5 more days, they reverted to small lymphocytes that were still cytotoxic.[3] It is thus evident that CL generated in vitro represent a rather heterogenous population, the size of which varies during the course of culture. These results are consistent with the findings that CL formed early in allograft responses are found in large, low-density cell populations, whereas they are smaller and more dense during later phases of the response.[16,24,25]

REPEATED ANTIGENIC STIMULATION OF MLC POPULATIONS

Most of the studies related to CL generated in vitro have concentrated on the effector cells obtained during the first week of MLC. In the mouse, as culture conditions have improved, it has recently been possible to investigate the effect of antigenic restimulation of MLC cells kept in vitro for 2 to 3 wk.[23] As mentioned above, MLC populations still contained CL on day 15, although at a lower relative frequency than on day 5. On day 21, cytotoxicity, although still detectable, was strongly reduced. When the day-15 MLC cells were reexposed to the same irradiated allogeneic spleen cells, it was found that cytotoxic activity reappeared, reaching levels similar to that observed at the peak of primary MLC (Fig. 1). Kinetics studies revealed that a rapid increase in cytotoxicity occurred already within the first 2 days after restimulation. Three weeks after secondary stimulation, the cytotoxic activity of the cultured cells was very low, but a third exposure to the same stimulating cells again resulted in rapid reappearance of high cytotoxicity. These findings thus indicate that mouse lymphoid cells can be stimulated several times in MLC and give rise to CL at each stimulation. Because cell separation studies[23] revealed that the cell fractions in day-15 MLC, which gave the highest cytotoxic activity on secondary MLC, also contained the residual CL generated during primary MLC, it is tempting to speculate that the latter cells functioned as precursors of CL formed on restimulation. Further studies are needed to establish the validity of this hypothesis. By using stimulating cells of different genotypes, it should also be possible to test whether or

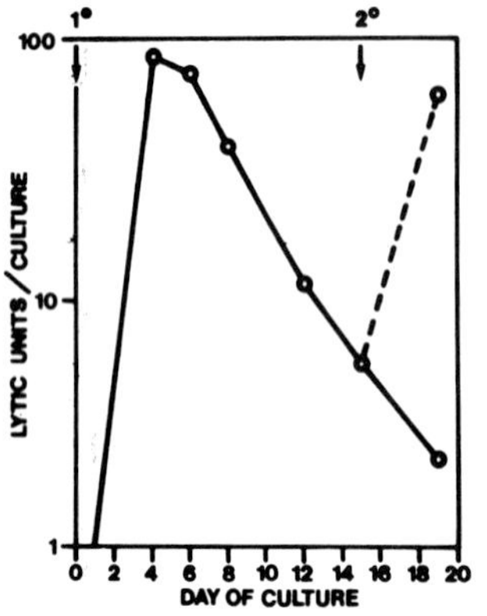

Fig. 1. Effect of antigenic reexposure of MLC cells on CL formation. C57BL/6 spleen cells were incubated with irradiated DBA/2 spleen cells and assayed for cytotoxicity on ^{51}Cr-labeled P-815 (DBA/2) tumor cells at different incubation time intervals. Lytic units were calculated as described in reference 12. On day 15, MLC cells were incubated with either DBA/2 or C57BL/6 irradiated spleen cells for 4 more days and tested for cytotoxicity on labeled P-815 cells. The dotted line shows the reappearance of cytotoxicity following reexposure of MLC cells to allogeneic stimulator cells.

not the responsiveness of lymphoid cells in secondary MLC is restricted to the antigenic structures of the stimulating cells used in primary MLC.

All these observations underline the fact that quantitative studies of CL formation in vitro are needed before any firm conclusion can be drawn as far as specificity of cell-mediated lysis is concerned. Characterization of responding and stimulating cells by use of physical procedures and antigenic markers should also provide useful information as to the cellular events required for successful induction of CL in vitro. Finally, a detailed comparative analysis of the properties of CL formed either in vitro or in vivo may give further insight into the possible relevance of in vitro findings to in vivo manifestations of allograft immunity.

REFERENCES

1. Häyry P, Defendi V: Science 168:133, 1970
2. Wagner H, Feldmann M: Cell Immunol 3:405, 1972
3. Häyry P, Andersson LC, Nordling S, Virolainen M: Transplant Rev 12:91, 1972
4. Cerottini J-C, Brunner KT: Adv Immunol (in press)
5. Freedman LR, Cerottini J-C, Brunner KT: J Immunol 109:1371, 1972
6. Eijsvoogel VP, du Bois MJGJ, Melief CH, et al: in: Histocompatibility Testing 1972, Copenhagen, Munksgaard, (in press)
7. Trinchieri G, Bernoco D, Curtoni SE, et al: in: Histocompatibility Testing 1972, Copenhagen, Munksgaard, (in press)
8. Alter BJ, Schendel DJ, Bach ML, et al: J Exp Med 137:1303, 1973
9. Schendel DJ, Alter BJ, Bach FH: Transplant Proc 5:1651, 1973
10. Bloom BR, Maillard J, Gaffney J, et al: Transplant Proc 4:329, 1972
11. Canty TG, Wunderlich JR: Transplantation 11: 111, 1971
12. Cerottini J-C, Brunner KT: in Bloom BR, Glade PR (eds): In Vitro Methods in Cell-mediated Immunity, New York, Academic, 1971, p 369
13. MacDonald HR: thesis, University of Toronto, 1972
14. Cerottini J-C, MacDonald HR, Engers HD, et al: Adv Biosciences (in press)
15. Wagner H, Harris AW, Feldmann M: Cell Immunol 4:39, 1972
16. MacDonald HR, Phillips RA, Miller RG: J Immunol 111:575, 1973
17. Marbrook J: Lancet 2:1279, 1967
18. Cerottini J-C, Engers HD, MacDonald HR, Brunner KT: manuscript in preparation
19. Wagner H, Feldmann M, Boyle W, Schrader JW: J Exp Med 136:331, 1972
20. Wagner H: manuscript in preparation
21. Wagner H, Wyss C: Eur J Immunol (in press)
22. Miller RG, Phillips RA: J Cell Physiol 73:191, 1969
23. MacDonald HR: manuscript in preparation
24. Pelet J, Brunner KT, Nordin AA, Cerottini J-C: Eur J Immunol 1:238, 1971
25. Shortman K, Brunner KT, Cerottini J-C: J Exp Med 135:1375, 1972

Cell-mediated Cytotoxicity In Vitro: Target-Cell Recognition and Effector-Cell Requirements

By P. Perlmann, G. Holm, and V. Stejskal

CELL-MEDIATED CYTOTOXICITY INVOLVING RECOGNITION OF IMMUNOLOGICALLY DEFINED ANTIGENS

CELL-MEDIATED cytotoxicity in vitro constitutes a model for elucidation of cellular effector mechanisms operative in vivo in tissue-destruction immune responses. When the effector cells are obtained from donors immunized against target-cell surface antigens, the latter are attacked and lysed, while nonantigenic bystander cells remain intact. More recently, similar specific reactions have been obtained with lymphocytes from nonimmune donors after sensitization in vitro.[1-3] Cell-mediated lympholysis (CML) is an example of this latter type in which the mixed lymphocyte reaction (MLC) provides for the sensitizing phase.[4-7]

Crucial for these reactions is their immunologically defined specificity, ultimately based on recognition of target-cell antigens by some cells in the effector-cell populations. It is also established that reactions of this type (1) may take place without participation of humoral antibodies, as demonstrable with available methods, and (2) may require thymus-derived lymphocytes (T cells) as initiator cells and effector cells. Such T-cell-requiring cytotoxic reactions have been shown primarily to play a role in the destruction of histoincompatible target cells involving the H-2 system of the mouse. However, there is also evidence indicating (1) that several cell types may exhibit immunologically specific cytotoxicity and (2) that it may comprise cooperation of several cell types. Thus T lymphocytes may be needed to start a reaction in which the effector cells are non-T, e.g., macrophages. The role of T cells may also be restricted to their helper function in inducing B cells to produce humoral antibody of IgG type. This antibody may then be instrumental in inducing cytotoxic reactions in a variety of different effector-cell types, including lymphocytes. Finally, even when cytotoxicity has been shown to be dependent on T cells exclusively, the T inducer cells may be different from the T effector cells.[8] For review of the extensive recent literature on these subjects, see references 2, 9, and 10.

CYTOTOXICITY OF LYMPHOCYTES AFTER NONSPECIFIC ACTIVATION

Lymphocytes activated by agents different from target-cell antigens may be cytotoxic for a wide variety of cells.[1] Since these findings have indicated that certain activating reactions may release cytotoxic effector functions independently of any obvious target-cell recognition, this type of cytotoxicity has been called nonspecific, a designation that is not entirely correct (see below). This model has been useful for the analysis of effector-cell types and of the different phases of cell-mediated cytotoxicity in general.

Mitogens such as PHA, which induce blast transformation and DNA synthesis in lymphocytes, also induce cytotoxicity. Mitogen doses optimal for transformation and DNA synthesis have also been found to be optimal for cytotoxicity. The extent of activation of a lymphocyte preparation has been seen to be correlated to cytotoxicity.

From the Department of Immunology, Wenner-Gren Institute, University of Stockholm, Stockholm, Sweden.

Supported by grants from the Swedish Medical Research Council (No. 16X-148) and the Swedish Natural Science Research Council (No. 2032–035).

© 1973 by Grune & Stratton, Inc.

However, although these different expressions of cell activation seem to be interrelated, blast transformation or DNA synthesis are no prerequisites for cytotoxicity.[1] With chicken erythrocytes as target cells, PHA may in fact induce cytotoxicity in human blood monocytes and granulocytes[11] or in fetal mouse (16-day) liver cells, freed of phagocytic cells and consisting of immature lymphoid and myeloid precursor cells.[12] In such cells PHA has no mitogenic activity. In regard to lymphocytes from adult donors, PHA induces cytotoxicity in T cells of both mouse and human origin.[12–15] This PHA-induced cytotoxicity of T cells may take place in the absence of B lymphocytes or macrophages, but cooperation between functionally different T-cell types can not be excluded.[12,14,15] On the other hand, T-cell-depleted mouse lymphocytes (including those from nude mice) and human peripheral blood lymphocytes, freed from T cells by removal of those cells that form rosettes with sheep erythrocytes, also develop a PHA-induced cytotoxicity toward chicken erythrocytes.[12,16]

Supernatants from cultures of activated lymphocytes are cytotoxic for tissue culture cells. The factor responsible for this effect is called lymphotoxin. Although different target cells vary in their susceptibility to lymphotoxin, no distinguishable pattern of specificities has been found.[17,18] However, when the cytotoxic experiment is performed with living, nonspecifically activated lymphocytes, a certain specificity of the lytic event is nevertheless detected. Thus human lymphocytes activated by means of PHA, PPD, etc., preferentially kill target cells of human origin. Conversely, mouse lymphocytes activated in the same way preferentially kill mouse target cells.[19,20] Taken together, the results cannot be explained on the basis of differential aggregating effects of the activating agents. Operationally, this species specificity of the cytotoxic interaction is quantitative rather than qualitative, and it is not detected when the supernatants from the activated lymphocytes are used for target-cell killing in a different experimental setup.[17–20]

The nature and specificity of the recognition step that is the basis for this phenomenon is not known. It probably does not comprise recognition of target-cell structures determined by the major histocompatibility locus, since nonspecifically activated lymphocytes have been shown to kill autologous or syngeneic target cells with high efficiency.[21–23] The relationship of this recognition phenomenon to the recognition of self-antigens described by Feldman et al.[10] is unknown. Clarification of these problems requires further investigation by strictly quantitative methods.

In summary, the results reviewed herein indicate, first, that several different cell types, including lymphocytes of different origin and function, possess the potential to develop into killer cells, a potential that can easily be set in motion by PHA or similar agents. In regard to lymphocytes, available evidence also indicates that this development of a killing potential requires energy-dependent activation of surface-bound processes in the effector cells.[1]

Second, these results also show that cytotoxicity after nonspecific activation of lymphocytes involves a recognition phase that registers genetically determined surface configurations on the target cells. They do not exclude participation of a nonspecific soluble lymphotoxin as a common cytotoxic effector molecule or some other nonspecific mechanism of the killing phase. However, they strongly suggest that a recognition phase, probably requiring contactual interaction between activated effector cells and target cells, greatly enhances the efficiency of killing. In the model discussed herein, this recognition phase may have a nonimmunologic basis but may nevertheless influence the outcome of a cytotoxic lymphocyte–target-cell interaction in various immune situations in which the effector cells are in addition equipped with receptors for immunologically defined structures on the target-cell surface.

CELL-MEDIATED CYTOTOXICITY DEPENDENT ON ANTIBODY

It has already been stated that cytotoxic T lymphocytes are equipped with a specific recognition factor for antigen on the target-cell surface. Cytotoxic reactions exhibited by such effector cells are not inhibited by antibodies against immunoglobulin from the species of the effector-cell donor, and the chemical nature of the recognition factors involved in these instances remains to be clarified.[2,10] However, work in many laboratories has shown that very minute amounts of humoral antibodies against target-cell surface antigens may induce strong cytotoxicity of apparently normal lymphoid cells from nonsensitized donors.[1,2] It has been shown that nonadherent, nonphagocytic cells with the ultrastructural appearance of lymphocytes may function as effector cells in these cytotoxicity models.[24,25] While an antibody-dependent effector function of certain T lymphocytes cannot perhaps be ruled out completely,[26] there is much evidence that this cytotoxicity may take place in the absence of T cells.[9,27,28] 7S IgG antibodies are required for induction of this cytotoxicity that is independent of complement, including its terminal lytic components C8 and C9.[29,30]

Antibody-induced cell-mediated lysis requires effector cells with Fc receptors that mediate the lytic contact with antibodies on the target cells.[1,2] Effector cells with adsorbed antigen–antibody complexes may also be cytotoxic to target cells with surface antigens reactive with the antibodies in these adsorbed complexes.[14] The reaction is easily inhibited by complexes of antibodies against irrelevant antigens, which emphasizes the importance of the cellular Fc receptors.[32] The effector cells also possess receptors for complement C3b.[9,32] However, the interaction between C3b on the target cells with the complement receptor on the effector cells in the absence of IgG antibody does not induce a lytic reaction, in spite of high-affinity binding. This suggests that the Fc/Fc-receptor interaction may be needed as the trigger for the cytolytic event.[32]

Fc and complement receptors are known to be expressed on the surface of B lymphocytes. However, mature B lymphocytes characterized by high concentrations of surface-bound immunoglobulin do not seem to be capable of exhibiting antibody-dependent cytotoxicity.[9,33,34] Some of the features mentioned above and others such as the properties of the Fc receptors also seem to distinguish the effector cells from mature monocytes.[35,36] The latter are also efficient cytolytic effector cells in antibody-dependent killing of certain target cells such as erythrocytes.[37] However, some nucleated target cells are lysed by antibody-dependent lymphoid cells with the above-mentioned properties but not by monocytes.[38,39] The nature of the effector cells in antibody-mediated cytotoxicity of lymphocytes therefore remains an open question. They may represent immature B lymphocytes, lymphocytes of unknown type, or precursor cells belonging to the monocyte series.

Knowledge of the facts briefly summarized above has been gained in experiments in which effector cells, target cells, and inducing antibodies were artificial mixtures, originating in donors from one or even several species, including man.[1,2] However, it has also been shown that cell-mediated cytotoxicity exhibited by lymphoid cells from immunized donors may be of the antibody-dependent type, most likely due to the presence of antibody-releasing cells in the effector-cell preparations.[40] Many different kinds of antigens, including transplantation antigens, may be involved.[1,2]

It has recently been found that humoral antibodies against serologically defined (SD) structures of the HL-A system may induce human lymphocytes from normal donors to lyse lymphocytic target cells of relevant antigenic types.[41,42] This is of special interest if the specificity of CML is considered. For induction, CML has been shown in both mouse and man to depend on the presence on the stimulator cells, of lymphocyte-defined (LD) structures different from the known SD structures but also genetically determined by the major histocompatibility locus. However, the ensuing cytolytic reaction seems to have specificity for the SD structures present on both stimulator and target cells.[41,43,44] It has also been stated that the proliferating cells triggered by MLC in the inductive phase are different from the cytotoxic cells in the effector phase of CML.[45] Therefore it would be tempting to assume that CML reflects a cell cooperation phenomenon in which the recognition factor for the lytic phase is a humoral antibody (recognizing SD) produced by activated B cells. However, available facts speak against such a mechanism. Thus, removal of B cells and cells with Fc receptors from the cells responding in an MLC reaction does not affect the ensuing CML.[23] Likewise, removal of such cells after completion of the MLC phase has no effect on CML.[46] These experiments indicate that B cells or cells with Fc receptors are not required for either the induction phase or the effector phase of CML. This is also compatible with experiments in mice, indicating that MLC-induced cytotoxic reactions within the H-2 system are exhibited by highly purified T cells.[47]

In conclusion, certain humoral antibodies may function as specific recognition factors in cell-mediated cytotoxicity in vitro. Various cell types, including lymphoid cells with Fc receptors, may act as effector cells, but the nature of the latter cells is unknown (although we know that they are distinct from peripheral T cells). The specificity of CML cannot be explained on the basis of participation of B cells or their products. However, this does not exclude that this may be the case in other cytotoxic situations involving products of the major histocompatibility locus, particularly after in vivo immunization (e.g., in transplant patients).

REFERENCES

1. Perlmann P, Holm G: Adv Immunol 11:117, 1969
2. Cerottini J-C, Brunner KT: Adv. Immunol (in press)
3. Häyry P, Andersson LC, Nordling S, Virolainen M: Transplant Rev 12:91, 1972
4. Häyry P, Defendi V: Science 168:133, 1970
5. Soliday S, Bach FH: Science 170:1406, 1970
6. Lightbody J, Bernoco D, Miggiano VC, Ceppellini R: J Bacteriol Virol Immunol 64:243, 1971
7. Miggiano VC, Bernoco D, Lightbody J, et al: Transplant Proc 4:231, 1972
8. Cohen IR: Cell Immunol (in press)
9. Perlmann P, Wigzell H, Lamon E, et al: Proceedings VIIth International Symposium of Immunopathology, Yugoslavia, 1973 (in press)
10. Feldmann M, Cohen IR, Wekerle H: Transplant Rev 12:57, 1972
11. Skottner A, Nilsson H, Perlmann P: to be published
12. Britton S, Perlmann H, Perlmann P: Cell Immunol (in press)
13. Möller G, Sjöberg O, Andersson J: Eur J Immunol 2:586, 1972
14. Perlmann P, Perlmann H, Wigzell H: Transplant Rev 13:91, 1972
15. Stejskal V, Härfast B, Holm G, Perlmann P: Proceedings Eighth Leucocyte Conference, 1973 (in press)
16. Perlmann H, Perlmann P: to be published
17. Williams TW, Granger GA: Cell Immunol 6:171, 1973
18. Rosenberg SA, Henrichon M, Coyne JA, David JR: J Immunol 110:1623, 1973
19. Stejskal V, Holm G, Perlmann P: Cell Immunol 8:71, 1973
20. Stejskal V, Lindberg S, Holm G, Perlmann P: Cell Immunol 8:82, 1973
21. Perlmann P, Perlmann H, Holm G: Science 160:306, 1968
22. Lundgren G, Möller G: Clin Exp Immunol 4:435, 1969
23. Stejskal V, Härfast B, Holm G, Perlmann P: Eur J Immunol (in press)
24. Biberfeld P, Perlmann P: Exp Cell Res 62:433, 1970

25. Biberfeld P, Biberfeld G, Perlmann P, Holm G: Cell Immunol 7:60, 1973

26. Gelfand EW, Resch K, Prester M: Eur J Immunol 2:419, 1972

27. Harding B, Pudfin DJ, Gotch F, MacLennan ICM: Nature [New Biol] 232:80, 1971

28. Van Boxel JA, Stobo JD, Paul WE, Green I: Science 175:194, 1972

29. Henney CH, Mayer MM: Cell Immunol 2:702, 1971

30. Perlmann P, Perlmann H, Lachmann P: Scand J Immunol (in press)

31. MacLennan ICM: Clin Exp Immunol 10:275, 1972

32. van Boxel JA, Paul WE, Frank MM, Green I: J Immunol 110:1027, 1973

33. Greenberg AH, Hudson L, Shen L, Roitt IM: Nature [New Biol] 242:111, 1973

34. Wislöff F, Fröland SS; Scand J Immunol 2:151, 1973

35. Larsson Å, Perlmann P, Natvig JB: Immunology (in press)

36. MacLennan ICM, Howard A, Gotch FM, Quie PG: Immunology (in press)

37. Holm G, Hammarström S: Clin Exp Immunol 13:29, 1973

38. Hersey P, MacLennan ICM: Immunology 24:385, 1973

39. Holm G: to be published

40. Schirrmacher V, Rubin G, Pross H, Wigzell H: J Exp Med (in press)

41. Trinchieri G, Bernoco D, Curtoni SE, et al: in: Histocompatibility Testing. Copenhagen, Munkgaard, 1972, p 509

42. Dickmeiss E: Scand J Immunol 2:251, 1973

43. Eijsvoogel VP, du Bois M, Melief C, et al: in: Histocompatibility Testing. Copenhagen, Munksgaard, 1972, p 501

44. Alter BJ, Schendel DJ, Bach ML, et al: J Exp Med 137:1303, 1973

45. Bach FH, Segall M, Stouber-Zier K, et al: Science 180:403, 1973

46. Svedmyr E, Wigzell H: (to be published)

47. Andersson LC, Nordling S, Häyry P: Scand J Immunol 2:107, 1973

Lymphocyte Antibody Lymphocytolytic Interaction (LALI) With Special Emphasis on HL-A

By G. Trinchieri, M. De Marchi, W. Mayr, M. Savi, and R. Ceppellini

AN inhibitory effect of humoral antibodies upon cell-mediated lysis is often observed in in vitro systems with rodent cells.[1,2] While attempting to induce such a type of inhibition in a human allogeneic system through the use of CML, the cell-mediated-lymphocytolysis test,[3] it was observed that HL-A antibodies against the target, added to the mixture (in the absence of any known source of C′) during the killing phase of CML, increased the target's damage.[4] It was soon realized that this lymphocyte–antibody lymphocytolytic interaction (LALI) was also obtained by the use as effectors of fresh lymphocytes that had not been exposed to MLC activation. Thus LALI corresponds to a well-known phenomenon studied in recent years by many authors, particularly by Perlmann and MacLennan (for a recent review see reference 5). While not claiming any particular originality for our observation, we present here additional data showing the use of PHA blasts as targets, which is of significant advantage for the study of allogeneic antibodies against polymorphic structures expressed on the membrane of human lymphoid cells. Data on the kinetics of the reaction and on the blocking effect on LALI and CML of protease inhibitors are also presented.

Special emphasis is given to the far greater complexity of the HL-A system as it is revealed by LALI in comparison to the complement-dependent lysis (CdL) currently used.

From the Basel Institute for Immunology, Basel, Switzerland, Istituto di Genetica Medica dell'Università, Torino, Italy, and Clinica Medica dell'Università, Parma, Italy.

The work done in Torino and Parma has been supported in part by NIH grant AI 08896 and in part by CNR contract Centro di Studio per l'Immunogenetica e l'Istocompatibilità.

© 1973 by Grune & Stratton, Inc.

MATERIALS AND METHOD

Panels of Lymphocytes and Antisera. The lymphocytes used in the experiments came from a panel of 700 donors typed for all HL-A specificities described at the Histocompatibility Workshop of 1972[6] and in part for four alleles of the SD3 locus.[7] Some of them were genotyped through family analysis. When possible they were selected for being full-house, i.e., with all the HL-A antigens identified.

The alloantisera employed were obtained from volunteers immunized by planned blood transfusion in Torino and Parma[8] or from multiparous women screened in Tübingen and Wien. The HL-A specificity of the sera had already been studied and classified as far as complement-dependent lysis (CdL) is concerned by means of population and family analysis and, for some of them, by absorption/elution techniques. A 50% cytotoxic unit of antibody (Ab U) is the quantity (expressed as reciprocal of titer or volume or Ig weight) that kills 50% of cells on standard (NIH) CdL technique in complement excess.

Terminology. HL-A specificities are indicated according to the Joint Report 1972.[6] The terms supertypic and subtypic,[9,10] for describing specificities (patterns of reaction) that are, respectively, more frequent in the population and include less frequent ones, are preferred to other designations in use (long, broad-reacting, short, partigens; for a more detailed discussion see Ceppellini[11]). These terms correspond to public and private specificities, respectively, of the H-2 system.[12]

Because of the reciprocal definition of antigens and antibodies, the terms supertypic and subtypic can also be extended to antisera. Thus an antiserum can be at the same time monospecific on the basis of absorption/elution analysis and supertypic because it reacts with more than one allelic variant. Conversely, polyspecific sera, i.e., heterogeneous populations of antibodies that can be separated by absorption/elution, may be a mixture of either supertypic and/or subtypic reagents. CYNAP are cytotoxicity-negative, absorption-positive reactions studied in CdL.[13]

Absorption/Elution. Absorption of sera has been done with platelets and/or leucocytes with overnight incubation at 4°C. The eluates were prepared from platelets according to an adaptation of the acid elution method described by Luzzati et al.[14] The platelets were incubated overnight with the serum, washed four times with 3% bovine serum albumin in phosphate-buffered saline (PBS), eluted with gly-SO_4 buffer (pH 3) for 7 min, and then spun down at 1,000 g for 15 min. The supernatants were neutralized with tris-HCl buffer (pH 9.8) and then dialyzed overnight against PBS.

Preparation of F(ab')$_2$ Fragments. F(ab')$_2$ fragments were prepared through digestion with pepsin of isolated IgG fractions from alloantisera, followed by chromatography on Sephadex G-150. The purity of the preparations was checked by immunodiffusion. Their activity was checked through inhibition of CdL by the corresponding intact cytotoxic IgG.[15]

Lymphocyte–Antibody Lymphocytolytic Interaction (LALI). The technique is derived from Trinchieri et al.[4] with only minor modifications for performing the test in microplates. The modalities here described have been chosen for current use on the basis of the experimental data discussed in the section Results.

Effector Cells. Effector cells were usually obtained from heparinized blood of healthy human donors after Ficoll Urovison sedimentation.[16] Mononuclear cells were contaminated with an average of 1 to 4% red cells and 2 to 5% granulocytes. After two washings with PBS at 4°C, they were resuspended in RPMI-Hepes at a concentration of 10^7 cells/ml and stored at 16°C until used. For selection of cell subpopulations, further purification methods, as indicated under Results, were used. Owing to variability of efficiency (see below) the use of three different donors of effectors is recommended.

Target Cells. Target-cell suspensions obtained by Ficoll Urovison sedimentation were cultured in plastic bottles (Falcon 3012, 2×10^6 cells/ml, 6 ml/bottle): medium RPMI-1640 supplemented with penicillin (100 U/ml), streptomycin (100 μg/ml), and 20% heat-inactivated fetal calf serum (FCS) in the presence of PHA (PHA-M, Difco, final concentration 1:100). At the end of the third day, the cultures were centrifuged and resuspended in 0.5 ml of medium (approximately 25×10^6 cells/ml) with 500 μCi of $Na_2{}^{51}CrO_4$ in a volume of 0.1 ml added (spec. activ. 100–500 Ci/mmole, Eidg. Institut für Reaktorforschung, Würenlingen, Switzerland); the mixture was incubated for 2 hr at 37°C in humidified 5% CO_2 atmosphere with frequent shakings. The cells were then washed three times with PBS at 4°C, resuspended in RPMI-1640 medium with Hepes buffer 0.03 M (RPMI-Hepes) at a concentration of 3.33×10^5 cells/ml, and stored at 4°C until used.

Cytotoxic Test. The cytotoxic test was performed in round-bottom microplates (M220-24Ar, Greiner, Nürtingen, Germany). In each well 10^4 target cells (0.03 ml) were mixed with 0.03 ml of the serum to be tested. All sera had been carefully inactivated at 56°C and diluted in FCS. Usually, for saving effector cells, logarithmic dilutions on a basis higher than two were used. After 30 min at 4°C, 0.1 ml of effector-cell suspension in RPMI-Hepes was added (usually 10^6 cells/well).

Controls. Controls were done on wells of each microplate used; 10^4 target cells were incubated with FCS in substitution of sera under test and the following assays were performed: (*a*) total release (T) for each target to be tested by adding to the well 0.1 ml of saponin (10% Zaponin, Coulter Electronics, in water); (*b*) spontaneous release in the presence of effectors (S) for each target–effector combination (10^4 target cells + 10^6 effector cells/well). T and S values were used for computation. As a further control, spontaneous release from the target in the absence of effector was also measured by adding 0.1 ml of RPMI-Hepes/well.

The plates containing both experimental and control assays were then incubated 4 hr at 37°C in humidified 5% CO_2 atmosphere.

At the end of incubation the plates were centrifuged at 400 g for 15 min at 4°C. From each well, 0.1 ml of supernatant was taken and counted for ^{51}Cr activity in a well-type gamma counter, with output on a punched tape, that can be used directly for computation of data and statistical analysis (Cintra Statistician 911).

Experimental release (E) is the actual number of ^{51}Cr c.p.m. obtained in experimental wells; specific ^{51}Cr release (R) is expressed as percentage of net experimental release over net total release, according to the formula:

$$R = (E - S/T - S) \times 100 \qquad (1)$$

All experimental and control values are the average of at least three replicates.

For practical use, the definition of a positive reaction is based on three criteria: (1) R should be $\geq 10\%$; (2) P of difference between E and S, as given by Student's t test (one-tailed), should be ≤ 0.005; (3) criteria 1 and 2 should be fulfilled with at least two out of three different effectors.

CML. Cell-mediated lympholysis (CML) is the specific destruction caused by lymphocytes activated in vitro through unidirectional mixed leucocytes culture (MLC) of PHA blasts as targets with no intervention of humoral antibodies. The technique has already been described in detail.[17]

CdL. Complement-dependent lysis (CdL) has been performed according to the standard NIH technique.[18] Furthermore, some sera have been studied by the identical procedure followed for LALI, including 4 hr incubation at 37°, but where 0.1 ml of rabbit C′ instead of effector cells was added to ^{51}Cr-labeled PHA blasts. C′ was carefully absorbed with human pooled red blood cells for removing xenoantibodies that otherwise would lyse PHA blasts. A 50% cytotoxic unit of C′ (C′ U) is the reciprocal of the titer that kills 50%

of cells on Cdl technique with standard lymphocytes coated with 8 Ab U of a standard anti-HL-A serum.

Proteinase Inhibitors. Proteinase inhibitors were dissolved in RPMI-Hepes and used for LALI and CML at the concentrations indicated under Results. *N*-α-tosyl-L-lysyl-chloromethane (TLCK) and Kunitz soybean trypsin inhibitor (STI) were obtained from Calbiochem, basic bovine pancreatic trypsin inhibitor (BPTI) from Bayer (Trasylol).

RESULTS AND DISCUSSION

Targets. Although fresh lymphocytes (FL) of the peripheral blood charged with ^{51}Cr may be satisfactory targets[19] for LALI, in our experience, with no exceptions, PHA blasts gave superior results because specific release (*R*) was always significantly higher, particularly for short incubation times.

The use of PHA blasts has been criticized on the ground of extra reactions, which indeed are observed while using blasts in comparison with fresh lymphocytes. This is true not only for LALI but also for CdL. This is, however, one of the points of merit in favor of PHA blasts, because the so-called extra reactions are not due to an unspecific greater fragility of the blasts in comparison to small lymphocytes. On the contrary, they can be explained in terms of antibodies that actually were fixed by the small lymphocytes but were not able to exert upon them their lytic action. PHA blasts may be compared to enzyme-treated red cells in regard to the so-called incomplete Rh antibodies, which can be fixed on untreated red cells (and detected by Coombs test or by immunofluorescence) but do not directly agglutinate them. In general, PHA-transformed blasts allow direct detection, even with standard CdL, of reactions that are CYNAP against fresh lymphocytes.

Table 1 gives the serotyping of a donor on fresh lymphocytes from the peripheral blood just after bleeding (FL) and on the same cells after 6 days in culture with PHA added on the third day (PHA-transformed blasts, PB). About 15% of the cultured cells appeared to be nonviable by dye-exclusion test, but these were easily removed by pronase treatment.[20] Thus controls were as good for PB as for FL suspensions (dead cells below 5%). In the cultured preparation, about 80% were typical PHA blasts according to morphological criteria. As shown in Table 1, all antigens detected in fresh lymphocytes were also present on PHA blasts. These, however, were positive with some other antisera labeled for defining other HL-A determinants that appeared to be negative on FL. However, when these sera were absorbed with fresh lymphocytes of the same donor, the reactivity against PHA blasts disappeared. The interpretation is that these antisera also contain, along with the operationally monospecific cytotoxic antibodies as they are recognized with standard CdL, antibodies (HL-A9 2 in serum 18.26; HL-A13 12 in serum 43.15) that are CYNAP for the cross-reacting de-

Table 1. Expression of HL-A Antigens on Fresh Lymphocytes and on PHA-transformed Blasts From the Same Donor

	HL-A Antisera													
	1	2	3	9a	9b	10	11	5	7	8	12	13	9b*	13*
Fresh lymphocytes	1	8	8	1	1	1	1	8	1	1	8	2	1	1
PHA blasts	1	8	8	1	6	1	1	8	1	1	8	8	1	1

Designation of HL-A determinants as in the Joint Report.[6]

Serum 9b (18.26) contains a monospecific cytotoxic anti-9 plus a cross-reacting 9 × CYNAP 2. Serum 13 (43.15) is cytotoxic anti-13 + CYNAP 13 × 12.9b* and 13* are the same sera after absorption with fresh lymphocytes from the same donor.

Cdl technique NIH.[18] Scores: 1 = negative; 2 = doubtful negative; 4 = doubtful positive; 6 = positive; 8 = strong positive.

terminants 2 and 12, respectively, when tested on fresh lymphocytes (in fact, FL are able to remove them on absorption), but that are cytotoxic when tested on PHA blasts. Of course the use of PHA blasts instead of FL obliges us to define de novo the specificity of antisera studied with the standard CdL technique. This is true, however, even when using other modifications, e.g., temperature. It is well known that the NIH CdL technique is more sensitive and therefore detects extra reactions in sera that have been defined according to the Kissmeyer-Nielsen technique.[21] This problem is also discussed elsewhere in this volume.[22]

In our experience, no loss of HL-A antigens has ever been observed in PHA blasts. In fact, they also allow the recognition by CdL of other non-HL-A antigens as A_1Se and Le[a], when cultured in autologous serum.[23–25]

The major sensitivity of PHA blasts over FL is, however, only a minor component for explaining the far higher sensitivity under appropriate conditions of LALI over CdL. As shown, for instance, in Fig. 1, CdL gives much lower titers even when exerted on ^{51}Cr-labeled PHA blasts. Comparison between relative efficiency of CdL and LALI will be discussed later.

From the practical point of view, the dose of 10^4 target cells/well was chosen mainly on the basis of: (*a*) the level of radioactivity that was practical to read and (*b*) the number of effector cells that it was practical to obtain.

Effector Cells. In our system, as in the ones described by Perlmann et al.[26] and MacLennan,[27] effector cells correspond to mononuclear cells of the peripheral blood. Efficiency of effectors, that is, the relative ability of different cell preparations to damage targets, is expressed, as explained under Kinetics, as the number of cells x in equation (2), when $x = k$. When the cell suspension obtained by Ficoll sedimentation was further purified by passage through a nylon-fiber column or by elimination of phagocytic cells (with carbonyl iron) or by elimination of adhering cells (by adherence on a glass surface), or by the three methods in sequence, the killing efficiency of the residual mononuclear, nonadherent, nonphagocytic cells was equal or even higher than the efficiency of the original cell suspension. On microscopic examination, such purified cells were represented only by small- and medium-size lymphocytes, with contamination of so-called monocytes less than 0.5%. Further studies are in progress for separating subpopulations of mononuclear cells endowed with maximal efficiency.

While in this series of experiments only target cells and antibodies of human origin were routinely used, a number of other species were also tested as donors of effector cells: chicken and sheep (peripheral

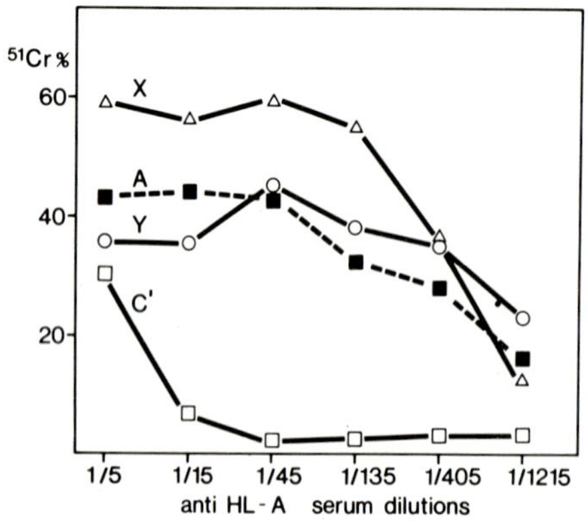

Fig. 1. Titration of serum BsSh by CdL and LALI. Serum BsSh (see text and Tables 4, 5, and 6); target: HL-A3, 7/–, 7 (genotyped). LALI: effectors used (10^6/well): A, from same donor used for target; X, HL-A2, W26, 5, 7; Y, HL-A1, 9, 12, W17. CdL (C′) of same ^{51}Cr-labeled PHA blasts used in LALI.

blood); mouse, rat, guinea pig, and rabbit (spleen). All preparations were definitely inferior to human lymphocytes and in some cases totally ineffective.

As shown in Fig. 1, lymphocytes autologous to target (line A) are effectors as efficient as allogeneic preparations (lines X and Y), thus proving the nonspecific role played by the cells in attacking the target. See below under Mode of Sensitization how to minimize consumption of antiserum by effectors.

Different effector preparations, as shown in Fig. 1 (lines X and Y), have different killing efficiencies. Rarely, but not exceptionally, peripheral blood lymphocytes of normal healthy adults may be very poor effectors. This variability among normal adult individuals has not been systematically studied, but it is large enough to recommend the use of at least two and possibly three different donors for a given experiment.

Studies in progress have shown that cells from thymus, liver, spleen, and bone marrow of young fetuses were totally inactive. Cell preparations from newborns and young infants are in general poor effectors, in agreement with other studies;[28] in individual cases, however, newborn cells may be as efficient as adult cells.

Killing efficiency of cells from two chronic lymphatic leukemias was studied. Cells from a first case (male, 71 yr old, first diagnosis 6 yr earlier, leucocytes 44,000/mm^3, more than 90% of lymphocytes positive with fluorescent anti-human Ig, under whole-body X-irradiation therapy) were totally inactive as effectors in LALI. Cells from a second case (female, 62 yr old, first diagnosis 9 yr earlier, leucocytes 28,000/mm^3, more than 40% of lymphocytes Ig-positive, under complex chemotherapy) showed a killing efficiency of about 1:10 in comparison to effectors from normal individuals used as controls in the same experiments.

Preparation of lymphocytes, even when kept under the best conditions (RPMI implemented with 20% autologous serum, incubation at 37°C in humidified 5% CO_2, strict sterility) lost a great part of their efficiency after 24 hr from bleeding and after 3 days were often inactive. By contrast, populations of cells after 6 days of unidirectional MLC maintained a good degree of LALI efficiency (see Table 2). It is likely that a trophic effect of dividing MLC cells

Table 2. (a) Action on LALI and CML of Protease Inhibitors; (b) Action on LALI and CML of an Allogeneic Antieffector Serum

Treatment of Effector Cells	LALI	CML	CML + LALI
None (control)	43.6	30.8	50.9
(a) TLCK	1.4	1.2	1.9
BPTI	18.7	*	*
STI	23.2	*	*
(b) Serum ToGn	2.1	27.7	28.6

Target cells: HL-A1, 3, 7, 8; effector cells: HL-A2, 3, 5, 12. CML: stimulator = target. Effector is activated through 6 days of mixed leucocyte culture (MLC). LALI: Effectors are fresh lymphocytes from the same donor used as effector in CML. Anti-target is serum BsSh, 1:50 in FCS. CML + LALI: MLC-activated effectors are added to target, which has been preincubated 30 min with BsSh 1:50 in FCS. Numbers represent percentage of specific ^{51}Cr release (*R*).

(a) Protease inhibitors are added at the beginning of the 4-hr incubation period between effectors and ^{51}Cr-labeled targets.

TLCK: *N*-α-tosyl-L-lysyl-chloromethane (0.5 mM)

BPTI: basic bovine pancreatic trypsin inhibitor (5,000 IU/ml)

STI: Kunitz soybean trypsin inhibitor (1 mM)

*Not done.

(b) Serum ToGn: anti-HL-A2, 5, 12, 4a, titer in CdL (NIH technique) > 1:10^4; effectors are incubated with serum ToGn (100 μl/10^6) 2 hr at 4°C, washed three times then added to target + BsSh serum.

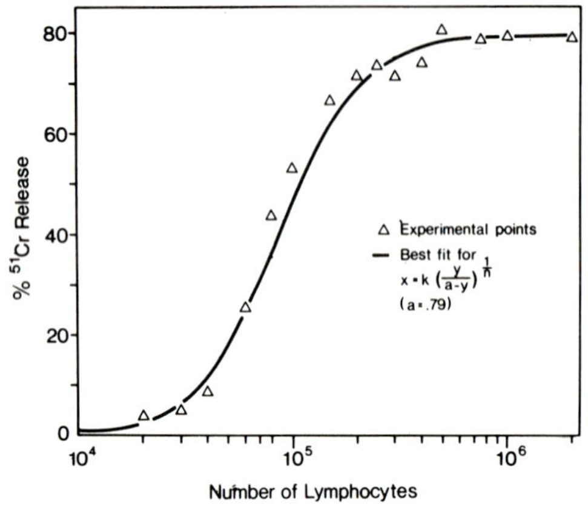

Fig. 2. Relation between number of lymphocytes (effector cells) and specific ^{51}Cr release (*R*). Target: lymphoblastoid line (HL-A1, 2, 5, 12, W4); serum: ToBu/64 anti-5, W4 (10 CdL units); incubation time: 4 hr.

protects the subpopulation of antibody-interacting non-T lymphocytes that are responsible for LALI. Other interpretations, however, cannot be discarded, and the equivalence of LALI induced by fresh lymphocytes and by MLC-activated cells remains to be proved.

Kinetics of Reaction. The main parameters of the reaction, i.e., efficiency of effector cells, time, temperature, and target sensitization by alloantibody, are here considered.

Efficiency: for minimizing additional sources of variability, comparisons among different effectors were performed using always the same target, i.e., an established lymphoblastoid line of phenotype HL-A1,2,5,12,W4, sensitized by a large excess of a standard alloantiserum (ToBu, 1.64; anti-HL-A5,W4; 100 μl/10^6 cells, corresponding to 10 Ab U in CdL). As effectors, only cells negative with this antiserum were studied. Notwithstanding these optimal conditions, the observed experimental ^{51}Cr release usually does not approach the level of total release, even when effector cells are used in large excess ($> 2 \times 10^6$).

The relation between the number of effectors and the value of specific ^{51}Cr release, *R* of equation (1), is not linear but follows a sigmoid curve when log of effector dose is plotted as shown in Fig. 2. This curve asymptotically approaches a maximal value of *R*, which is, however, always less than 100% and varies in different experimental systems from 60% to 90%. For a given system where all other variables have been constant (individual fragility of target, sensitizing dose of Ab, temperature, and incubation time), it is rather characteristic and compares well in different replicates. With the 4 hr incubation and effectors of average efficiency, this maximal value of *R* is approached with a number of cells below 10^6 (see also Fig. 3). For this reason, 10^6 effector cells/well have been chosen for routine.

As for hemolysis by complement, a good mathematical model for the sigmoid reaction curve is given by van Krogh, equation (29), but where 1 in the denominator is substituted by *a*

$$x = k\left(\frac{y}{a - y}\right)^{1/n} \qquad (2)$$

In equation (2), x represents the number of effector cells and $100y$ the corresponding value of specific ^{51}Cr release in (1) (i.e., $y = R \times 100$). By means of the least-square fit to equation (2), a value of a is found on the basis of correlation coefficients that represents the asymptote of the sigmoid curve. As depicted in Fig. 2, experimental data show a good fit with the curve described by equation (2).

The constant k is the number of effectors able to give a specific ^{51}Cr release $y = \frac{1}{2}a$. Then

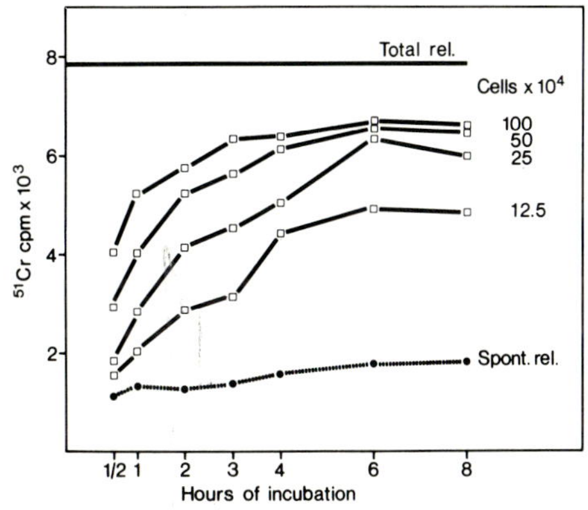

Fig. 3. Time courses of lysis by LALI with different numbers of effector cells. Target: lymphoblastoid line (HL-A1, 2, 5, 12, W4); serum: ToBu/64 anti-5, W4 (10 CdL units); squares connected by line represent experimental ^{51}Cr release (E) observed for different numbers of effectors.

$$\left(\frac{y}{a - y}\right)^{1/n} = 1 \quad \text{and} \quad x = k$$

Thus k is a useful measure of efficiency of different effectors in a given system. Logarithmic transformation of (2) gives

$$\log x = \frac{1}{n} \log \frac{y}{a - y} + \log k \qquad (3)$$

which, if $\log x$ is plotted against $\log [y/(a - y)]$, allows the transformation of the sigmoid curve into a straight line, with slope $1/n$ and intercept $\log k$. This function may be used for a graphic extrapolation of experimental points.

A similar description of the relation between number of effectors and cell damage has already been given by MacLennan[27] for his system using Chang cells as target, but where a constant value of a can be used.

Time: Time is another important variable, related in a complex way to efficiency and number of effector cells. With effectors of average efficiency, in amounts around 10^6/well, the reaction reaches in the first few hours a plateau that does not rise further even after long incubation times. Under these conditions, values of $R > 50\%$ are often already obtained after 30 min. Thus 4 hr as incubation time for routine use was chosen because it allows reliable results in the majority of experiments.

With a target-to-effector ratio around 1:10 (or with effectors of poorer than average efficiency), the dynamics of the reaction are quite different. As shown in Fig. 3, the rate of lysis in the first hours is poor, and a plateau is often not approached, at least in the limited range of time allowed by the ^{51}Cr-release methodology.

Temperature: 37°C, as physiological temperature, has been chosen. At 4°C the reaction is totally blocked, as well as ^{51}Cr release.[30] At variance with CML, LALI still induces at 20°C some lysis, but at a very low rate, and good levels of R are reached only after impracticably long incubation periods. Temperatures in between 20°C and 37°C should be systematically explored. It is well known that 37°C is not the optimal temperature for CdL in every system.[31]

Role of Proteases in Cell-mediated Lysis. Alloantibodies coating living lymphocytes are partially digested in vitro, and this process can be blocked by protease inhibitors.[32] This suggests that proteolytic enzymes, possibly linked to cell membranes,[33] may play an important role on a number of lymphocyte activities. It was thus decided to test whether protease inhibitors would also prevent cell damage by LALI. As shown in Table 2(a), BPTI and STI (two naturally occurring inhibitors) decrease R significantly but not completely. TLCK, an active-site titrant, completely prevents target damage without impairing cell viability. In the CML test, too, TLCK prevents target destruction by MLC-activated effectors. This suggests that the specific phase of target recognition, due in one case (LALI) to alloantibodies and in the other case (CML) to an intrinsic property of educated effector cells, activates a nonspecific mechanism for target destruction that seems to be due in both cases to similar enzymatic systems.

In both cases, CML and LALI, this lytic action seems to require close cell contact, because in repeated experiments: (*a*) in both cases supernatants do not exert any cytotoxic effect and (*b*) Ab-negative ^{51}Cr-labeled PHA blasts mixed with Ab-positive nonlabeled PHA blasts do not undergo any damage in LALI. Survival of the innocent bystander in CML has already been reported.[34]

Mode of Sensitization of Target Cells. Because of the sensitivity of LALI, which unravels in many sera specificities undetected by CdL (see below), it is impossible to predict on the basis of the usual HL-A typing whether a given effector is negative with the serum to be tested. Should the effector be positive, in view of the 100:1 effector-to-target ratio used in routine, a significant part of antibodies would be fixed on the effector at loss of target sensitization, and false negative results could be obtained. It is therefore an important detail of the method here described that antiserum should be incubated for 30 min at 4°C with target alone before adding effector. This temperature has been chosen for obtaining a good fixation of antibodies and at the same time for blocking spontaneous ^{51}Cr release[30] and preventing desensitization.[22] With this precaution, variation of results due to different HL-A phenotypes of effectors is partly removed.

Antibodies Against Effector Cells. Preincubation of target with antiserum also obviates in part the damaging effect on efficiency brought about by some potent alloantisera that are able to react against effector. A typical example is serum ToGn, positive on NIH CdL with 90% of random donors up to dilutions $\sim 10^{-4}$. The main recognized specificities are anti-HL-A2,5,12,W4, but the presence of alloantibodies against some other polymorphic structures of the lymphocyte membranes is suspected. As shown in Table 2(b), when effector is sensitized (2 hr at 4°C) with ToGn, washed, and then added to target + Ab, ^{51}Cr release from target is totally abolished. The additive effect of LALI on CML[4] is also removed (*R*, 28.6% against 50.9% in control). CML per se, however, is not affected (*R*, 27.7% against 30.8% in control).

This differential inhibition suggests that MLC-sensitized effectors are not impaired by serum ToGn, whose damaging action seems to be limited to LALI effectors. A generic damage of viability, limited to the lymphocyte subpopulation active in LALI, cannot be excluded. More likely explanations seem to be specific impairment of the cell mechanisms that are necessary for LALI, e.g.: (*a*) Ag/Ab complexes formed at the effector-cell surface may be fixed by the Fc receptors of the same cell; (*b*) activated Fc of the Ag/Ab complexes on effector-cell surface may block Fc receptors of neighboring cells; (*c*) Ag/Ab complexes are shed in the medium and then may inactivate effectors.[22] MacLennan has in fact shown that antibody-dependent cell-mediated cytotoxicity is inhibited by immune complexes and aggregated IgG.[27]

In this regard, immune complexes that might be present in the serum have not represented for us a major problem. In fact, ultracentrifugation of our sera in conditions that are known to eliminate immune complexes has never modified their reactivity in LALI. It should be noted, however, that we were mainly working with antisera obtained from healthy volunteers, while serious problems may arise when working with sera from patients.[35]

Characteristics of Active Antibodies. A number of authors[36,37] have shown in similar systems that only IgG are able to interact with the Fc receptor of a lymphocyte subpopulation, which thus acquires lytic properties. Particularly IgM are in this respect totally inactive. This is also confirmed by our experience with LALI. A typical example is serum PR12, the only case observed by us of an HL-A antibody that was strongly positive in CdL (anti-HL-A3, titer 1:128) but completely inactive in LALI. Fractionation of this serum by DEAE and Sephadex chromatography showed that the cytotoxic activity, as recognized in CdL, was limited to 19 S fraction only.

A number of anti-A and anti-Le^a sera[25] that were clearly cytotoxic with the standard CdL technique were negative in LALI. Although we have not yet studied them for their physicochemical characteristics, it is well known that these types of antibodies often belong to IgM or IgA classes. We do not have direct experience about a differential efficiency of IgG subclasses in participating to LALI.

Panlymphocytotoxins found in pregnant women and in a number of autoimmune diseases, particularly SLE as described by Naito et al.,[38] were studied in LALI, always with negative results. It is to be noted that some of these sera showed a strong blocking effect on MLC activation.[11] With these types of antibodies, not only the class but the thermal optimum probably plays an important role in making them ineffective in the LALI test, which is carried on at 37°C.

As shown in Table 3, integrity of the Fc fragment of the IgG molecule is necessary for LALI. Moreover, as already shown by Larsson and Perlmann[39] for xenogeneic antibodies, $F(ab)_2$ fragments obtained by pepsin digestion are able to compete with intact IgG antibodies for the antigenic sites at the lymphocyte surface. An exploration of antigen topography with this method in LALI, following the approach used by Richiardi et al.[15] for CdL, would be of extreme interest for understanding the nature of the interactions taking place in LALI between target, antibody, and effector, and the possible differences with CdL.

Table 3. Inhibition in LALI of Anti-HL-A Antibody by Its $F(ab')_2$ Fragment

	IgG mg/ml			
$F(ab')_2$ mg/ml	–	0.01	0.1	1.0
–	0	22.6	52.3	45.4
0.1	−1.2	24.0	38.3	37.8
1.0	−0.6	−0.8	5.6	13.2
5.0	−1.7	1.5	1.7	7.2

Anti-HL-A antibody: ToBu/64, anti-5, W4. Cdl titer > 1:100. Target cells: HL-A2, W26, 5, 7, W4, W6. Target cells preincubated with $F(ab')_2$ 30 min at 4°C, IgG added, further incubation 30 min at 4°C, then effector cells (10^6/well) added. Numbers represent percentage of specific ^{51}Cr release (R).

Authors working with xenogeneic systems have observed in LALI extensive prozones, up to very high dilutions of sensitizing serum.[40] We have likewise observed prozone with allogeneic antisera but rather on a limited range. In general, no serum that would be positive at higher dilutions was completely negative already at 1:5. On further dilution, however, R was increased.

In our experience, prozone was not due to immune complexes. Other possible causes may be impairment of effector (as discussed for serum ToGn) or competition of IgM and/or IgA molecules with IgG molecules sharing the same Ab specificity.

HL-A Seen Through LALI. A number of sera obtained from parous women and by planned transfusions have been comparatively studied with LALI and standard CdL techniques. With the exceptions previously discussed (antibodies of the IgM/IgA class, cold pancytotoxins), LALI has shown to be of far higher sensitivity. For instance Carbonara et al.,[41] while screening for warm alloantibodies against husband's lymphocytes the sera of primiparae collected 6 days after delivery, found 21% positivities on CdL but 48% on LALI. Titers of alloantibodies are also much higher, usually by two orders of magnitude. A few exceptions on the low side (i.e., similar titers with the two techniques) could be explained by assuming in the serum the presence of a mixture of IgG and non-IgG antibodies with identical specificities. Much more frequently, sera were found with very high titers on LALI, while totally negative on CdL, even when tested against ^{51}Cr-labeled PHA blasts obtained from the specific immunizer (husband or blood donor).

When the sera had already been studied for HL-A specificities with standard CdL procedures, including absorption/elution, the HL-A specificity or specificities defined in CdL were also recognized in LALI. All HL-A antigens studied could easily be detected. Mayr et al.[7] report the segregation in a family studied with LALI of three alleles of the SD3 (AJ) locus.

As a general rule, however, the specificity of the antisera appeared with LALI to be much broader than with CdL. In our experience, however, the great majority of extra reactions can be explained on the basis of known cross-reactivities of the HL-A system. This is best shown by a close scrutiny of the results obtained with a few sera that could be studied in detail (Table 4).

Serum BsSh. Serum BsSh is from a biparous woman HL-A1,3,8,W17: type of husband and children unknown; last pregnancy 23 yr before the bleeding studied; never transfused. The serum was referred to us as a typical anti-HL-A7. This specificity was confirmed by us with a titer of 1:2 in CdL and a titer in LALI of 1:300–1:1,000 (dilutions × $\frac{1}{3}$). With this last technique, however, many A7-negative cells of the panel were positive. Some of these were positive at a much lower dilution (1:3–1:10) and will be discussed later. Some other A7-negative cells, however, gave almost the same titer as A7-positive cells, with individual variations between 1:100 and 1:1,000. As shown in Table 4, all the cells of this second group were W27, W10, or W22 positive.

Absorption/elution products studied in LALI (Table 5) and in CdL showed with this last technique some typical CYNAP reactions: e.g., W27 and W10 cells, although negative with the original serum, removed anti-A7 reactivity. Note that eluates were sometimes CdL-positive with cells that were negative with the original serum. Evidently CdL works with serum BsSh at the limits of its sensitivity, and the increased concentration of Ab molecules in eluates may explain these results. Likewise, two heterozygous cells W27/W22 and W22/W10 were CdL-positive with BsSh, suggesting an additive effect between sublytic doses (in CdL) of Ab populations with different specificity.

Analysis by LALI is clearer and obliges us to admit the existence in serum BsSh of at least four different Ab populations. In fact, four different patterns of reaction are obtained by absorption: while A7-positive cells absorb out all reactivity, each of the other three types exhausts reactivity against itself but leaves behind antibodies that react with all other cell types. Differences in titers and in amounts of platelets necessary for total absorbtion are not significant. Eluates are very active and show that from each

Table 4. HL-A Specificities and Titers of Some Alloantisera as Shown in CdL and LALI

	CdL		LALI	
Serum	Specificity*	Titer	Specificity*	Titer
BsSH	A7	1:4	A7,W27,W10,W22	1:400
PR2.24	–	0†	A14	1:100†
PR8.19	A5,W5	1:4†	A5,W5	1:100†
PR10.15	W18	1:2†	W18,A5,W5	1:400†
ToBn	–	0†	W16	1:10,000†

*Specificities proved by population analysis from $p < 0.01$.

†Titer against immunizing blood donor.

Table 5. Components of Serum BsSh Analyzed by Absorption/Elution as They Appear in LALI and CdL

	Titer on Target Cells							
	A7		W27		W10		W22	
	L	C	L	C	L	C	L	C
Original	1000	4	1000	0	300	0	300	0
Absorbed with A7	0	0	0	0	0	0	0	0
Eluted from A7	1000	4	1000	2	1000	2	300	*
Absorbed with W27	300	0	0	0	100	0	100	*
Eluted from W27	1000	1	1000	2	300	0	300	*
Absorbed with W10	300	0	300	0	0	0	300	*
Eluted from W10	1000	2	1000	0	1000	1	30	*
Absorbed with W22	300	1	300	1	300	1	0	*
Eluted from W22	300	1	300	0	30	0	300	*

Numbers are reciprocals of dilutions:
LALI (L) 1:3, 10, 30, 100, 300, 1000
CdL (C) 1:1, 2, 4; 0 = negative
*Not done.

type of cell, antibodies can be recovered that react with all cell types. A certain quantitative difference in cross-absorbing ability seems to exist between W10 and W22.

Our interpretation is that these antibody populations obtained by absorption/elution react with a multiplicity of determinants (different areas of the antigen molecule[11,15] that are all present on HL-A7 (a, b, c, d) and are in part shared by the related mutants W27 (a, c, d), W22 (a, b, d), and W10 (a, b, c).

The alternative view of an antibody population characterized by a continuous type of variability in regard to determinants of similar conformation cannot be ruled out. Competition studies between $F(ab)_2$ fragments and intact Ig from the different eluates should be attempted, following the approach of Richiardi et al.,[15] if this can be applied to LALI.

A third interpretation, i.e., that the observed cross-reaction between the four antigens detected by BsSh may be due to a very strong linkage disequilibrium between these antigens and the product of a new SD locus, has been ruled out by applying the lysostrip technique.[22] A7, W27, W10, W22 are all stripped by BsSh, which, however, leaves unaffected other HL-A antigens.

While the composite nature of BsSh could be a peculiarity of that individual serum, it was of extreme interest to see that a similar mixture of specificities could be found in all sera randomly collected and studied only because the CdL technique had recognized in them an anti-A7 activity (Table 6).

Note that in LALI all the six sera show

Table 6. Specificities and Titers by CdL and LALI of Different Anti-HL-A7 Sera

	CdL		LALI: Titer on Target Cells			
Serum	Specificity	Titer*	A7	W27	W10	W22
BsSh	A7	1:4	1:400	1:400	1:400	1:400
Hum	A7	1:4	1:400	1:400	1:400	1:400
Wim	A7,W27	1:4	1:400	1:400	1: 50	1:400
Bau	A7,W27	1:2	1:100	1:100	1:5	1:100
Dit	(A7,W22)†	0	1:100	1:100	0	1: 50
Spi	A7,W10	1:4	1:400	1:400	1:400	0

*Against HL-A7-positive cells.
†Previous bleedings

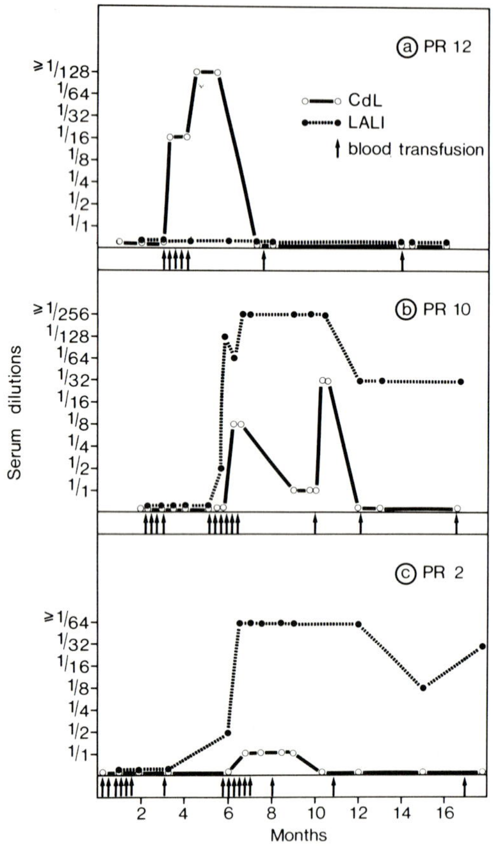

Fig. 4. Immunization courses studied comparatively in CdL and LALI. Immunization of three volunteers by repeated transfusions of whole blood.[8]

the same titer against A7 and W27, while there is some heterogeneity in regard to reactivity against W10 or W22. These findings confirm and extend the dimension of a family of similar antigens, probably related in evolution. Moreover, they show that the pattern of antibody response, when studied with appropriate methods, is less specific than it was thought. In other words, recipients, if they do respond to an immunogen of the A7 family, produce antibodies against many (all) determinants of the allogeneic antigen foreign to them. This is reminiscent of the broad cross-reactivity found in CML[4] and will be further discussed below.

Serum PR 2.24 was obtained by planned transfusions: recipient HL-Al, W29, 8, 12; blood donor HL-Al, W29, 8, W14. According to donor–recipient typing, an anti-W14 should have been produced, but as shown in Fig. 4a, besides a transient period when weak reactions against the specific donor's lymphocytes were observed, no cytotoxic activity could be detected in CdL. By contrast, with LALI the presence of a W14 antibody could be ascertained on a selected sample of 20 full-house donors (typed, however, only for SD1 and SD2). All six W14-positive individuals were positive at 1:100 (p by Fisher exact method 0.006), but four other cells of various HL-A phenotypes were also positive at the same titer. The important point is that all W14-positive cells, besides the specific blood donor, were able to absorb out reactivity against the W14-negative cells. Thus either a new unexpected cross-reacting family centered around W14 is detected by this serum or the four PR2-positive, W14-negative samples carry some other antigen that is in strong linkage disequilibrium with W14, and serum PR2 would be directed against such new antigens. For the moment, however, strip studies[22] have not been carried out.

Serum PR8.19 was obtained by planned transfusions: recipient 1, W19.6, 7, 8; blood donor 1, 11, 8, W5. Besides titers, both techniques agree in assigning to the serum the specificity A5 + W5 (Table 4). The small selected panel did not include W18+, W5−, A5− cells. Thus it cannot be excluded that the serum is a long Rafter.[42]

Serum PR10.15 was obtained by planned transfusions (see also Fig. 4): recipient HL-A9, W30, W15, 13; donor HL-A9, W31, 13, W18. As expected, a specific anti-W18 was detected in CdL. In LALI, however, the serum was reacting at about the same titer with all A5-positive and W5-positive cells. It was thus behaving in LALI as a typical Rafter.

Because absorption studies were not done, it is impossible to say how many components are present. On the basis of experience in our laboratory and others[42] with similar sera, PR10.15 could be a monospecific supertypic serum, CdL-active only with W18 but CYNAP with A5 and W5 (which would remove by adsorption anti-W18 activity). Alternatively, it could be a composite mixture of antibodies as shown for BsSh. Here again LALI in comparison with CdL detects a broader but not inconsistent spectrum of related specificities.

Serum ToBn was obtained by skin grafts followed by planned transfusions between two siblings differing by one haplotype. It is a serum of extreme interest, and a detailed study will be published elsewhere (A.O. Carbonara, in preparation). Here it is only mentioned because it represents an extreme case of a serum that over the course of many years has never reacted in CdL, even against the specific donor. It shows, however, a very high titer in LALI ($\sim 10^{-4}$) against all W16-positive cells. Thus the different efficiencies of CdL and LALI in detecting alloantibodies cannot be explained only on a quantitative basis of sensitivity.

Nature of Weak Extra Reactions. In many of the antisera studied by us in LALI, besides reactions missed by CdL that could easily be explained on the basis of HL-A cross-reactivity, a number of other reactions were observed, usually with a high frequency, against the panel of unrelated donors and with variable but rather low titers (1:5–1:20). Owing to the labor required, no extensive population or family studies have been carried on up to now, and we do not have definite evidence whether they are related to HL-A or not.

In principle there is no reason to think that any antigen expressed at the surface of PHA blasts, if able to induce appropriate IgG antibodies active at 37°C, should not be a competent target for the very sensitive LALI test.

Our preliminary experience, however, suggests that some of these weak reactions may indeed be related to HL-A. In fact, a number of HL-A7-positive cells from different unrelated donors were able to absorb out all extra reactions from serum BsSh. The same was true for W14-positive cells in regard to serum PR2 and for W16-positive cells for serum ToBn.

It may be that allogeneic anti-tissue immunization may produce, aside from antibodies against the strong SD antigens of the major histocompatibility complex, an array of antibodies of low titer and poor avidity with a broad specificity. This concept has already been forwarded by Terasaki and coworkers[38,43,44] for pancytotoxins, which, however, belong to IgM class with a low thermal optimum and therefore all LALI-negative as already discussed. Owing to the sensitivity of LALI, it is possible that an analogous family of antibody of the IgG class that is poorly active even at 37°C is detected. On the other hand, there is a strong desire, recently further stimulated by reports concerning the mouse,[45] to detect by serologic methods products of other loci of the HL-A complex, such as MLC and possibly the equivalents of Ir, if they are expressed at the surface of immunocytes. LALI seems to be a good candidate, and studies are in progress for comparing it systematically with other sensitive methods for detecting alloantibodies against such products and other polymorphic components of the cell membrane.

Alloimmunization Studied by LALI. Curtoni et al.[8] reported the disappearance of CdL-active cytotoxic antibodies, from the serum of recipients of planned blood transfusions, not overcome by further boosts. They commented that close investigation of the sera with different methods (block of lymphocyte activation, immunofluorescence) was necessary before an irreversible establishment of unresponsiveness could be accepted. Figure 4 (b and c) shows indeed that an apparent state of tolerance could be unmasked by LALI. Recipient PR12, however, has not shown reappearance of Ab, even when studied in LALI. It may not be fortuitous that the antibody initially produced by this recipient was IgM.

CONCLUSIONS

The data here presented emphasize the importance of the LALI test under different points of view. This is an in vitro test, which probably has an important counterpart in vivo for the immune mechanisms of defense by joining the recognition specificity of humoral antibodies with the destructive power of some types of cells that may be different and in some case more effective than the lytic effect of complement. It also measures a new function of some subpopulation of lymphoid cells, and its efficiency deserves to be carefully followed in some pathological conditions.[46] In our experience, for instance, lymphocytes from patients with chronic lymphatic leukemia were totally inefficient. As an in vitro test, however, its major merit seems to be the far higher sensitivity in comparison with CdL for some allogeneic systems.

Obviously it is futile to discuss interactions in transplantation and in tumor immunology between humoral and cellular immunity until antibodies that can be recognized only by their cooperation with lymphocytes have been systematically studied.

In regard to HL-A, this test has already shown great merit. Even if the role in vivo of Ab, which cannot be detected by standard CdL, is not yet known, LALI should already be included among the cross-matching procedures. Moreover, its great sensitivity will certainly help, when used in parallel with other recent techniques,[15,47] to clarify the complexity of HL-A antigens, their cross-reactions, and the course of immunization.

Other points that deserve to be emphasized are the analogies between CML and LALI. As already discussed, both are blocked by protease inhibitors, thus suggesting that the final mechanism of target destruction may be the same for both types of effectors. Another important analogy is that alloantisera studied in LALI show a broad cross-reactivity of the same order as that observed in the CML test for MLC-activated T cells.[4] This has a bearing on the nature of the structures that are first recognized and then subjected to damage in the two cases and suggests that antigen recognition is similar for the two compartments of immunity, at least in regard to histocompatibility systems.

SUMMARY

^{51}Cr-labeled PHA-transformed blasts from lymphocytes of the peripheral blood of man are a sensitive target for the lytic interaction between noneducated effectors (mononuclear, nonphagocytic, nonadherent cells of human peripheral blood) and allogeneic antisera for antigens expressed at the lymphocyte surface. The adaptation of this test to human allogeneic systems (LALI) is very sensitive and is able to detect antibodies of the IgG class that are missed by current C′-dependent lymphocytotoxic assays. LALI particularly has been shown to be a powerful tool for unraveling the complexities of the HL-A system and is recommended for cross-matching.

The kinetics of the reaction have been analyzed, and it has been shown that the destructive phase of LALI as well as of CML can be completely blocked by protease inhibitors. The significance in vivo of lymphocyte–antibody interaction has not yet been systematically analyzed, but it is thought to be important for the immune mechanism of defense.

ACKNOWLEDGMENTS

We are greatly indebted to Prof. S.E. Curtoni for the generous gift of sera and for important information concerning the immunization schedules. We acknowledge the excellent technical assistance of Mrs. Dorothy Mayr, Miss Mary Oliver and Mr. Roberto Boccardo. Our deep gratitude is due to the blood donors of AVIS of Vigatto.

REFERENCES

1. Mauel J, Rudolf H, Chapuis B, Brunner KT: Immunology 18:517, 1970

2. Harder F, De Marchi M, Trinchieri G, Thiel G: in preparation

3. Lightbody J, Bernoco D, Miggiano VC, Ceppellini R: G Batteriol Virol Immunol 64:243, 1971

4. Trinchieri G, Bernoco D, Curtoni ES, et al: in Dausset J, Colombani J (eds): Histocompatibility Testing, 1972. Copenhagen, Munksgaard, 1973, p 509

5. Cerottini JC, Brunner KT: Adv Immunol (in press)

6. Joint Report of the Fifth International Histocompatibility Workshop, in Dausset J, Colombani J (eds): Histocompatibility Testing, 1972. Copenhagen, Munksgaard, 1973, p 619

7. Mayr W, Bernoco D, De Marchi M, Ceppellini R: Transplant Proc 5:1581, 1973

8. Curtoni ES, Scudeller G, Mattiuz PL, et al: Tissue Antigens 2:415, 1972

9. Mi PM, Morton NE: Vox Sang 11:434, 1966

10. Ceppellini R, Curtoni ES, Mattiuz PL, et al: in Histocompatibility Testing, 1967. Copenhagen, Munksgaard, 1967, p 149

11. Ceppellini R: Progress in Immunology. New York, Academic, 1971, p 973

12. Amos DB: Ann NY Acad Sci 97:69, 1962

13. Ferrone S, Tosi RM, Centis D: in Histocompatibility Testing, 1967. Copenhagen, Munksgaard, 1967, p 357

14. Luzzati AL, Carbonara AO, Tosi RM; J Immunol Methods 1:101, 1971

15. Richiardi P, Carbonara AO, Mattiuz PL, Ceppellini R: in Dausset J, Colombani J (eds): Histocompatibility Testing, 1972. Copenhagen, Munksgaard, 1973, p 455

16. Bøyum A: Scand J Clin Lab Invest [Suppl 97] 21:1968

17. Miggiano VC Bernoco D, Lightbody J, et al: Transplant Proc 4:231, 1972

18. Brand DL, Ray GJ Jr, Hare DB, et al: in Histocompatibility Testing, 1970. Copenhagen, Munksgaard, 1970, p 357

19. Wunderlich JR, Rosemberg EB, Connolly JM: Progress in Immunology. New York, Academic, 1971, p 473

20. Tiilikainen A, Kaakinen A, Amos DB: Transplantation 10:361, 1970

21. Kissmeyer-Nielsen F, Thorsby E: Transplant Rev 4:121, 1970

22. Cullen SE, Bernoco D, Carbonara AO, et al: Transplant Proc 5:1835, 1973

23. Jeannet M, Bodmer JG, Bodmer WF, Schapira M: in Dausset J, Colombani J (eds): Histocompatibility Testing, 1972. Copenhagen, Munksgaard, 1973, p 493

24. Dorf M, Eguto SY, Cabrera G, et al: Vox Sang 22:344, 1972

25. Mayr W, Bernoco D, Rovis L, Ceppellini R: in preparation

26. Perlmann P, Perlmann H, Wigzell H: Transplant Rev 13:91, 1972

27. MacLennan ICM: Transplant Rev 13:66, 1972

28. McConnachie PR, Rachelefsky G, Stiehm ER, Terasaki PI: Pediatrics. (in press)

29. Van Krogh M: J Infect Dis 19:452, 1916

30. Berke G, Sullivan KA: Transplant Proc 5:421, 1973

31. Kabat EA, Mayer MM: Experimental Immunochemistry (2nd ed). Springfield, Thomas, 1961

32. Jacot-Guillarmod H, Carbonara AO, Ceppellini R: in XXI Bruges Colloquium on Protides of Biological Fluids. (in press)

33. Ferber E, Resch K, Wallach DFH, Imm W: Biochim Biophys Acta 266:494, 1972

34. Bach ML, Alter BJ, Lightbody JJ, Bach FH: Transplant Proc 4:169, 1972

35. MacLennan ICM: Clin Exp Immunol 10:275, 1972

36. MacLennan ICM, Loewi G, Howard A: Immunology 17:887, 1969

37. Perlmann P, Perlmann H: Cell Immunol 1:300, 1970

38. Naito S, Mickey MR, Hirata A, Terasaki PI: Tissue Antigens 1:219, 1971

39. Larsson A, Perlmann P: Int Arch Allergy 43: 80, 1972

40. Möller G, Svehag SE: Cell Immunol 4:1, 1972

41. Carbonara AO, Massobriø M, Trinchieri G: in Proceedings International Congress on Immunology in Obstetrics and Gynecology, Padua, June 1973. (in press)

42. Albert ED, Mickey MR, Terasaki PI: Tissue Antigens 1:47, 1972

43. Mottironi VD, Terasaki PI: in Histocompatibility Testing, 1970. Copenhagen, Munksgaard, 1970, p 301

44. Terasaki PI, Mottironi VD, Barnett EV: N Engl J Med 283:724, 1970

45. Hauptfeld V, Klein D, Klein J: Science 181:167, 1973

46. Campbell AC, MacLennan ICM, Snaith ML, Barnett IG: Clin Exp Immunol 12:1, 1972

47. Bernoco D, Cullen S, Scudeller G, et al: in Dausset J, Colombani J (eds): Histocompatibility Testing, 1972. Copenhagen, Munksgaard, 1973, p 527

On Cell-mediated Cytotoxicity as an Effector-Cell Assay in Transplantation Immunity

By Jonathan C. Howard

IT WAS recognized from the beginning that specific cell-mediated cytotoxicity reactions in vitro could represent the effector phase of the homograft reaction,[1,2] both because of the association with immunization and because both reactions, tissue rejection and target-cell cytotoxicity, had the aspect of specific target destruction in common. Nevertheless, from an observational point of view, homograft rejection differs substantially from target-cell destruction in vitro, so that it would be impossible at present to draw up a chart of parallel occurrences in the events leading to graft rejection and the events leading to target-cell destruction as evidence that these were two expressions of the same process. It therefore remains possible that cell-mediated cytotoxicity is a precise in vitro expression of the cytopathic changes that afflict a rejecting homograft, or at the other extreme, that the two forms of degenerative change are totally unrelated.

In recent years results have been reported that constitute evidence against the identity of in vivo and in vitro criteria for the activity of effector cells. These experiments demonstrate graft rejection in situations where cell-mediated cytotoxicity reactions are not detected. Klein and Murphy[3] demonstrated cross-reaction in skin homograft immunity between three congenic-resistant mouse strains carrying the H-2 alleles b, d, and k. For example, a B10.D2 ($H\text{-}2^d$) mouse sensitized by a primary graft from B10 ($H\text{-}2^b$) rejects a graft from B10.BR ($H\text{-}2^k$) in an accelerated fashion, even though B10 and B10.BR share only a single public antigen in H-2 lacked by B10.D2. These in vivo results, as emphasized by Klein and Murphy,[3] clearly contradict the in vitro studies of Brondz[4] and others.[5] Following in vivo immunization in the same strain combinations, cytotoxicity in vitro was fully specific for the products of the immunizing H-2 chromosome. Thus with respect to transplantation immunity involving incompatible mouse H-2 chromosomes, there is a clear inconsistency between accelerated graft rejection and in vitro cytotoxicity as assays for a state of sensitivity.

A similar conclusion follows from analysis of cell-mediated lympholysis (CML) following mixed lymphocyte culture (MLC) in congenic-resistant mouse strains. In the AQR–B10.T(6R) combination, vigorous reciprocal MLC occurs[6] and there is no detectable CML,[7] but grafts are rejected rapidly in at least one direction.[8] In this combination, CML as an index of in vitro cytotoxic activity is clearly dissociated from graft rejection as an index of the activity of effector cells.

Analogous results have been obtained in human kidney grafting experience and in experimental human skin grafting. HL-A-identical unrelated pairs that stimulate in the MLC have been shown to produce significant CML activity only very occasionally against the stimulating cell donor,[9] yet skin grafts exchanged in such combinations are invariably rejected[10] and kidney grafts frequently so.[10] Naturally it is not possible to exclude the role of minor transplantation antigens in causing these rejections, but since the kidney grafts are rejected despite massive immunosuppression, it seems that major incompatibilities are involved.

Clearly, therefore, when in vitro or in

From the Medical Research Council Cellular Immunology Unit, Sir William Dunn School of Pathology, Oxford University, Oxford, England.

©1973 by Grune & Stratton, Inc.

vivo immunized cell populations fail to show cytotoxicity in vitro, it is not a valid conclusion that the immunization ipso facto failed to generate effector cells, if effector cells are to be defined as the specific cellular component active in the rejection of incompatible tissue grafts.

It seems that the simplest resolution of these inconsistencies lies in the nature of the in vitro cytotoxic assay. When, as is usual, the assay depends either on directly observed cell death or on the release of ^{51}Cr-labeled intracellular protein over a few hours, it seems probable that an extreme consequence of effector-cell activity is being observed. That this effect is a special case is suggested by the difficulty of finding normal target cells that show a satisfactory degree of sensitivity. Wide variations that are clearly target-dependent are noted in the ease with which different targets can be killed.[11] Much of the analysis of T-cell cytotoxicity has depended on the fortuitous finding that the P-815 X-2 mastocytoma of Dunn and Potter[12] shows an extreme sensitivity to cell-mediated cytotoxicity.[11] Indeed, it has been a problem to find suitable control targets in experiments on the specificity of killing in the P-815 system.

A provocative aspect of in vitro cytotoxicity, especially as measured by the CML assay following MLC, has been the finding that to a great extent only serologically defined (SD) determinants of the major histocompatibility complex will serve as adequate cytotoxic targets.[7,13] This has led to the view that effector cells are members of a distinct cell lineage largely restricted in specificity to the SD range of determinants or to the products of genetic regions thus far inseparable from the regions specifying these determinants.[7,9] A number of objections to this conclusion has been discussed in a previous contribution to this volume.[14] The simplest interpretation of the findings to date is that the majority of lymphocyte-defined (LD) determinants that cause lymphocyte stimulation also provoke the formation of effector cells but normally provide an inappropriate target for in vitro cytotoxicity as an expression of effector-cell activity. Nevertheless, in vivo these effector cells are able to cause sufficient prejudice to grafted tissues to result in gross rejection. Such properties as determinant density, turnover, or aggregation could all contribute to the adequacy of a determinant as a cytotoxic target.

New in vitro effector-cell assays are clearly at a premium. An assay is needed that correlates better with the grafting results and in particular that detects effector cells whose activity is directed against LD determinants. There seem to be three kinds of approach to this problem. One is to keep to the current cytotoxic assay methods of ^{51}Cr release or cell death, but to search for more sensitive targets than are presently available. A second approach is to search for less extreme manifestations of target-cell damage than death or the disemboweling implied by ^{51}Cr release. ATP release and the release of $^{86}Rb^{+}$ as a K^{+} analog have recently been monitored as extremely rapid (30-min) assays for cytotoxic cells using the P-815 mastocytoma as target.[15] It would be of the greatest interest to employ these assays with cell targets that did not show cytotoxicity by ^{51}Cr release. The third approach is to search for properties of effector cells that distinguish them from other T lymphocytes but that are not apparently direct expressions of their effector function. Perhaps such a property is permissiveness to growth of RNA virus studied by Bloom and colleagues.[16,17] This approach has the advantage of universality but lacks internal evidence for immunologic specificity.

In conclusion, it seems that there is an inconsistency between in vitro and in vivo assays for effector-cell activity in transplantation immunity. The inconsistency is asymmetrical in that rapid graft rejection can occur in situations where no in vitro cytotoxicity is detectable, while the reciprocal case has not been described. Either it must be concluded that the in vitro assay detects the activity of a cell that is not involved in graft rejection or that the two assays are differentially sensitive, the in vitro assay detecting only an extreme consequence of effector-cell activity not required for graft rejection. This possibility seems the more likely since only few potential target-cell types are sufficiently sensitive for in vitro cytotoxic assays, and these show wide variations in sensitivity among themselves. It is argued that failures to detect in vitro cytotoxic activity against LD determinants, even when the target cell is known to be sensitive to cytotoxicity via SD determinants, is due to the nature of the LD determinants themselves, their density or distribution, and is not due to an absence of effector cells with specificity for LD determinants. Three approaches to the development of new in vitro effector-cell assays are mentioned.

REFERENCES

1. Govaerts A: J Immunol 85:516, 1960

2. Rosenau W, Moon HD: J Natl Cancer Inst 27:471, 1961

3. Klein J, Murphy DB: Transplant Proc 5:261, 1973

4. Brondz BD: Folia Biol (Praha) 14:115, 1968

5. Mauel J, Rudolf H, Chapuis B, Brunner KT: Immunology 18:517, 1970

6. Bach FH, Widmer MB, Bach ML, Klein J: J Exp Med 136:1430, 1972

7. Alter BJ, Schendel DJ, Bach ML, Bach FH: J Exp Med 137:1303, 1973

8. Livnat S, Klein J, Bach FH: Nature [New Biol] 243:42, 1973

9. Bach FH, Segall M, Zier KS, et al: Science 180: 403, 1973

10. Van Rood JJ, Koch CT, van Hooff JP, et al: Transplant Proc 5:409, 1973

11. Brunner KT, Mauel J, Rudolf H, Chapuis B: Immunology 18:501, 1970

12. Dunn TB, Potter M: J Natl Cancer Inst 18:587, 1957

13. Eijsvoogel VP, du Bois R, Melief CJM, et al: Transplant Proc 5:1301, 1973

14. Howard JC: Transplant Proc 5:1647, 1973

15. Henney CS: J Immunol 110:73, 1973

16. Jimenez L, Bloom BR, Blume MR, Oettgen HF: J Exp Med 133:740, 1971

17. Kano S, Bloom BR, Howe ML: Proc Natl Acad Sci USA 70:2299, 1973

The Involvement of LD- and SD-Region Differences in MLC and CML: A Three-Cell Experiment

By Dolores J. Schendel, Barbara J. Alter, and Fritz H. Bach

LYMPHOCYTES from one inbred mouse strain confronted with cells from a genetically different inbred strain respond to foreign histocompatibility antigens. This response can be studied in vitro using cell culture techniques; different assays assess various component parts of the total reaction. The initial recognitive event in the response leads to enlargement and proliferation of the responding cell. This proliferative phase is the basis of the mixed leukocyte culture (MLC) test. Lymphocytes that have been stimulated in MLC by foreign histocompatibility antigens can lyse target cells bearing these antigens. This destructive phase is studied in the cell-mediated lympholysis (CML) assay.

A single chromosomal region designated the major histocompatibility complex (MHC) plays an important role in the control of lymphocyte reactivities. At least two types of histocompatibility antigens are associated with the MHC: SD antigens are defined serologically and act either as the targets in CML or serve as genetic markers for the CML target; LD antigens are defined by their ability to induce lymphocyte responses in MLC and perhaps in the in vivo graft-vs.-host (GvH) response.[1]

Using congenic strains of mice, it has been possible to investigate how LD and SD differences affect lymphocyte reactivities in vitro. Widmer et al. showed that LD differences of the MHC are primarily responsible for MLC activation;[2] they also stimulate GvH reactivity[1] or skin graft rejection.[2,3] SD differences, on the other hand, are weak or nonstimulatory in MLC.[2] The regions important for CML are, in some cases, different than those controlling MLC reactivity. This article reviews our findings concerning the role of LD and SD differences in CML.

From the Departments of Medical Genetics and Surgery, University of Wisconsin, Madison, Wisc.

Supported by NIH grants GM-15422, AI-08439, AI-06525; NF-MOD grant CRBS 246, and ONR grant N00014-67-A-0128-003.

D. J. Schendel is an NIH Trainee supported by NIHGMS grant GM-00398.

This paper is No. 1690 from the Laboratory of Genetics, University of Wisconsin, Madison, Wisc.

©1973 by Grune & Stratton, Inc.

MATERIALS AND METHOD

Mice used in these studies were raised in our own colony; breeding pairs were obtained from J. Klein and J. Stimpfling. The strains differ for various regions of the MHC and have been discussed in detail.[2] All strains, except AQR, are congenic; however, the effects seen with AQR in MLC seem attributable to the MHC.[2] We refer to the four regions on the MHC chromosome—H-2K, Ir, Ss, and H-2D from left to right—with four capital letters, one for each of the four regions (i.e., strain B10.A is designated KKDD). MLC tests are performed using the micro method of Widmer et al.[4] Responding cells (1×10^6) are mixed with an equal number of mitomycin-C-treated stimulating cells; when two different stimulating populations are used in a three-cell culture, 0.5×10^6 of each stimulating type is used. The CML assay used is that of Alter et al.[5]

RESULTS

The CML studies involving the various strain combinations can be divided into three categories: CML with LD-different strains, CML with SD-different strains, and CML with strains having both LD and SD differences.

LD Differences in the MHC

We have previously reported our findings on the role of LD differences in the generation of effector cells for CML.[5] We have examined three strain combinations: AQR–B10.T(6R), B10.A(4R)–B10.A(2R), and C57BL/6–H(zl). The animals of the first two combinations have LD differences because of recombinational events in the MHC. AQR (QKDD) and B10.T(6R) (QQQD) are SD-region-identical but differ in the Ir and Ss-Slp regions. These strains show strong reciprocal MLC responses;[2] however, MLC sensitization does not generate CML effector cells. B10.A(4R) (KKBB) and B10.A(2R) (KKDB) show a significant MLC response in only one direction—B10.A(4R) responds to stimulation by B10.A(2R).[2] The CML response is analogous to that of AQR–B10.T(6R)—negative in both directions. The C57BL/6 and H(zl) strains differ by a spontaneous mutation in the MHC, located somewhere to the left of the Ss-Slp region. There is reciprocal MLC activation, skin graft rejection, and CML between these strains.[6] Although it is possible that these strains differ for SD antigens, extensive cross-immunization has failed to detect such differences.[3]

SD Differences in the MHC

Three combinations with only SD-region differences in either the H-2K or H-2D ends of the MHC have been tested for their in vitro lymphocyte reactivities. These SD-different pairs show a variable pattern of response in both MLC and CML. Repeated testing of the same combination will sometimes reveal CML effector cells and at other times fail to detect them. An example of such a pattern is shown in Table 1 with the B10.G–B10.T(6R) combination that has SD differences in the H-2D region. In two of the three experiments there is positive CML; the third experiment, however, failed to produce effector cells, although activation of B10.G by AQR indicated that the B10.G responding population could produce effector cells in that experiment. When a CML response does occur with an SD-different combination, the percentage cytotoxicity can be very high, as is seen in Table 1. The reason for this sporadic responsiveness is unclear at present. The ability to generate effector cells may be related to a proliferative event, and further investigations may reveal some correlation between the occurrence of a significant MLC response and the production of CML effector cells.

Combined LD and SD Differences in the MHC

In a previous report we presented evidence for an interaction between LD- and SD-region differences in CML.[5] We found situations where an SD-region difference

Table 1. Variation in SD-Region-Different Responses

MLC Sensitization		CML Assay	
Responding Cell (Effector)	Stimulating Cell (Sensitizing)	Target Cell	% CML
1. B10.G (QQQQ)	B10.T (6R) (QQQD)	B10.G (QQQQ)	− 3.7
		B10.T (6R) (QQQD)	69.0
B10.G (QQQQ)	B10.G (QQQQ)	B10.G (QQQQ)	− 6.7
2. B10.G (QQQQ)	B10.T (6R) (QQQD)	B10.G (QQQQ)	−26.6
		B10.T (6R) (QQQD)	58.9
3. B10.G (QQQQ)	B10.T (6R) (QQQD)	B10.G (QQQQ)	− 2.3
		B10.T (6R) (QQQD)	−14.0
B10.G (QQQQ)	AQR (QKDD)	B10.G (QQQQ)	5.8
		AQR (QKDD)	29.9
B10.G (QQQQ)	B10.G (QQQQ)	B10.G (QQQQ)	− 2.0

The percentage CML is based on the following spontaneous-release (SR) and maximum-release (MR) values for each target cell (mean of triplicates ± SD): (1.) B10.G, SR = 561 ± 9, MR = 1428 ± 40; B10.T(6R), SR = 440 ± 23, MR = 1101 ± 46; (2.) B10.G, SR = 542 ± 44, MR = 1336 ± 31; B10.T(6R), SR = 584 ± 39, MR = 1204 ± 33; (3.) B10.G, SR = 524 ± 42, MR = 1554 ± 80; B10.T(6R), SR = 511 ± 11, MR = 1444 ± 35; AQR, SR = 308 ± 21, MR = 843 ± 35.

alone failed to produce CML; however, another cell having this same SD-region difference, as well as an LD difference, could generate a positive CML response to the target cell carrying both the LD and SD determinants, as well as to a target cell carrying only the SD-region determinants.

Such a collaborative interaction between LD and SD can be further investigated in the three-strain combination of AQR–B10.T(6R)–B10.A, as we have previously reported.[5] AQR (QKDD) and B10.T(6R) (QQQD) differ for LD; AQR (QKDD) and B10.A (KKDD) differ for SD. Table 2 shows representative data from CML studies with these strains. When AQR is sensitized in MLC to B10.T(6R), there is a strong MLC response, but no CML. When AQR is sensitized to B10.A, there is neither significant MLC nor CML. However, when AQR is sensitized to both B10.T(6R) and B10.A in a three-cell MLC, effector cells are generated that can lyse the target cell bearing the SD determinant (B10.A) to which AQR was sensitized in MLC. These results further indicate a kind of collaborative interaction between LD and SD in CML. The need for an LD-region difference is not strictly obligatory; one can sometimes obtain CML responses with the AQR–B10.A combination. However, in the six times that this three-strain combination has been tested, the addition of the LD stimulus to the SD stimulus in each case strongly enhanced the CML response. Eijsvoogel et al. have independently done a three-cell experiment in man, and their results have been confirmed by Mawas et al.[7,8]

DISCUSSION

The results reviewed here suggest that the target for CML is either the SD antigen itself or the phenotypic product of a very closely linked gene. Furthermore, LD differences are generally not recognized as targets for CML, although LD differences can be involved in an interaction in the response leading to the generation of CML effector cells. These results are consistent with the findings of Eijsvoogel et al. in man.[9]

A number of general considerations must be examined in evaluating these roles of LD and SD. First, why is the LD difference that is effectively recognized in MLC not recognized as a target for CML? Several explanations may be proposed: (1) LD differences may not be expressed on PHA-blast target

Table 2. A Three-Cell Experiment

MLC Sensitization			CML Assay		
MLC (Mean c.p.m. + SD)	Responding Cell (Effector)	Stimulating Cell (Sensitizing)	Target Cell	^{51}Cr Released (Mean c.p.m. + SD)	% CML
53,163 ± 4812	AQR (QKDD)	B10.T(6R) (QQQD)	AQR (QKDD)	571 ± 23	−31.2
			B10.T(6R) (QQQD)	432 ± 26	− 6.6
			B10.A (KKDD)	598 ± 22	−11.9
			C57BL/10 (BBBB)	425 ± 13	−19.5
21,920 ± 1518	AQR (QKDD)	B10.A (KKDD)	AQR (QKDD)	368 ± 21	−31.9
			B10.T(6R) (QQQD)	363 ± 32	−14.1
			B10.A (KKDD)	630 ± 18	− 7.1
			C57BL/10 (BBBB)	402 ± 26	−22.9
	AQR (QKDD)	B10.T(6R) (QQQD)	AQR (QKDD)	424 ± 20	−20.1
74,357 ± 1143		+	B10.T(6R) (QQQD)	536 ± 31	4.7
		B10.A (KKDD)	B10.A (KKDD)	1346 ± 45	102.0
			C57BL/10 (BBBB)	693 ± 15	21.1
19,283 ± 1639	AQR (QKDD)	AQR (QKDD)	AQR (QKDD)	403 ± 26	−24.4

The percentage CML is based on the following spontaneous-release (SR) and maximum-release (MR) values for each target cell (mean of triplicates ± SD): AQR, SR = 519 ± 40, MR = 993 ± 43; B10.T(6R), SR = 493 ± 20, MR = 1409 ± 15; B10.A, SR = 677 ± 23, MR = 1333 ± 47; C57BL/10, SR = 554 ± 10, MR = 1215 ± 66.

cells; (2) LD may not be expressed on the surface of a cell at all, or not in a way that an effector population can be sensitized to recognize it as a foreign target; or (3) LD may be clonally expressed in a population of cells so that the number of target cells being lysed in CML would be too small to detect with our assay system.

Second, is an SD antigen the actual target for CML? Clearly, something segregating in either the H-2K and/or H-2D regions is recognized in the CML response, but further investigation will be required to determine whether this target is actually the SD antigen itself or some other difference determined by genes closely linked to those determining the SD antigens. It must be stressed that when we speak of two strains having SD differences we are speaking of strains that differ for SD regions, and possibly only part of the genetic material contained in such a region is coding for SD antigens. We have discussed earlier the findings of CML response with C57BL/6–H(zl), strains having apparent serological identity.

Third, why is there a discrepancy between the lack of CML with the AQR–B10.T(6R) and B10.A(4R)–B10.A(2R) combinations and the positive CML response with C57BL/6–H(zl)? There are several models that can explain this difference: (1) The SD differences are in fact the actual targets for CML, and C57BL/6–H(zl) may have a serological difference which has not been detected to date. (2) There are two types of LD differences, one causing the proliferative MLC response and the second serving as the actual target for CML. The genes controlling the LD-target difference segregate with the SD loci. Thus the AQR–B10.T(6R) and B10.A(4R)–B10.A(2R) combinations would not have an LD-target difference, whereas the mutation in H(zl) could have affected both kinds of LD loci. (3) One may be dealing with at least two mechanisms of killing, with the CML seen with C57BL/6–H(zl) qualitatively different from that seen with the other combinations.

Finally, what is involved in the interaction between LD and SD? LD differences cause strong proliferative responses in MLC; M. Bach et al. showed that early abrogation of this MLC response subsequently abolishes the CML response.[10] Hence one could postulate that the role of LD in the interaction is to provide a proliferative stimulus. Whether this is an essential event or only a helper effect has not yet been critically determined. Clearly SD-region differences alone can, at times, lead to CML, but it must be emphasized that SD-region differences are not totally incapable of activating MLC responses. MLC testing among SD-region-different pairs reveals a MLC range of 0.8 to 5.4 when stimulation is expressed as a ratio of c.p.m. in allogeneic cultures to c.p.m. in isogeneic cultures.[2] The SD regions may themselves contain quantitatively weaker LD loci that stimulate low-level proliferation; such responses may not even lead to increases above background incorporation detectable by our techniques. Alternatively, SD antigens themselves may cause low levels of proliferation. It is even possible that some culture-medium component such as fetal calf serum or human plasma can substitute for LD as a stimulus for proliferation.

Despite the capability of SD-region differences alone to lead to CML responses, they are enhanced by inclusion of LD differences. Furthermore, the three-cell experiment presented here shows a case of interaction between the LD- and SD-region differences that causes a response that neither alone can cause.

These CML studies provide evidence for an interaction of antigenic determinants in the generation of effector cells. An intriguing possibility to consider is that the complexity of the genetic control for MLC and CML responses (i.e., the existence either of more than one type of LD locus, an LD activating locus and an LD target locus, or of the LD and SD loci) may be paralleled by a dual cell system. LD differences of the MHC may activate a proliferating helper cell, which in turn facilitates the activation of a second population that responds to SD-region differences. This second population would provide the effector cells for CML.[11]

Recent work from our laboratory has provided evidence consistent with the existence of two cell populations; one population responds in MLC, as measured by incorporation of tritiated thymidine, while the other is the effector cell in CML.[12] If two such populations exist, the work by Häyry et al. in this volume demonstrating that the effector cell in CML is a T cell would suggest T–T-cell collaboration. Work from other groups has also suggested the existence of two T-cell populations.[13,14]

ACKNOWLEDGMENT

We are grateful to Drs. Jan Klein and Jack Stimpfling for providing us with breeding pairs of some of the mouse strains used in these studies.

REFERENCES

1. Livnat S, Klein J, Bach FH: Nature [New Biol] 243:42, 1973

2. Bach FH, Widmer MB, Bach ML, Klein J: J Exp Med 136:1430, 1972

3. Bailey DW, Snell GD, Cherry M: in Proceedings Symposium of Immunogenetics of the H-2 System. Basel, Karger, 1971, p 155

4. Widmer MB, Bach FH: J Exp Med 135:1204, 1972

5. Alter BJ, Schendel DJ, Bach ML, et al: J Exp Med 137:1303, 1973

6. Widmer MB, Alter BJ, Bach FH, et al: Nature [New Biol], 242:121, 1973

7. Eijsvoogel VP, du Bois RS, Meinesz A, et al: Transplant Proc 5:1675, 1973

8. Mawas C, Sasportes M, Christen Y, et al: Transplant Proc 5:1683, 1973

9. Eijsvoogel VP, du Bois RS, Melief CJM, et al: Transplant Proc: 5:1301, 1973

10. Bach ML, Alter BJ, Lightbody JJ, Bach FH: Transplant Proc, 4:169, 1972

11. Bach FH: Transplant Proc, 5:23, 1973

12. Bach FH, Segall M, Zier KS, et al: Science 180:403, 1973

13. Bloom BR, Kano S, Howe ML: Transplant Proc 5:1705, 1973

14. Cantor H, Asofsky R: J Exp Med, 135:764, 1972

Further Studies on the Genetic Basis for Cell-mediated Lymphohysis in Mice

By S. Freiesleben Sørensen

THE antigens belonging to the major histocompatibility system may be subdivided into those that are serologically defined (SD) and those that are defined by their ability to stimulate lymphocytes in mixed lymphocyte culture (MLC) and graft-vs.-host (GvH) reactions. The latter are usually called MLC determinants or lymphocyte-defined (LD) antigens.[1] The distinction between these two types of antigens is probably not absolute. Recent studies indicate that the LD antigens may be detected by serologic methods,[2] and, vice versa, it cannot be excluded that the SD antigens may cause some stimulation in MLC.

However, a further distinction between these two types of antigens has been provided from studies employing the cell-mediated lympholysis (CML) technique. In this test, normal lymphocytes are sensitized in MLC, and the effector-cell activity of the in vitro sensitized cells is measured, using phytohemagglutinin (PHA) blasts as target cells.[3] It has been shown that MLC between cell donors who are SD-identical, differing only for LD antigens in spite of strong MLC activation, fail to produce a specific killing potential as measured in CML.[4-6] The reason appeared to be that the effector phase in CML is directed not against the strongly stimulating LD antigens but against antigens that map together with (or are identical to) the SD antigens.[4,5,7,8]

In the present study, the genetic control of CML in mice has been investigated in order to obtain further information on the relative role of the SD and LD antigens in the in vitro immune response. A preliminary account of this study has been published in a previous article.[7]

MATERIALS AND METHOD

The mice used were provided by Dr. Peter Démant of the Czechoslovak Academy of Sciences in Prague. All strains (except the A.TH strain[7]) were congenic on a C57BL/10ScSnPh background, i.e., differing with respect to only the major histocompatibility complex. For the congenic strains, the following abbreviations have been used: C57BL/10ScSnPh: B10; B10.D2: D2; B10.A: A; B10.HTT: HTT; B10.A(2R): 2R; B10.A(5R): 5R; B10.BR: BR.

The H-2 locus can be subdivided into four regions termed H-2K, Ir, Ss-Slp, and H-2D. The H-2K and H-2D regions carry the genetic information for the SD antigens, the Ss-Slp region codes for a serum protein, and the Ir region contains genes determining the immune response to certain antigens.[1] In the individual recombinant strains these regions may be designated according to their origin, as previously described.[7] For example, the HTT strain may be termed H-2K^{s}, Ir^{k}, Ss-Slp^{k}, H-2D^{d}, or abbreviated to skkd.

The Tla locus or region that is closely linked to the H-2D region but localized outside the H-2 locus has been shown to have histocompatibility effects,[9] and it is therefore reasonable to include this region in the major histocompatibility complex. For this marker the following terminology has been used: a: TL1,2,3; b: TL minus; c: TL2. The gene products of this region will be considered incompatible if the two strains in question have different Tla regions.

When considering the possible incompatibility in a given strain combination, it should be emphasized that the current knowledge on the H-2 complex is incomplete. If, for example, a strain combination is different with respect to the H-2D and Tla regions, these two strains differ not only for the currently detectable H-2D and Tla antigens but almost certainly also for an unknown amount of genetic material localized between and on both sides of these two markers. Furthermore, since the precise crossover positions in the various recombinant alleles are unknown, the precise limits of the various regions cannot be deduced. For this reason, the rather unprecise terms K-end and D-end[10] have been used in some contexts for the left-hand and right-hand parts of the H-2 complex.

From the Tissue Immunology Unit, London Hospital Medical College, London, England.

Supported by the Danish Medical Research Council, the Novo Foundation, the London Hospital Medical College, and the Cancer Research Campaign.

© *1973 by Grune & Stratton, Inc.*

The MLC and CML techniques have been described in detail previously.[7] In brief, lymph node lymphocytes were cultured in RPMI-1640 with Hepes, antibiotics, and 10% fetal calf serum (FCS). Flat-bottomed culture tubes were used, each containing 0.75×10^6 responding and 0.75×10^6 stimulating lymphocytes in 0.5 ml of culture medium. Cells from the appropriate F_1 hybrids were used as stimulating cells. The MLC activation was assessed by incorporation of radioactively labeled thymidine. Effector cells for the CML were collected after 5 days of culture.

The CML test was carried out in flat-bottomed culture tubes, the ratio between effector and target cells usually being 50:1. However, in experiments 3 and 4, round-bottomed tubes were used and the ratio was increased to 100:1. The specific chromium release was calculated according to the formula[3]

$$\frac{\text{experimental release} - \text{spontaneous release}}{\text{total release} - \text{spontaneous release}} \times 100$$

RESULTS AND DISCUSSION

The LD genes in mice are associated with two independently segregating chromosomal regions. One is the M locus,[11] which so far has not been shown to contain SD markers, and the other is the H-2 complex. The number and precise localization of the LD loci within the H-2 complex are unknown. Most studies indicate that these loci are spread out over the entire chromosomal region but that the LD loci associated with the Ir region in general cause considerably stronger stimulation than the remaining LD loci of the H-2 complex.[1,10,12,13] Incompatibility for the D-end alone may, nevertheless, in some strain combinations lead to MLC stimulation of similar magnitude as that observed when incompatibility for the Ir region is involved (see experiment 3).

The general scheme of the present series of experiments has been to sensitize responding cells in MLC against stimulating cells that are incompatible with respect to the whole or a part of the H-2 complex and to test the resulting effector-cell activity against (1) target cells syngeneic to the stimulating cells, (2) target cells syngeneic to the responding cells (syngeneic control), and (3) third-party target cells sharing with the stimulating cells one or more H-2 chromosomal regions that are lacking in the responding cells, i.e., carrying the corresponding gene products against which sensitization could have occurred.

What Are the Targets for the Effector Cells?

Experiment 1 demonstrates that cells sensitized against the whole H-2 complex not only kill target cells syngeneic to the stimulating cells but also target cells (5R) that carry either the H-2K and Ir regions *or* the Ss-Slp, H-2D, and Tla regions in common with the stimulating cells. This experiment has been repeated twice, and the 5R cells have consistently been lysed to the same degree by the two kinds of MLCs. This finding indicates that the gene products of the K end and the D end act equally well as targets for the CML.

In experiments 2 and 3, cells were sensitized against the gene products of the K end and the D end, respectively, and in both cases a specific killing potential developed, as is shown by the lysis of target cells syngeneic to the stimulating cells in the cultures. In addition, third-party target cells were lysed, provided these carried either the H-2K region or the H-2D region in common with the stimulating cells. However, target cells carrying only the Ir region, the Ir and Ss-Slp regions, or the Ss-Slp region in common with the stimulating cells failed to be lysed.

This finding indicates that the specificity of the effector phase in CML is determined either by the SD genes or by genes that are closely linked to the SD genes. The additional possibility that the gene products of the Tla region could act as targets has not been investigated in the present experiments.

The lack of killing of target cells, which share with the stimulating cells the chromosomal region (Ir) responsible for the bulk of the stimulation in the sensitizing MLCs, is not understood. It should be stressed that this finding has so far been reported using only PHA blasts as target cells. It cannot

Table 1. CML in Mice

Exp. No.	Responding Cells	Stimulating Cells	^{14}C Thymidine Uptake Increment / Ratio	Target Cells	% Spec. Release
1	A kkdda	B10 *bbbbb*	9,800 / 4.1	A kkdda	−1.0
				5R *bb*dda	23.3
				B10 *bbbbb*	26.9
	B10 bbbbb	A *kkdda*	10,000 / 4.9	A *kkdda*	21.2
				5R bb*dda*	21.8
				B10 bbbbb	−2.2
2	D2 ddddc	A *kkdda*	8,200 / 3.5	A *kkdda*	37.6
				BR *kk*k*a*	42.6
				HTT s*kk*dc	−1.8
				A.TH sssd?	2.9
				D2 ddddc	−0.8
	D2 ddddc	HTT s*kk*dc	7,700 / 3.3	A k*k*dda	4.5
				BR k*kk*ka	6.3
				HTT s*kk*dc	22.5
				A.TH sssd?	28.7
				D2 ddddc	2.7
3	B10 bbbbb	5R bb*dda*	7,400 / 3.4	B10 bbbbb	2.3
				HTT skk*d*c	59.2
				2R kk*d*bb	8.1
				5R bb*dda*	64.1
	5R bbdda	B10 bb*bbb*	2,900 / 1.9	B10 bb*bbb*	18.9
				HTT skkdc	0.9
				2R kkd*bb*	16.9
				5R bbdda	0.5
4	A kkdda	B10 *bbbbb*	6,500 / 2.9	A kkdda	1.6
				2R kkd*bb*	44.2
				B10 *bbbbb*	65.6
	A kkdda	2R kkd*bb*	−300 / 0.9	A kkdda	−1.5
				2R kkd*bb*	34.5
				B10 bbb*bb*	34.9

The H-2 chromosomal regions of the cell partners in the MLCs and of the target cells have been designated according to the description given in Materials and Method. For example, the A strain being H-2K^k, Ir^k, Ss-Slp^d, H-2D^d, Tla^a is designated kkdda. In the stimulating cells, the chromosomal regions that are different from the corresponding regions in the responding cells are in italics, indicating that sensitization against the gene products of these regions may have occurred. The H-2 chromosomal regions in the target cells that are shared with the stimulating cells but absent from the responding cells are in italics, indicating that the target cells carry the corresponding gene products against which sensitization may have occurred. Cell proliferation in the MLCs has been estimated by ^{14}C thymidine uptake (in experiments 1 and 2 at day 4–5; in experiments 3 and 4 at day 3–4). Calculations are based on c.p.m. per culture (median of the triplicate determinations), and results are expressed as increment of stimulation, i.e., MLC minus mean controls and as ratio between MLC and mean controls.

The specific chromium release has been calculated according to the formula given in Materials and Method. Basis of calculations have been c.p.m. (median of the triplicate determinations, which never exceeded ±5% of the mean). Values for total and spontaneous release are not given, but the spontaneous release ranged between 15 and 35% of the total release.

All experiments have been repeated at least once, and the results have in all cases been reproducible.

be excluded that these cells fail to express the LD antigens (although they do express the SD antigens[3]) and therefore escape the killing. The finding that the H-2-identical M-locus-incompatible BALB/c stimulated by DBA/2 strain combination fails to kill PHA blasts from DBA/2 but nevertheless does kill P-815 mastocytoma cells (of DBA/2 origin)[6,14] could perhaps be interpreted along this line.

It has been shown that the effector cells produced after both in vitro and in vivo sensitization are T cells.[15] The finding that the targets in the CML test may be the SD antigens themselves has nevertheless raised the possibility that antibody could be involved in this particular system. Therefore it was investigated whether antibody against mouse Fab (produced in sheep and provided by Dr. Frank Hay, Middlesex Hospital, London) could inhibit the CML system.

The effector cells were incubated with the crude antiserum at room temperature for ½ hr before they were mixed with the target cells, and the antiserum remained in the system during the entire period of effector–target-cell incubation (in final dilution 1:10 and 1:100). In four independent experiments no inhibition was seen (not shown). The antiserum was subsequently tested by Dr. MacLennan, Oxford, in the antibody-dependent cell-mediated cytotoxicity system, and here almost complete inhibition was observed when the antiserum was added in final dilution 1:50 (to be published). This finding speaks against, but naturally does not exclude, the involvement of antibody in CML.

Is Lymphocyte Activation Due to LD Antigens a Necessary Requirement for the In Vitro Sensitization?

In the previous report,[7] two D-end-incompatible strain combinations, which showed no or only minimal stimulation in MLC, were tested in CML, and no significant killing was observed. However, another D-end-incompatible combination (B10 responding to 5R) showed rather strong MLC activation, and positive killing occurred in CML (see also experiment 3). This finding is in accordance with other findings in man[4] and mice[5,13] that SD-incompatible combinations that fail to stimulate in MLC fail to produce a specific killing potential as measured in CML.

The question is whether lymphocyte activation by LD antigens is necessary for the development of the killing potential, which, as discussed above, is directed against some other cell surface structures (the SD antigens?). This possibility was investigated by testing two other D-end-incompatible combinations that were known in advance to give no or only minimal MLC stimulation,[13] namely 5R responding to B10 and A responding to 2R. In order to facilitate the possibility of cell-to-cell contact during the effector–target-cell incubation, the method was slightly modified as described above. In both cases significant killing occurred (see experiments 3 and 4). Admittedly, in the 5R responding to B10 combination low but clearly positive MLC activation was observed, but in the A responding to 2R combination no measurable MLC activation occurred (in another experiment a ratio between mixtures and controls of 1.4 was observed). The latter finding would thus support the contention that MLC activation is not a necessary requirement for the in vitro sensitization. However, two points must be considered before this conclusion can be drawn.

First, in virtually all D-end-incompatible combinations, some MLC activation can be demonstrated, at least on repeated testing.[13] This is true even if there is incompatibility for the H-2D region alone. It is not known whether this weak activation is due to stimulation by the SD antigens themselves or by the products of LD genes in the H-2D region. The sensitization could thus be ascribed to the action of weakly stimulating LD antigens associated with the D end that for technical reasons escaped detection in these experiments.

Second, the FCS in the culture media causes varying and sometimes rather high stimulation itself. The sensitization could thus be explained if the lymphocyte activation by FCS could substitute for the lymphocyte activation by LD antigens. The finding that strong lymphocyte activation due to M-locus incompatibility fails to produce a killing potential between cell donors who in addition are incompatible for SD antigens of the H-2 complex,[16] however, speaks strongly against the possibility that lymphocyte activation per se should have a nonspecific helper effect in the sensitization phase.

Disregarding for the moment the two possibilities mentioned above, it could tentatively be concluded that sensitization can occur without LD incompatibility. This, naturally, would not exclude a participation of LD (or LD-linked) genes in the sensitization phase. Although dose–response studies so far have not been carried out, the result of experiment 4 suggests that the H-2D- and Tla-incompatible target cells (2R) are lysed to a greater degree by effector cells sensitized against the whole H-2 complex (including the strongly stimulating LD antigens), as compared to effector cells sensitized against the H-2D and Tla regions only.[5] Since lymphocyte activation per se fails to exert a nonspecific helper effect,[16] this finding suggests that the H-2 complex contains genes that have a more specialized function as amplifiers in the sensitization phase. It remains to be shown whether these genes are identical to the LD genes of the H-2 complex or rather are new types of H-2 genes that are closely linked to the LD genes.

SUMMARY

The genetics of cell-mediated lympholysis (CML) in mice was investigated employing congenic strains carrying recombinant alleles of the H-2 complex. The results can be summarized as follows: (1) The specificity of the effector phase is determined by the serologically detectable (SD) antigens or by the products of genes that map together with the SD genes. (2) Evidence has been produced that incompatibility for the lymphocyte-defined (LD) antigens is not an absolute requirement for sensitization to occur. However, LD (or LD-linked) genes of the H-2 complex may have amplifier effects in the sensitization phase.

REFERENCES

1. Bach FH, Widmer MB, Bach ML, Klein J: J Exp Med 136:1430, 1972

2. Klein J, et al: (in press)

3. Lightbody J, Bernoco D, Miggiano VC, Ceppellini R: J Bacteriol Virol Immunol 67:243, 1971

4. Eijsvoogel VP, duBois R, Melief CJM, et al: Transplant Proc 5:1301, 1973

5. Alter BJ, Schendel DJ, Bach ML, et al: J Exp Med 137:1303, 1973

6. Abbasi K, Festenstein H: Eur J Immunol (in press)

7. Sørensen SF, Hawkes SP: Transplant Proc 5:1361, 1973

8. Nabholz M, Vives G, Shreffler D, et al: (in preparation)

9. Snell GD, Graff RJ, Cherry M: Transplantation 11:525, 1971

10. Rychlíková M, Démant P, Iványi P: Folia Biol (Praha) 16:218, 1970

11. Festenstein H, Démant P: Transplant Proc 5:1321, 1973

12. Meo T, Vives J, Miggiano V, Shreffler D: Transplant Proc 5:377, 1973

13. Abbasi K, Démant P, Festenstein H, et al: Transplant Proc 5:1329, 1973

14. Häyry P: personal communication

15. Golstein P, Blomgren H, Svedmyr EAJ, Wigzell H: Transplant Proc 5:1441, 1973

16. Festenstein H: Transplant Proc (in press)

The H(Tla) Histocompatibility Locus: A Study of In Vitro Lymphocyte Reactivity

By Michael B. Widmer, Dolores J. Schendel, Fritz H. Bach, and Edward A. Boyse

ONE in vitro technique that has been useful in rat,[1] mouse,[2] and man[3] for detecting disparity associated with the major histocompatibility complex (MHC) is the mixed lymphocyte culture (MLC) test. The MLC measures the proliferation of lymphocytes obtained from one individual in response to foreign histocompatibility antigens present on the lymphocytes of a second individual. We have recently demonstrated that the mouse MHC, designated H-2, contains loci responsible for MLC reactivity that are genetically separable from the serologically defined (SD) H-2K and H-2D loci.[4,5] MLC studies involving intra-H-2 recombinant mouse strains have suggested that there are a minimum of two such lymphocyte-defined (LD) loci in the MHC, one of which can be formally positioned within the chromosomal region between the two SD loci.[6]

Another in vitro technique, cell-mediated lympholysis (CML), measures the ability of MLC-activated effector lymphocytes to lyse ^{51}Cr-labeled target lymphocytes.[7] Those regions of the MHC responsible for CML are, in some cases, different from those controlling MLC reactivity. Although killing has been observed in one mouse strain combination presumed to be only LD-different,[8] results obtained from one family in man,[9] five unrelated SD-identical humans,[10] and other mouse strain combinations[11] suggest that the target for CML segregates with the SD loci.

It has not been determined from the studies involving intra-H-2 recombinants whether there are LD and/or CML target determinants controlled by regions of mouse linkage group IX outside of the H-2 region. The Tla (thymus-leukemia-antigen) locus, determining the presence (TL^+) or absence (TL^-) of thymus leukemia antigen on thymocytes, is separated from the H-2D locus at the distal end of the H-2 region by a recombination frequency of approximately 2%.[12] Boyse et al. have recently described a histocompatibility locus that presumably is linked to Tla.[13] The new locus is tentatively called H(Tla), signifying a histocompatibility locus (H) in the neighborhood of a second known locus (Tla). Two pairs of congenic strains that differ for the Tla region are available. Our interest in the present study was to examine the MLC and CML reactivity between the congenic TL-different mice.

The two inbred strains C57BL/6 (B6/TL^-) and A (A/TL^+) differ by a variety of genetic determinants, including both H-2 and Tla. The region near and including the Tla^a locus of the A strain has been placed onto the C57BL/6 background by serial backcrosses for 26 generations from a mouse bearing a crossover between $H\text{-}2^b$ and Tla^a, resulting in a congenic strain that has the genetic background of the C57BL/6 strain, including identity at H-2, but that carries the Tla region of the A strain. This strain is designated as B6/TL^+. Likewise, the Tla^b locus of the C57BL/6 strain is available on the A background in the A/TL^- strain, derived from a reciprocal

---

From the Departments of Medical Genetics and Surgery, University of Wisconsin, Madison, Wisc., and Sloan-Kettering Institute for Cancer Research, Cornell Medical College, New York, N.Y.

Supported by NIH grants AI-08439 and GM 15422, ONR grant N00014-67-A-0128-0003, National Foundation–March of Dimes grant CRBS 246, and NCI CA 08748.

D. J. Schendel is an NIH Trainee supported by NIH training grant GM 00398.

This paper is No. 1641 from the Laboratory of Genetics, University of Wisconsin, Madison, Wisc.

© 1973 by Grune & Stratton, Inc.

crossover of the type H-2^a/Tla^b that was backcrossed for 15 generations.[12] Reciprocal skin grafts exchanged between A/TL^+ and A/TL^- or B6/TL^+ and B6/TL^- are rejected despite the failure to obtain cytotoxic or agglutinating antibodies by cross-immunization.[13] This skin graft rejection is relatively slow (survival time ranging from 15 to 90 days) and unusual in that many second-set grafts are not rejected.[14]

The MLC method has been described elsewhere in brief.[5] Five separate experiments testing the MLC reactivity of both sets of congenic TL-different strains were performed. The results are summarized in Table 1 as the average ratio of stimulation (c.p.m. in allogeneic cultures/c.p.m. in isogeneic cultures) for each combination, as well as the range of ratios observed in the given number of experiments. In addition there is an enumeration of the various levels at which stimulation was significant by t tests performed on $\log_{10}$-transformed data. The greatest average stimulation ratio obtained with congenic TL-different partners was 1.13 for the B6/TL^+ $(B6/TL^-)_m$ combination. The c.p.m. in cultures containing this mixture were not significantly different (p > 0.05 in t test) from c.p.m. in isogeneic control B6/TL^+ $(B6TL^+)_m$ cultures in any of the five experiments. In only 1 instance of 20 was stimulation significant across only the Tla-region difference. Varying the cell concentration and times of assay did not result in detection of stimulation between congenic strains. In contrast to this reciprocal lack of reactivity, the stimulation between noncongenic H-2-different strains was significant: 4 times at $p < 0.01$ and 32 times at $p < 0.001$. In addition, there were no apparent differences in the average stimulation ratio for a given responder with stimulating cells from strains noncongenic to the responder but carrying either the same or a different Tla region, e.g., average ratio for B6TL^+ $(A/TL^+)_m$ = 14.99 and for B6TL^+ $(A/TL^-)_m$ = 13.36.

Table 2 shows the results of an experiment testing the involvement of H(Tla) in CML. Effector cells cultured in MLC with

Table 1. Summary of MLC Studies in Mice With Tla-associated Histocompatibility Differences

Mixture	Average Ratio*	Range	Number of Experiments	Significance† NS	p <0.01	p <0.001
A/TL^+ $(A/TL^-)_m$	1.04	(0.61– 1.54)	5	5		
A/TL^+ $(B6/TL^-)_m$	14.59	(2.33–37.71)	5		2	3
ATL^+ $(B6/TL^+)_m$	17.94	(7.28–46.10)	4		2	2
A/TL^- $(A/TL^+)_m$	0.92	(0.60– 1.28)	5	5		
A/TL^- $B6/TL^-)_m$	15.97	(9.27–30.50)	4			4
A/TL^- $(B6/TL^+)_m$	16.67	(6.67–45.82)	5			5
B6/TL^- $(B6/TL^+)_m$	1.09	(0.64– 1.93)	5	4	1	
B6/TL^- $(A/TL^+)_m$	14.96	(4.74–33.99)	5			5
B6/TL^- $(A/TL^-)_m$	15.73	(5.53–34.76)	4			4
B6/TL^+ $(B6/TL^-)_m$	1.13	(0.59– 1.92)	5	5		
B6/TL^+ $(A/TL^+)_m$	14.99	(5.40–40.28)	4			4
B6/TL^+ $(A/TL^-)_m$	13.36	(4.37–43.49)	5			5

*Average ratio of allogeneic c.p.m./isogeneic c.p.m. for all tests on a given combination.

†Number of times stimulation was significant at various levels of probability by a t test. (NS, not significant).

MLCs are performed by culturing 10^6 spleen cells of one mouse strain with 10^6 mitomycin-C-treated stimulating spleen cells of either the same or a different strain in 0.2 ml of 95% RPMI-1640:5% heat-treated (56° C for 30 min) human plasma. After 72 hr incubation at 37° C in a humidified 5% CO_2:95% air atmosphere, 2 μCi ^{3}HTdR (sp. act. 1.9 Ci/mole) is added to replicate cultures. Sixteen hours later, cultures are precipitated onto glass-fiber filters and assayed for uptake of ^{3}HTdR by liquid scintillation spectrophotometry. In one experiment, 2.5 × 10^5 responding and stimulating lymph node cells were substituted for spleen cells in this protocol.

Table 2. CML in Congenic Tla-different Mice

MLC (Mean c.p.m. ± SD)	Mixture	Target	^{51}Cr released (Mean c.p.m. ± SD)	% CML
9934 ± 1715	A/TL^{+}(A/TL^{-})$_m$	A/TL^{+}	351 ± 35	− 4.6
		A/TL^{-}	192 ± 21	− 5.6
		B6/TL^{+}	192 ± 19	−10.7
		B6/TL^{-}	244 ± 13	− 5.2
9575 ± 1498	A/TL^{-}(A/TL^{+})$_m$	A/TL^{-}	232 ± 50	0.0
		A/TL^{+}	360 ± 32	− 3.6
		B6/TL^{+}	197 ± 9	− 9.9
		B6–TL^{-}	217 ± 10	− 8.6
8003 ± 678	B6/TL^{+}(B6/TL^{-})$_m$	B6–TL^{+}	197 ± 23	− 9.9
		B6/TL^{-}	236 ± 5	− 6.2
		A/TL^{+}	360 ± 1	− 3.6
		A/TL^{-}	217 ± 10	− 2.0
8779 ± 1642	B6/TL^{-}(B6/TL^{+})$_m$	B6/TL^{-}	226 ± 16	− 7.5
		B6/TL^{+}	193 ± 13	−10.4
		A/TL^{+}	346 ± 14	− 5.2
		A/TL^{-}	186 ± 2	− 6.4
15831 ± 3124	A/TL^{+}(A/TL^{+})$_m$	A/TL^{+}	375 ± 6	− 1.8
16289 ± 1667	A/TL^{-}(A/TL^{-})$_m$	A/TL^{-}	202 ± 6	− 4.2
13703 ± 1654	B6/TL^{+}(B6/TL^{+})$_m$	B6/TL^{+}	214 ± 14	− 7.2
13509 ± 1129	B6/TL^{-}(B6/TL^{-})$_m$	B6/TL^{-}	229 ± 4	− 7.1
31349 ± 2817	A/TL^{+}(B6/TL^{-})$_m$	A/TL^{+}	370 ± 2	− 2.4
		A/TL^{-}	229 ± 14	− 0.4
		B6–TL^{+}	361 ± 12	15.5
		B6–TL^{-}	450 ± 39	20.0
91412 ± 16717	A/TL^{-}(B6/TL^{+})$_m$	A/TL^{-}	248 ± 17	2.4
		A/TL^{+}	418 ± 34	3.1
		B6/TL^{+}	540 ± 7	43.1
		B6/TL^{-}	668 ± 19	46.9
71232 ± 10156	B6/TL^{+}(A/TL^{-})$_m$	B6/TL^{+}	282 ± 9	3.2
		B6/TL^{-}	225 ± 36	− 7.6
		A/TL^{+}	961 ± 24	65.3
		A/TL^{-}	701 ± 26	66.6
85567 ± 7658	B6/TL^{-}(A/TL^{+})$_m$	B6/TL^{-}	294 ± 15	0.9
		B6/TL^{+}	223 ± 15	− 5.8
		A/TL^{+}	996 ± 26	65.8
		A/TL^{-}	719 ± 26	69.1

Lymph node cell suspensions from the same animals used for MLC sensitization were cultured in RPMI containing 10% fetal calf serum (FCS) at 3×10^6 cells/ml in metal-closed glass tubes (1 ml per tube). After 24 hr of incubation 25 ml of PHA-M (Difco) were added to each tube. PHA-stimulated lymph node cells harvested at the end of culture (day 4) were incubated in 0.5 ml autochthonous media containing 250 μCi $^{51}Cr(Na_2CrO_4$, New England Nuclear) at 37°C for 60 min. Labeled cells were washed three times in ice-cold Hanks balanced salt solution and suspended in 5% FCS in RPMI. Target-cell concentration was adjusted to give 1×10^4 viable cells per 0.1 ml of suspension; 7.5×10^5 viable effector cells from MLC were combined with 10^4 labeled target cells in a final volume of 0.2 ml in Linbro (No. IS-MRC-96TC) microtiter plates and incubated for 3 hr in 5% CO_2 and air at 37°C. Aliquots of released ^{51}Cr removed from triplicate cultures were counted in a Nuclear-Chicago gamma counter. Percentage CML is calculated as follows:

$$\frac{\text{c.p.m. (released in CML)} - \text{c.p.m. (spontaneous release)}}{\text{c.p.m. (freeze-thaw release)} - \text{c.p.m. (spontaneous release)}} \times 100^{7}$$

Spontaneous release of target: A/TL^{+} = 391 ± 16; A/TL^{-} = 231 ± 36; B6/TL^{+} = 261 ± 8; B6/TL^{-} = 287 ± 30.
Maximum release of target: A/TL^{+} = 1264 ± 28; A/TL^{-} = 937 ± 9; B6/TL^{+} = 908 ± 16; B6/TL^{-} = 1100 ± 19.

congenic TL-different stimulating cells were unable to cause significant ^{51}Cr release from target cells isogeneic or allogeneic to the stimulating cells. Thus the H(Tla) difference did not, by itself, result in the production of cytotoxic cells. However, studies in both man[9] and mouse[11,15] suggest that there are some MHC determinants that by themselves can neither cause proliferation in MLC nor effectively sensitize for CML, but that may be recognized as CML targets if a proliferative stimulus is provided during the MLC sensitization. The possibility that H(Tla) might be a target for CML, provided the effector cells were significantly activated in MLC, was investigated by sensitizing effector cells in MLC to non-congenic TL-different stimulating cells and testing for CML on target cells differing from the effector cells at only the Tla region. The results indicate that this region is not a target for CML. For example, $B6/TL^-$ cells sensitized in MLC to A/TL^+ stimulating cells did not lyse $B6TL^+$ target cells (−5.8% in CML), although this same $B6TL^-(A/TL^+)_m$ mixture was able to kill both A/TL^- (65.8% CML) and A/TL^+ (69.1% CML) target cells.

It is clear that Tla is linked to H-2, although available genetic evidence does not permit the precise localization of the associated histocompatibility locus—it could map between H-2D and Tla or it could lie to the right of Tla. Because of this linkage, the histocompatibility functions formerly attributed to the D end of H-2 have not yet been distinguished from the combined effects of H-2D plus H(Tla).

A comparison of the present results with those of previous studies indicates that there is a difference between H-2 and H(Tla) in the ability to determine in vitro lymphocyte proliferation. Although the serologically undetected H(Tla) differences do result in skin graft rejection, they do not cause lymphocyte reactivity as measured by MLC or CML. In the strain combinations B10.T(6R)–AQR, in which known MHC differences have been difficult to detect serologically,[16] and C57BL/6–H(zl), whose MHC differences have as yet been serologically undetectable,[17] there is both skin graft rejection and MLC activation.[5,8]

We feel that the MHC should not be defined exclusively by the ability to generate in vitro lymphocyte reactivity. It is possible that there are other loci to the right of H-2D that can cause MLC or CML, or that loci analagous to H(Tla) that determine skin graft rejection but not MLC or CML may be found in the region between the H-2 SD loci as more recombinant strains become available. The results presented here neither extend nor restrict the D-end boundary of the MHC.

REFERENCES

1. Silvers WK, Wilson DB, Palm J: Transplantation 5:1053, 1967
2. Dutton RW: J Exp Med 123:665 1966
3. Bach FH, Amos DB: Science 156:1506, 1967
4. Bach FH, Widmer MB, Segall M, et al: Science 176:1024–1027, 1972
5. Bach FH, Widmer MB, Bach ML, Klein J: J Exp Med 136:1430, 1972
6. Widmer MB, Peck AB, Bach FH: Transplant Proc 5:1501, 1973
7. Lightbody JJ, Bernoco O, Miggiano VC, Ceppellini R: Gr Batt Virol Immunol 64:273, 1971
8. Widmer MB, Alter BJ, Bach FH, et al: Nature [New Biol] 242:239, 1973
9. Eijsvoogel VP, du Bois MJGJ, Melief CJM, et al: in: Histocompatibility Testing 1972. Proceedings of the Fifth International Histocompatibility Workshop Conference, Evian, 1972 (in press)
10. Bach FH, Segall M, Zier KS, et al: Science 180:403, 1973
11. Alter BJ, Schendel DJ, Bach ML, et al: J Exp Med, 137:1303–1309, 1973
12. Boyse EA, Old LJ, Stockert E: in Grabar P, Miescher P (eds): Immunopathology. IVth International Symposium. Schwabe, 1965
13. Boyse EA, Flaherty L, Stockert E, Old LJ: Transplantation 13:431, 1972
14. Flaherty LA: PhD thesis, Cornell University, 1973

15. Schendel DJ, Alter BJ, Bach FH: Transplant Proc 5:1651, 1973
16. Livnat S, Klein J, Bach FH: Nature [New Biol] 243:42, 1973
17. Bailey DW, Snell GD, Cherry M: in Proceedings Symposium of Immunogenetics of the H-2 System. Basel, Karger, 1971, p 155

Cellular Immunity in the Mouse: III. In Vitro Kinetic Studies on the Relationship Between Recognition and Effector Phases

By S.M. Phillips, C.B. Carpenter, and T.B. Strom

THE mixed lymphocyte culture (MLC) and subsequent lymphocyte-mediated alloimmune cytotoxicity (LAC) are thought to represent useful functional in vitro analogues of the in vivo afferent and efferent phases of the immune response.[1] However, the relationship between the two in vitro reactions and their analogy to the in vivo events is not clearly defined.[2] We have been studying the reactions using precise kinetic measurements and defined antibodies to functionally compete with the cell-surface receptors in an attempt to more fully elucidate the stoichiometry of the reactions.[3,4]

MATERIALS AND METHOD

Antibody. Enhancing antibody was prepared in A/J mice by multiple immunization with C57BL/6 mouse cells and assayed in vivo as previously described.[5]

Mixed Lymphocyte Culture. MLCs were performed as previously described, with modifications.[6] 50×10^6 responding splenic mononuclear cells (7–9μ in diameter) were incubated with 50×10^6 irradiated (1200 R ^{60}Co) target cells in upright tissue-culture flasks (Falcon No. 3012) in 25 ml vol under 10% O_2. Media consisted of RPMI-1640, Hepes buffer (0.005 *M*) 10% fresh heat-inactivated normal human serum (40 min at 56°C, obtained from fasting donor), penicillin and streptomycin, with 25% v:v exchanged every 48 hr. Proliferation was assessed by ^{3}H-thymidine incorporation.

Lymphocyte Alloimmune Cytotoxicity (LAC). The effector cells were prepared from the MLCs by layering the cell population upon a 1.081 s.g. Ficoll Hypaque gradient. Media consisted of RPMI-1640, 0.005-*M* Hepes buffer, and 10% heat-inactivated fetal calf serum (4 hr at 56°C). The target cells were prepared from the thymus of an exsanguinated 6-wk-old mouse. This was excised and pressed through a 60-gauge stainless-steel screen. The nonadherent cell suspension, prepared by incubation on a plastic petri dish, a procedure resulting in the removal of 15% of the total cells, was further purified on a Ficoll Hypaque density gradient. After washing, the thymic cells (> 98% small lymphocytes) were suspended in a concentration of 1×10^7 thymocytes/ml, in the presence of 250 μCi of ^{51}Cr (sodium chromate, Amersham-Searle) and incubated for 90 min prior to washing twice with media. Lymphocyte-mediated alloimmune cytotoxicity was determined by modification of the method of Brunner.[7] All incubation consisted of 2×10^4 target cells suspended in 2 ml of RPMI-1640 containing 0.005-*M* Hepes and 10% heat-inactivated fetal calf serum in disposable 12- × 75-mm capped glass tubes. Target cells were cultured in the presence of media alone, with the addition of the 2×10^5 to 4×10^6 MLC cells, or frozen and thawed four times in an acetone–dry-ice bath. After an incubation (30 min at 37.3°), all tubes were centrifuged at 50 g for 5 min. Mixtures were then further incubated for 3½ hr at 37.3°C. Incubations were then terminated by centrifugation at 400 g for 10 min. Supernates were decanted into disposable 12- × 75-mm glass test tubes and counted for ^{51}Cr release. Percentage specific chromium release (% Sp.Cr.R.) was determined by the formula: c.p.m. experimental minus c.p.m. control divided by c.p.m. freeze-thaw minus c.p.m. control × 100. Total cytotoxic potential per culture was determined by dividing the total number of MLC-derived cells by the number of cells required to release 30% of the total releasable chromium in 4 hr (30% LAC units).

RESULTS

The relationship between cell division and cytotoxic activity is shown in Fig. 1. Both isotope incorporation and subsequent effector-cell capability evolved in a log-linear manner relative to time. Additional experiments demonstrated that LAC activity was first detectable approximately 18 hr after the onset of blastogenesis.

Table 1 illustrates the specificity and sensitivity of the lymphocyte alloimmune

From the Department of Immunology, Division of Communicable Diseases and Immunology, Walter Reed Army Institute of Research, Washington, D. C., and the Immunology Laboratory, Cardiorenal Section, Department of Medicine, Peter Bent Brigham Hospital, Harvard Medical School, Boston, Mass.

Dr. Carpenter is an investigator for the Howard Hughes Medical Institute.

Supported in part by USNIH grant No. AI-00301.

© 1973 by Grune & Stratton, Inc.

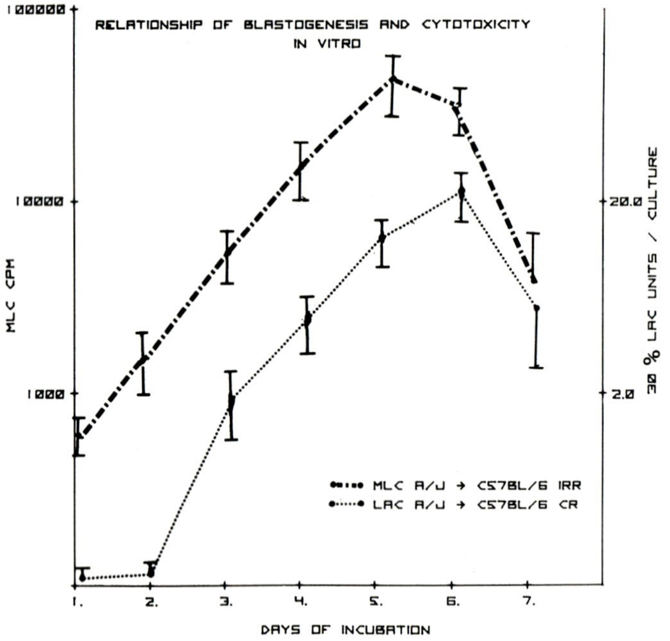

Fig. 1. Relationship of blastogenesis and lymphocyte-mediated alloimmune cytotoxicity (LAC) in vitro. Cytotoxic activity was first observed 18 hr following the onset of blastogenesis. Both phenomena developed in a log-linear manner, relative to time. 30% LAC units (see text) were measured against cells syngeneic to those serving as MLC targets. CPM of unmixed MLC controls were 1306 ± 236 on day 1 and 837 ± 120 on day 2.

cytotoxicity (LAC) reaction. Maximum specific release of chromium was found when using the cell population that was syngeneic to the target cells of the MLC. As a measurement of cross-reactivity, a specificity ratio was defined: LAC using cells syngeneic to the MLC target cells/LAC using cells allogeneic to the MLC target cells. Although the specificity of this reaction using ^{51}Cr-labeled PHA blast cells[8] is similar to that shown by normal thymocytes,[9] we have found the latter cell source superior for three reasons: (1) The spontaneous release rate of ^{51}Cr relative to the maximum releasable ^{51}Cr is lower, allowing a greater range for quantitative discrimination. (2) The addition of syngeneically sensitized cells does not lead to as much negative specific ^{51}Cr release (often observed to exceed 20 to 40% with PHA-

Table 1. Specificity of Lymphocyte Alloimmune Cytotoxicity

	Chromium-labeled Normal Thymocytes		
	C57BL/6	C3H/He	A/J
Freeze-thaw × 4	2130 ± 45*	2020 ± 30	2410 ± 61
C†	486 ± 15	453 ± 17	506 ± 21
A/J → C57BL/6^{ir} ‡	1660 ± 36	831 ± 11	438 ± 18
% Sp.Cr.R.§	+71	+24	−4
S.R.¶	3.0		
A/J → A/J^{ir} ‖	−6	−7	−9

*c.p.m. ± SD.

†Cells incubated at 37.3°C for 4 hr with soft spin.

‡Effector cells derived from MLC A/J → C57Bl/6 (irradiated) 100:1 effector/target ratio.

§Percentage specific chromium release: c.p.m. E − c.p.m. C/c.p.m. FT − c.p.m. C

¶ Specificity ratio.

‖ Effector cells derived from MLC A/J → A/J (irradiated).

Table 2. Sequential Development of Lymphocyte Alloimmune Cytotoxicity

	Day of Incubation			
	3	4	5	6
Cytotoxic units*	1.6	3.1	8.3	10.2
Specificity ratio†	1.4	2.4	3.7	4.2
Antibody‡	50.	43.	36.	16.

*Number of effector-cell units releasing 30% Sp. Cr. from 2 × 10^4 specific cells.

†Sp. Cr. R. cells (syngeneic/allogeneic) to target of MLC.

‡Percentage suppression of cytotoxic reaction by antibody (1/50 v:v).

labeled blast cells). This negative ^{51}Cr release observed with thymocytes can be compensated for by the addition of syngeneic normal cells to control-cell cultures. (3) Autotoxicity is less frequently observed. In addition, the thymocytes represent a theoretically more normal cell population relative to blast cells. They are preferable to spleen and lymph node cells due to a greater sensitivity to attack by effector cells.[9]

The cytotoxic reaction was immunologically specific and evolved kinetically, as illustrated in separate experiments by Table 2 and Fig. 2. Both the specificity ratio and the total specific chromium release increased with time of cultures. This is analogous to that observed for antibody formation, akin perhaps to evolving titer and specificity. The change in ratio was primarily a result of increasing LAC directed against specific target cells with a relatively lesser increase in LAC against third-party cells (Fig. 2). This implies an active selection phenomenon. No cytotoxicity was directed against the responding cell population (autotoxicity) until conditions for cell proliferation and total specific cytotoxicity were no longer optimal.

Additional support for increasing specificity and functional avidity was provided by utilizing A/J anti-C57BL/6 antibody produced by animals syngeneic to those that provided in vitro cells and directed against cells syngeneic to those serving as targets of the in vitro assays (Table 2). These studies indicate that the effectiveness of a fixed concentration of enhancing antibody in inhibiting the observed in vitro LAC reaction decreased with time. This effectiveness pattern was the inverse of that observed for the development of total cytotoxicity and specificity.

Further information on the relationship

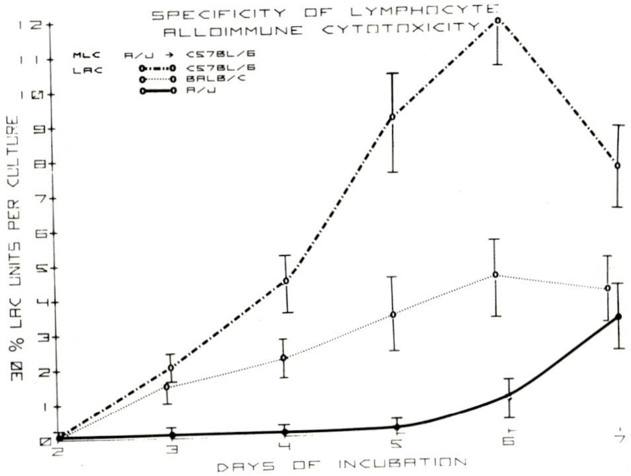

Fig. 2. Specificity of lymphocyte alloimmune cytotoxicity. Mixed lymphocyte cultures (A/J → C57BL/6) were terminated at 24-hr intervals and assayed for cytotoxicity against C57BL/6 (specific), BALB/c (third-party), A/J (autologous) ^{51}Cr-labeled thymocytes. Total specific cytotoxicity increased with time at a rate greater than that observed for third-party cells, resulting in an increased specificity ratio (see text). Significant autotoxicity was not observed until after conditions for proliferation and allotoxicity were no longer optimal.

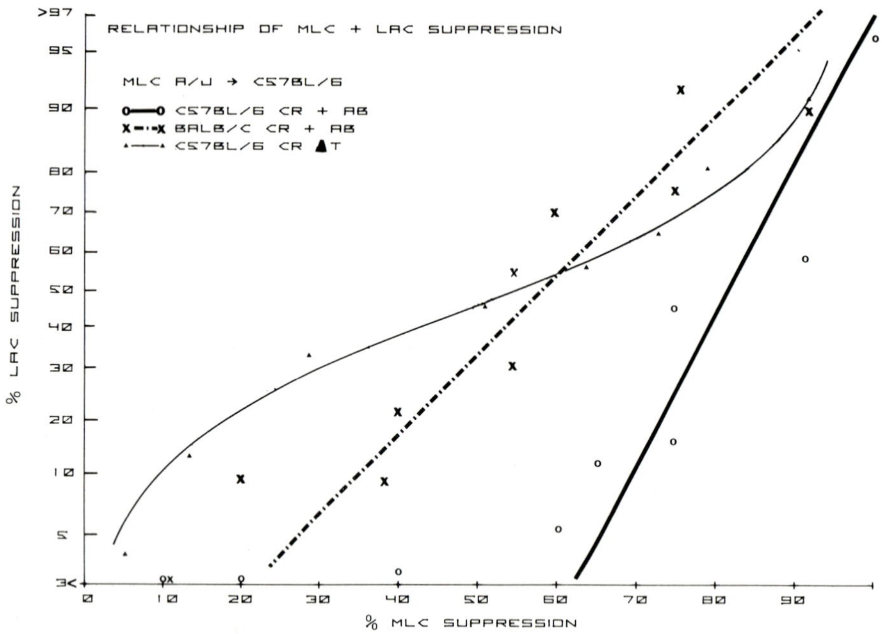

Fig. 3. Relationship of MLC and LAC suppression. Antibody (A/J anti-C57BL/6 1:200–1:3200) and temperature manipulation (35.0 to 39.0°C) were used to suppress and A/J → C57BL/6 MLC assayed by isotope incorporation. The degree of suppression of LAC against C57BL/6 and third-party BALB/c cells was determined (note linear probit plot). Up to 60% of total blastogenesis could be impaired before any significant impairment of specific LAC activity was noted when antibody was utilized. However, 50% of LAC directed against third-party cells was lost at this level of MLC suppression. Conversely, the two phenomena were equally impaired by the use of temperature manipulation.

between suppression of MLC and LAC activity by enhancing antibody is shown in Fig. 3. The subsequent LAC development against both specific C57 and third-party BALB/c cells is shown following addition of various concentrations of A/J anti-C57BL/6 antibody to the original MLC. In both instances, a considerable portion of the total blastogenesis could be suppressed before any impairment of the subsequent development of LAC directed against the specific or third-party cells was observed. However, suppression of LAC against third-party cells occurred when total blastogenesis was much less impaired (20%) than that which would have been required to cause an equivalent suppression of the development of LAC against specific target cells (60%). These results demonstrate that a considerable portion of total blastogenesis was not directly germane to effector-cell generation and may imply that several populations of proliferating cells are involved in that effector-cell generation. In contrast, when MLCs were incubated at various temperatures, the development of blastogenesis and effector-cell potential varied in parallel. Thus the differential selective suppression induced by antibody appeared to be a specific effect.

Further evidence to be presented in detail elsewhere for the dissociation of blastogenesis and effector activity was provided by the separation of the MLC-derived effector cells on a 12-step discontinuous gradient of Ficoll Hypaque (density 1:100–1.050) prepared on an Isco Dialograd model 382 programmed gradient pump. Fractions were analyzed for isotope incorporation, effector capability, and cell size profile using a Coulter model Z plotter. These results indicated that effector-cell activity was initially associated with the fraction of morphologically transformed large dividing cells. With time, however, effector activity became associated with a population of smaller cells with less total mitotic activity.

DISCUSSION

These studies indicate that the cytotoxic effector cells that result from an MLC reaction evolve in a manner analogous to that observed for antibody formation in vivo, with both specificity and total cytotoxicity potential increasing with time. A prediction stemming from this analogy to antibody formation is that at any given point in time the observed cytotoxic effect would be the result of the summation of the individual effects of a heterogeneous population of cells of differing specificity, affinity, and avidity for target-cell antigens. In addition, the development of this heterogeneous population of effector cells is in turn dependent upon cell division. The relationship between MLC and LAC is nevertheless complex and probably dependent either upon multiple precursor subpopulations of cells[10] and/or multiple possible pathways of differentiation for a given cell population. The role of additional modulating populations of cells or their products must also be relevant.

These and other studies[3,4] have also shown that the specificity and effectiveness of these reactions (MLC and LAC) can be titrated by the use of appropriate antibody, which competes for available antigenic determinants or possibly through direct interaction with responding cells per se. Significant differences in the specificity and functional avidity of the cells involved in the two reactions have already been shown.[3,4] In addition, the observation that cross-reacting cytotoxicity was more easily inhibited than specific cytotoxicity is of special interest. This finding is compatible with the involvement of either a more limited number of cells or a population of cells with lower affinity receptors in the cross-reacting vs. direct system. The observation of greater cytotoxicity against specific cytotoxicity compared to third-party or cross-reacting target lymphocytes (Fig. 1) is consistent with either of these possibilities.

Since the antibody involved is polyspecific and may contain activity against SD, LD,[11] or other antigens, the mechanism of suppression is far from clear. However, this technique would permit the analysis of antibody with more limited specificity. In addition, it would permit a more careful dissection of the cell subpopulations involved in the reactions. The use of antibody titrations to inhibit the cellular response, when coupled to more sophisticated methods of subpopulation separation, should, therefore, allow for a fuller understanding of cell-receptor–target-cell interactions in the recognition and effector phases of the immune response.

ACKNOWLEDGMENT

We thank Dr. J. P. Merrill for many suggestions and support, Dr. J. M. Corson for kindly supplying the antibody used in this study, and Ms. R. N. Speer and Rick O'Guin for excellent technical assistance.

REFERENCES

1. Eijsvoogel VP, du Bois R, Melief CJM, et al: Transplant Proc 5:1301, 1973
2. Festenstein J, Démant P: Transplant Proc 5:1321, 1973
3. Phillips SM, Strom TB, Corson JM, et al: Proceedings of the VIIth Leucocyte Culture Conference, 1973, p. 601
4. Phillips SM, Strom TB, Corson JM, et al: Transplant Proc 5:577, 1973
5. Corson JM: Transplantation 10:491, 1970
6. Phillips SM, Carpenter CB, Merrill JP: Cell Immunol 5:235, 1972
7. Brunner KT, Mauel J, Cerottini JC, Chapuis B: Immunology 14:181, 1968
8. Lightbody J, Bernoco D, Miggiano VC, Ceppellini R: Gr Batt Virol Immunol 64: 243, 1971
9. Phillips SM: unpublished observations
10. Feldmann M, Nossal GJV: Transplant Rev 13:3, 1973
11. Bach FH: Transplant Proc 5:23, 1973

The Specificity and the Activation Mechanism of Cell-mediated Lympholysis (CML) in Man

By V. P. Eijsvoogel, M.J.G.J. du Bois, A. Meinesz, A. Bierhorst-Eijlander, W.P. Zeylemaker, and P.Th.A. Schellekens

WE HAVE previously reported CML studies performed in families with children revealing recombination either between the first and second loci of HL-A or between the second locus and the major MLC locus (or loci).[1] These investigations demonstrated that MLC incompatibility between the stimulator and the responder cells (resulting in lymphocyte activation of the latter) is a prerequisite for subsequent cytotoxicity by the responder cell. The specificity of this cytotoxicity, however, was found not to be directed toward the MLC-inducing determinant of the stimulator cell but toward the HL-A antigens (or antigens determined by very closely linked loci) present on the stimulator cell and absent on the responder cell. These data are summarized in Table 1. These findings seem to be in agreement with the studies of Trinchieri et al.[2] regarding CML specificity when investigating combinations of unrelated individuals. By virtue of the presence of children with recombination between the first and second loci of HL-A in the families we studied, we could also investigate whether cytotoxicity would occur on the basis of incompatibilities for only the first locus or only the second locus, respectively.

The antigens of the first series that could be tested in this respect for their immunogenicity in CML (HL-A1, HL-A3, HL-A11, W28) were found to elicit no or only weak cytotoxicity. The antigens of the second series that could be tested in these families (HL-A8, HL-A5, W5) all induced pronounced cytotoxicity. These findings suggested to us that possibly the antigens of the second series are considerably more important targets for the specific destruction in vitro than the antigens of the first series, but since this conclusion was based only upon testing the four above-mentioned antigens of the first series, experiments have been performed between unrelated individuals having either the phenotypes HL-A1, 3, 7, 8 or HL-A1, 2, 7, 8. In MLC-positive combinations between these individuals, the CML test was performed, the results of which are given in Table 2. These data seem to demonstrate the following:

(1) Since in the previous studies HL-A8 was shown to be a good immunogen, the absence of destruction in the 15 combinations tested here of 1.3.7.8 stimulator cells by unrelated 1.3.7.8 responder cells demonstrates a great homogeneity of this antigen for CML, regardless of the fact that all combinations were between unrelated individuals. If the generalization holds that all antigens of the second series are good immunogens, then a similar homogeneity for HL-A7 in these individuals has to be assumed.

(2) As HL-A1 was shown in the previously mentioned studies to be a poor immunogen for CML, if so at all (at least for the responders used in these investigations), no conclusion can be drawn now about its homogeneity in this group of unrelated individuals. The antigen HL-A3, however, could not be tested in our previous family studies.

(3) On the basis of the absence of any significant cytotoxicity in the 1.3.7.8 + 1.3.7.8 combinations, we must postulate either a great homogeneity or a nonimmunogenicity of this antigen as well.

From the Laboratory for Experimental and Clinical Immunology, University of Amsterdam, and the Central Laboratory of the Netherlands Red Cross Blood Transfusion Service, Amsterdam, The Netherlands.

©1973 by Grune & Stratton, Inc.

Table 1. Relationship of HL-A, MLC, and CML

Responder vs. Stimulator Cell: MLC Locus	Responder vs. Stimulator Cell: HL-A Locus	Destruction in CML With Target: Stimulator Cell	Destruction in CML With Target: Third-Party Cell With Following Determinants Common Between Stimulator and Target Cell, but Absent in Responder Cell: MLC Determinants	Destruction in CML With Target: Third-Party Cell With Following Determinants Common Between Stimulator and Target Cell, but Absent in Responder Cell: HL-A Determinants
≠	≠	+(25/25)*	−(0/3)	+(3/3)
≠	=	−(0/3)	−(0/3)	
=	≠	−(0/3)		−(0/2)

=, identical for that particular system; ≠, incompatible for that particular system.
*The number of positive reactions over the total number of combinations tested are within parentheses.

(4) In the five combinations 1.2.7.8 + $1.2.7.8_m$ → 1.2.7.8, two were found to be negative and three revealed cytotoxicity ranging from 8 to 20%. This may indicate specific destruction in some combinations based upon limited heterogeneity and immunogenicity of the antigen HL-A2.

(5) In the 14 combinations of 1.2.7.8 + $1.3.7.8_m$ → 1.3.7.8, the mean cytotoxicity of 1.9% confirms that HL-A3 is indeed a poor immunogen, since it is not recognized and/or destroyed by cells not carrying this determinant.

(6) The significant destruction (mean 20.5%) detectable in the combinations 1.3.7.8 + $1.2.7.8_m$ → 1.2.7.8 clearly demonstrates that the antigen HL-A2 can indeed be a good immunogen. The cytoxicity measured here cannot be explained on the basis of heterogeneity of HL-A7 or HL-A8, since that would have been detected in the previously discussed combinations as well.

These data imply that although some antigens of the first series (HL-A1, HL-A3, HL-A11, W28) are poor immunogens for CML (for the responders tested), other antigens like HL-A2 can clearly elicit cytotoxicity. In the case of the antigen HL-A2, this seems to parallel the in vivo findings of Curtoni et al.[3] In broader sense this seems to indicate that one cannot generalize and say that all antigens of the second series are important in CML and that no antigens of the first series are, but rather that this has to be determined for each antigen separately, taking into account that the findings obtained may well be influenced by the responder cell used as well.

In the studies reported here, very little evidence is obtained in the total of 31 combinations (15 + 14 + 2) for a possible heterogeneity of the antigen HL-A8. In our previous studies[1] in which the (unrelated) parents of one family shared this antigen, we postulated such a heterogeneity based on the fact that cells carrying the HL-A8 of the mother did destroy cells carrying the HL-A8 of the father. (The other haplotype

Table 2. Specific CML Between Unrelated Individuals

Responder Cell	Stimulator Cell	Number of Combinations	% Destruction of Target: 1.**3**.7.8. (n = 6)	% Destruction of Target: 1.**2**.7.8. (n = 4)
1.**3**.7.8.	1.**3**.7.8.	15	1.3	
1.**2**.7.8.	1.**2**.7.8.	5		8.8.
1.**2**.7.8.	1.**3**.7.8.	14	1.9	
1.**3**.7.8.	1.**2**.7.8.	13		20.5

$p < 0.001$ (1.3 vs. 20.5)
$p < 0.001$ (1.9 vs. 20.5)

Only MLC-positive combinations are included and are tested with target cells being the same as the stimulator cell. For further explanation see text.

could not interfere, as it was present in both the stimulator and responder cells.) However, the antigen HL-A8 from the father belonged to the haplotype HL-A2–HL-A8. In view of our new findings, the question must be raised whether the HL-A2 may not have participated in eliciting this cytotoxicity. The heterogeneity of the antigen W5, however, as postulated previously,[1] cannot be explained on the basis of an accompanying first-locus incompatibility.

The conclusion reached in previous studies that MLC activation is a prerequisite for subsequent destruction with the specificity of HL-A (or antigens of closely linked loci) raises the question of whether the MLC-stimulating determinant and the antigen(s) to which the subsequent destruction is directed must be present on the same (stimulator) cell. The family KA, containing the recombinant children, allowed us to study this in more detail. Mixing one responder cell with two different stimulator cells, one of which differs with the responder cell only for MLC (thus by itself only eliciting activation, but no destruction by lack of HL-A incompatibility) and another differing with the responder cell only for HL-A and not for MLC (by itself not eliciting activation, thus excluding subsequent destruction) was found to lead, in this three-cell experiment, to sensitization and to subsequent destruction of the HL-A-incompatible target cell. This seems to indicate that the activating MLC determinant and the antigens to which the subsequent destruction is directed do not necessarily have to be present on the same cell. Similar findings have been made recently in man by Mawas[4] and in mice by Schendel.[5] Festenstein,[6] on the other hand, reported that activation on the basis of M-locus incompatibility does not allow sensitization to and destruction of H-2-incompatible cells. It might be postulated that activation by incompatibilities of the major MLC locus (loci) may represent an allogeneic effect allowing sensitization to antigens present in the culture.

We performed further experiments to investigate whether this phenomenon could be reproduced in a different model. In 1970 we described[7] that lymphocytes treated for 60 min at 45° C maintained their HL-A antigens but lost their MLC-activating capacity. In the experiment shown in Table 3, such heat-treated cells were used as innocent-bystander cells in MLC to investigate whether this would induce additional cytotoxic specificities in the responder cell. The experiments were performed with three different bystander cells, of which the mean destruction (with the range), is given. It should be noted that only heat-treated cells were used in the culture but that normal PHA-transformed cells of the same donor were used as the target. The bystander cells (A^1, A^2, and A^3) were so chosen that $X + Y_m$ did not result in cross-killing of A^1, A^2, or A^3 (mean

Table 3.

Responder Cell	Stimulator Cell	Bystander Cell	MLC Reaction	% Destruction of X	% Destruction of Y	% Destruction of Bystander Cell A*
X	Y_m	–	+	1.6	40.9	4.3 (1.8–6.2)
X	–	A^{*45}	–	0		0 (–3.2–0.8)
X	Y_m	A^{*45}	+	0.1	58.3	20.0 (16.9–22.7)

*Three different bystander cells have been tested, the mean of which is given; 45 means treated for 60 min at 45°C (see text).

destruction of 4.3%). As can be seen, the bystander cells themselves never did induce any destruction (by lack of MLC activation). When, however, the bystander cells were co-cultured with the normal X + Y_m mixture, a clear destruction of bystander cells was found in subsequent CML, suggesting that the mere presence of these cells with their HL-A antigens (or possibly antigens determined by closely linked loci) is sufficient to induce in the responder cell X, in combination with the activation by Y_m, an additional specificity of destruction. This artificial third-cell experiment seems to confirm the above-described genetic third-cell experiment, in both of which one cell type induced the activation while the other presented the specificity for CML.

The induction of CML specificity by an innocent (not MLC-activating) bystander cell also enabled us to investigate whether the activation phase required for CML could also be induced by nonspecific mitogens, such as PHA. So far we have been unable to elicit any cytotoxic potential in cells stimulated with PHA for 6 days at concentrations of 100 μg/ml or 12.5 μg/ml when co-cultured with heat-treated bystander cells. The question can certainly be raised whether the binding of the mitogen by the responder cell may have prevented the subsequent recognition of the antigens on the bystander cell, or that the activation of the effector cell for CML has very specific requirements, such as the cell subpopulation involved or a particular mechanism. Preliminary experiments with stimulation by antigen (PPD and tetanus toxoid) seem to suggest that such activation may allow subsequent CML in the bystander model.

SUMMARY

In CML experiments between unrelated individuals with the phenotypes 1.3.7.8 and 1.2.7.8 it was shown that in contrast to the antigens HL-A3, HL-A1, HL-A11, and W28, which seem to have a very poor immunogenicity for CML, the antigen HL-A2 appears to be a good immunogen. This also indicates that antigens of the first segregant series can elicit specific destruction. No indications were obtained in these studies for a pronounced heterogeneity of the antigens HL-A8 or HL-A7 among unrelated individuals. Furthermore, it was shown in two different models that the MLC-activating determinant and the antigen(s) toward which the CML is directed do not necessarily have to be present on the same (stimulator) cell during the sensitization in MLC. The latter specificity can be provided by a cell that on its own cannot stimulate the responder cell either by virtue of MLC identity (recombinant) or because of heat treatment, which abolishes its MLC-activating capacity but maintains its HL-A antigens. Activation of the responder cell by PHA instead of by a MLC-incompatible cell has so far, in the latter model, not resulted in CML induction.

REFERENCES

1. Eijsvoogel VP, du Bois R, Melief CJM, et al: Transplant Proc 5:1301, 1973

2. Trinchieri G, Bernoco D, Curtoni SE, et al: in Dausset J (ed): Histocompatibility Testing 1972. Copenhagen, Munksgaard, 1973

3. Curtoni ES, Mattiuz PL, Scudeller G: Tissue Antigens 3:108, 1973

4. Mawas et al: Transplant Proc 5:1683, 1973

5. Schendel DJ: Personal communication

6. Festenstein, et al: Transplant Proc 5:1329, 1973

7. Schellekens P Th A, Eijsvoogel VP: Clin Exp Immunol 7:229, 1970

SD vs. LD Antigens as Targets for Lymphocyte-Mediated Cytotoxicity: Study of a Family Presenting a Recombination Event Within the MHR

By G. D. Bonnard,* M. Chappuis, A. Glauser, W. Mempel, P. Baumann, H. Grosse-Wilde, and E. D. Albert

THE separate assessment of cellular proliferation and lymphocyte-mediated cytotoxicity (LMC) at the end of a unidirectional mixed lymphocyte culture (UMLC) reaction in man was described recently.[1,2] The observed LMC was directed against the serologically defined (SD) antigens on the target cells or against sites genetically linked with the major histocompatibility region (MHR).[3] Eijsvoogel[4,5] most clearly defined the relevance of the MHR as the target for LMC by studying two families with children recombinant within the MHR. The lymphocyte-defined (LD) antigens were a prerequisite for cellular proliferation and for the induction of LMC. On the contrary, LD antigens were not the target of the LMC.[4] The SD antigens, more precisely the the SD2 antigens, were established as the target for LMC. These remarkable findings were analyzed in detail, and their possible in vivo correlates were outlined.[4,5]

The present data on the in vitro induction of LMC and on its target were obtained using another family with a recombination event within the MHR. They confirm the preponderant role of the SD region as the target for LMC. The functional dichotomy of the SD and LD antigens was emphasized by the successful induction of LMC with SD antigens and LD antigens present on two different stimulating cells (three-cell experiment).

From the Immunogenetics Laboratory, Hôpital Cantonal Universitaire, Service de Pédiatrie, Lausanne, Switzerland, and the Immunologic Department, Institut für Haematologie der GSF, Munich, West Germany.

**Currently at the Cellular and Tumor Immunology Section, National Cancer Institute, Bethesda, Md.*

Supported by grant 3.695.71 from the Swiss National Foundation for Scientific Research and by Sonderforschungbereich.

©1973 by Grune & Stratton, Inc.

MATERIALS AND METHOD

The recombination event in family L has been presented before.[6] Blood was obtained from sibs M and R and from the recombinant sib W. An unrelated donor E was chosen for sharing the SD2 specificities of the sibs; E had also a SD1 specificity in common with sib M. An unrelated donor F had no known SD identities or cross reactions with the L family. The SD genotypes or phenotypes and the presumed mapping of the LD determinants of the participants in the experiment are shown in Table 1.

The LMC test, involving the sensitizing UMLC, the assessment of thymidine incorporation (TI), the measurement of ^{51}Cr release, and the calculation of the percentages of LMC on the various target cells, was done as described previously.[7] Thymidine incorporation was measured during a 16-hr overnight incubation (day 5 to 6). LMC was assessed twice for most cultures, i.e., on day 5 and again on day 6, with qualitatively the same results. The incubation time was 6 hr. The effector cells were not counted, and LMC tests were done on a per culture basis. On day 6, the effector cells were also tested at dilutions of 1:3 and 1:10.

RESULTS

Table 2 shows the results of TI and LMC on day 6 for the reactions involving the three sibs and the control F. The irradiated stimulating cells are designated here with x. The absence of LD differences between effector cells and stimulating cells (WMx, MWx) was inferred from the absence of TI. In these reactions, no LMC was detected. The presence of LD differences between effector cells and stimulating cells was characterized by high TI, and the results of LMC on the specific target cells depended on the SD difference. In effector cell/target cell combinations with no SD difference

Table 1. Presumed Mapping of the MHR in Sibs* and in Unrelated Controls†

Partners	Presumed Mapping of MHR	Code for the Haplotypes
Sibs		
R	W19–W15–A/11–W5–C	ac
W	W19–W15–A/11–W5–D	ac/d
M	W19–W15–A/3–W5–D	ad
Unrelated		
E	2-W15-X/3-W5-Y	xy
F	1, 12, V, 28, 7, Z	vz

*Genotypes according to Mempel et al.[6]

†The capital letters next to the SD antigens are the presumed LD antigens.

(LD difference only: RWx, WRx), no significant lysis occurred. In effector cell/target cell combinations with a SD difference in addition to the LD difference (RMx, MRx, F, and all others), lysis was readily demonstrable.

Table 2 also gives the results of LMC tested on different target cells having either SD or LD antigens in common with the specific target cells (study of cross lysis). When the target cells were similar for LD only (RMx on W) no lysis occurred. When the target cells were similar for SD only (MRx on W) the lysis was as important as

Table 2. TI and LMC After Various UMLCs

Responding Cells		Stimulating Cells		TI	Dilution of Effector Cells	LMC Percentage of Cytotoxicity			
						R	W	M	F
Partner	Genotype	Partner	Genotype	c.p.m.	Suspension	ac	ac/d	ad	vz
W	ac/d	Mx	ad	442	none	−4.0		2.3	
					1 to 3	−4.0		1.0	
					1 to 10	−0.2		7.2	
M	ad	Wx	ac/d	749	none	3.6	−2.4		
					1 to 3	−1.6	−5.2		
					1 to 10	−4.9	−5.9		
R	ac	Wx	ac/d	10,738	none	0.3	2.4	7.6	
W	ac/d	Rx	ac	8,738	none	0.7		3.7	
					1 to 3	−3.3		7.2	
					1 to 10	−4.9		5.2	
R	ac	Mx	ad	14,072	none		0.0	31.1	
					1 to 3			22.5	
					1 to 10			18.0	
R	ac	Mx + Wx	ad + ac/d	26,204	none		0.1	19.1	
					1 to 3		3.9	13.7	
					1 to 10		6.0	12.1	
M	ad	Rx	ac	13,964	none	47.4	52.1		
					1 to 3	30.8	27.3		
					1 to 10	12.6	17.4		
M	ad	Rx + Wx	ac + ac/d	26,409	none	40.8	38.0		
					1 to 3	29.1	24.8		
					1 to 10	12.1	11.1		
F	vz	Rx	ac	39,450	none	37.7	52.0	36.6	
F	vz	Wx	ac/d	41,302	none	36.4	43.0	32.2	
F	vz	Mx	ad	38,788	none	35.2	30.5	43.0	
R	ac	Fx	vz	55,852	none				80.0
W	ac/d	Fx	vz	37,837	none				65.3
M	ad	Fx	vz	77,671	none				68.4
W	ac/d	Mx + Rx	ad + ac	9,500	none	3.2		26.6	

LMC was assessed on day 6 for 6 hr on a per culture basis with three dilutions of the effector cell suspensions. The mean autokilling was subtracted (i.e., 8.6% for R; 5.9% for W, 1.7% for M, and 5.0% for E).

Table 3. TI and LMC After Various UMLCs

Responding Cells		Stimulating Cells		TI	LMC Percentage of Cytotoxicity				
					R	W	M	E	F
Partner	Genotype	Partner	Genotype	c.p.m.	ac	ac/d	ad	xy	vz
F	vz	Ex	xy	37,044	47.5	28.2	44.5	56.5	3.7
F	vz	Rx	ac	39,450	43.1			33.2	
F	vz	Wx	ac/d	41,302		24.9		39.7	
F	vz	Mx	ad	38,788			33.9	49.5	
E	xy	Rx	ac	21,076	7.0	4.7	0.5	4.3	
E	xy	Wx	ac/d						
E	xy	Mx	ad	20,892	1.5	−2.1	2.7	−4.3	
E	xy	Fx	vz	31,648					31.6
R	ac	Ex	xy	31,608	−1.4	−3.5	19.9	42.4	
W	ac/d	Ex	xy	44,636	2.0	−2.8	26.7	39.5	
M	ad	Ex	xy	50,531	4.4	−1.6	0.6	31.3	
R	ac	Mx + Wx	ad + ac/d	14,072	1.4	−3.4	12.9	14.2	
M	ad	Rx + Wx	ac + ac/d	26,409	20.4	18.5	0.5	4.7	

LMC was assessed here on day 5 for 6 hr on a per culture basis (effector cell/target cell ratio about (100:1). The auto-killings were not subtracted and are also indicated.

on the specific target cells. Finally, in one three-cell experiment, effector cells of the recombinant W were cultured with a mixture of stimulating cells of her two sibs, Mx and Rx. LMC against M (SD difference only) was now demonstrable (26.6% lysis), whereas no lysis against R (LD difference only) could be detected.

Table 3 shows part of the results of TI and LMC done on day 5. In these reactions, E was introduced. E shared with all sibs the phenotypes W15 and W5 at the SD2 locus. The target cells from E were lysed like those from the sibs when the control F was the effector. Further, E did not become cytotoxic to either R or M (W not tested). These findings are in favor of a prevalent role of the SD2 antigens as the target for LMC,[5] but they are not conclusive, as discussed below. Indeed, in mixtures with effector cells from the sibs, target cells from E were lysed. They shared specificities with M but not with R or W.

DISCUSSION

This study of a family with a recombinant child confirmed the main findings of Eijsvoogel.[4,5] The LD antigens were necessary for the induction of LMCs but were not their target. The SD antigens were the obvious target under the conditions of the test. Further analysis on the timing of the cytotoxic responses might provide useful information on the SD and LD antigens as target. In this family, positive LMCs were low at day 5 and high at day 6.

The three-cell experiment suggested that the LD and SD antigens provided two functionally separate stimuli. Similar findings in three-cell experiments have now been reported in man[8-10] and mice.[11] F. Bach et al. have further provided evidence that the LD and SD recognition steps could be due to two different populations of lymphocytes in man.[12] PHA-stimulated blasts are not the best target cells for such experiments, since nothing is known on the relative concentration of SD and LD antigens on the cell surface after this treatment. We could not use fresh lymphocytes as target cells on day 6 because the observed cytotoxicities on PHA blasts were too low on day 5.

Eijsvoogel pointed out the prevalent role of the SD2 antigens as the target for LMC.[5] The present experiments were in favor of the importance of the SD2 antigens (Table 3 when F or E respond). However, the haplotypes 11–W5 of R or W and 3–W5 of M were distinct targets. The presence of HL-A3 in M and E cells, which cross-reacted, suggested a possible role for the SD1 antigens as target or co-target in this particular family. This prevented us from drawing any conclusion as to the heterogeneity or identity of the W5 specificities on the c or d haplotype in this family. For this reason, the precise location of the crossing-over remained unclear. This point is presently under study.

SUMMARY

The target of in vitro–induced lymphocyte-mediated cytotoxicity was studied using cells of a family presenting a recombination event within the MHR. The LD antigens were necessary for the induction of LMC, but the SD antigens were the obvious target under these experimental conditions. In a three-cell experiment the LD antigens of a sib effectively triggered the recombinant to respond toward the SD antigens of the other sib. The present data did not allow any conclusion as to the relative importance of SD2 and SD1 specificities as target for LMC.

ACKNOWLEDGMENT

We thank Dr. M. Jeannet, Histocompatibility and Transplantation Unit, Geneva, for typing the controls E and F, and Prof. E. Gautier, head of the Pediatric Department, Lausanne, for constant support.

REFERENCES

1. Lightbody JJ, Bernoco D, Miggiano VC, Ceppellini R: G Batt Virol Immunol 64:243, 1971

2. Bonnard GD, Lemos L: Transplant Proc 4:177, 1972

3. Miggiano VC, Bernoco D, Lightbody JJ, et al: Transplant Proc 4:231, 1972

4. Eijsvoogel VP, du Bois MJGJ, Melief CJM, et al: Histocompatibility Testing 1972 (in press)

5. Eijsvoogel VP, du Bois R, Melief CJM, et al: Transplant Proc 5:1301, 1973

6. Mempel W, Albert E, Burger A: Tissue Antigens 2:250, 1972

7. Bonnard GD, Lemos L, Chappuis M: Scand J Immunol (in press)

8. Eijsvoogel VP: personal communication, 1973

9. Eijsvoogel VP, et al: Transplant Proc 5:1675, 1973

10. Mawas C, et al: Transplant Proc 5:1683, 1973

11. Schendel DJ, Alter BJ, Bach FH: Transplant Proc 5:1651, 1973

12. Bach FH, Segall M, Zier KS, et al: Science 180:403, 1973

Cell-mediated Lympholysis (CML) in the Absence of LD2 Mixed Lymphocyte Reaction and CML in the Presence of SD1–SD2 Identity in Two HL-A-genotyped Families

By C. Mawas, M. Sasportes, Y. Christen, A. Bernard, J. Dausset, B. J. Alter, and M. L. Bach

THE operational meaning of three types of unconventional MLR activation in the in vitro generation of cytotoxic effectors was investigated using HL-A genotyped families where the father and the mother share one identical HL-A haplotype. The results of the unexpected MLR in two of these families are presented and discussed in another article in this issue.[1] A third family, with an LD2 recombinant outside SD2, already published,[2] is included in our CML study. Therefore, besides the LD2 MLR activation, three uncommon types of lymphocyte activation were studied in the CML assay: (1) positive MLR between SD–LD2 heterozygous cells responding against SD–LD2 homozygous cells; (2) borderline positive MLR between two SD–LD2 heterozygous cells, SD–LD2 phenotypically identical between them; (3) positive MLR between cells identical for SD and negative MLR against different SD in a case of LD2 recombinant.

The data are largely in agreement with mouse[3] and human data,[4] but provide additional facts: (1) a positive MLR may not be a prerequisite for the generation of CML cytotoxic effectors in certain conditions; (2) specificities physically linked or not linked to SD1 and SD2 may be suitable CML targets; (3) any positive MLR reaction may provide a nonspecific event that acts as a starter for the generation of cytotoxic effectors toward SD-different target cells.

From the Laboratoire d'Immuno-Hematologie, INSERM U93, Institut de Recherches sur les Maladies du Sang, Hôpital Saint-Louis, Paris, France, and the Department of Pediatrics, University of Wisconsin, Madison, Wisc.

Supported in part by grant AI-CA-9293, National Institutes of Health, Bethesda, Md.

B. Alter is a recipient of a fellowship of Le Ministère des Affaires Etrangères, France.

M. L. Bach is a Faculty Research Awardee of the American Cancer Society.

© 1973 by Grune & Stratton, Inc.

MATERIALS AND METHOD

Family Col (No. 0110), Fig. 1. The father A (a^Fb) and the mother B (a^Md) share the haplotype a (HL-A1,8); b is W32,W10 and d is W23,HL-A12. Sibs D and E (a^Mb) are phenotypically identical to the father (a^Fb); sib C is homozygous for the haplotype HL-A1,8 (a^F a^M). The immunization schedule of A by D and the skin graft survival of D, E, and C on A is described in an accompanying article.[1] CML studies were performed 40 mo after the last immunization.

Family Le (No. 0225). Father A (a^Fb) and mother B (a^Md) share the haplotype HL-A3,7; b is HL-A2,12 and d is W24,X. Sibs C and D are homozygous (a^Fa^M) for the haplotype HL-A3,7. Sib E (a^Mb) is phenotypically identical to his father A (a^Fb), and sib F (a^Fc) is phenotypically identical to his mother. Furthermore, MLR data between the mother B and sibs F, C, and D are consistent with an LD2 recombinant in sib F, who therefore behaves as LD2 homozygous, like sibs C and D. The immunization schedule of the father A can be found in the accompanying paper.[1]

Family Ba (no. 0168). The father A (ab) is W28,W14/W30,HL-A13; the mother B (cd) is HL-A2,W10/HL-A3,W5. Sib D is the recombinant shown in Fig. 2; a crossing-over between the paternal LD2 rendered sib D LD2-identical to sib E, although SD-different; sibs D and E, although SD-identical, are LD2-different.

The CML test was performed according to Lightbody et al.,[5] but adapted to a micromethod.[3] In short, the sensitization phase was done according to the MLR microtechnique described by Hartzman et al.[6] After Ficoll Hypaque purification, 1–2 × 10^5 peripheral blood lymphocytes were cultivated with 4 × 10^5 mitomycin-C-treated stimulating lymphocytes (25 μg/ml, 30 min at 37°C). To a triplicate of each combination, ^{3}H-thymidine was added 16 hr before the termination of the culture; MLR were harvested by precipitation with a microprecipitator (Otto-Hiller, Madison, Wisc.). Results are expressed as mean c.p.m. Cells to be used as effector cells in CML

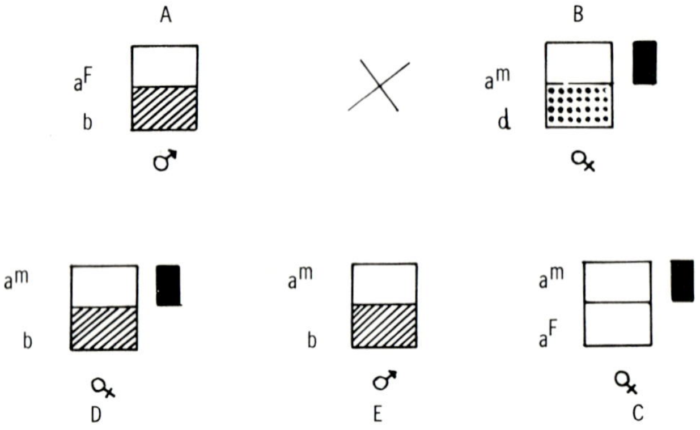

Fig. 1. Family Col. Distribution in the family of the additional maternal determinant, which is different from SD1 and SD2 (HL-A1,8). The white boxes stand for the shared haplotype HL-A1,8; the paternal haplotype is designed a^F and the maternal a^M. The black rectangle stands for the additional maternal specificity and is outside the HL-A1,8 haplotype because it may or may not be coded for by the HL-A chromosome.

were collected, pooled, and adjusted to 0.7–1 × 10^7 trypan blue negative lymphocytes per milliliter. Target cells were prepared on the same day as the MLR cultures; 10 × 10^6 were cultured in a Falcon bottle (No. 3020) at a concentration of 1 × 10^6/ml). After 3 days PHA M (Gibco No. R150576) was added to each bottle at a final concentration of 1:100.

On the day of the CML test, targets were incubated in 1 ml of the PHA culture medium with 200 μCi of ^{51}Cr (C.E.A., Saclay, France) for 1 hr at 37°C. After three washes, they were adjusted to a concentration of 1 × 10^5 trypan blue negative lymphoblasts per milliliter. The CML test was performed in round-bottom Linbro microplates No. IS.MCR-96TC, usually in triplicate samples, consisting of 0.7–1 × 10^6 effector cells and 1 × 10^4 target cells in a total volume of 0.2 ml. Controls consisted always of autologous combination on autologous target cells and/or spontaneous release of target cells in the absence of effector cells. After 4 hr at 37°C, 0.05 ml of medium was added to all wells, except to the maximum release determined by freeze-thawing (3×). The plates were centrifugated at 800 g for 10 min; the supernatants were collected in tubes and counted in an Intertechnic gamma counter. Results were calculated as

$$\frac{\text{experimental release} - \text{spontaneous release}}{\text{total release} - \text{spontaneous release}} \times 100$$

and expressed as percentage of specific cytotoxicity. Bicarbonate-buffered RPMI-1640 medium supplemented with 20% human plasma heat-inactivated (56°C, 30 min) was used in all MLR sensitization; MEM (F14, Gibco) supplemented with 20% human plasma heat-inactivated and buffered with Tris was used for the CML test.[4]

RESULTS

Family Col (No. 0110). Table 1 shows that when the combination ABm is tested on target C, the homozygous child, there is a positive CML (16.3% cytotoxicity). This indicates that A has become sensitized to a maternal determinant that is present on C. The fact that ABm is also cytotoxic for D (a^Mb) indicates that D also carries this determinant. However, E (who types identically to D) is affected weakly by the ABm cytotoxic effectors and therefore is totally

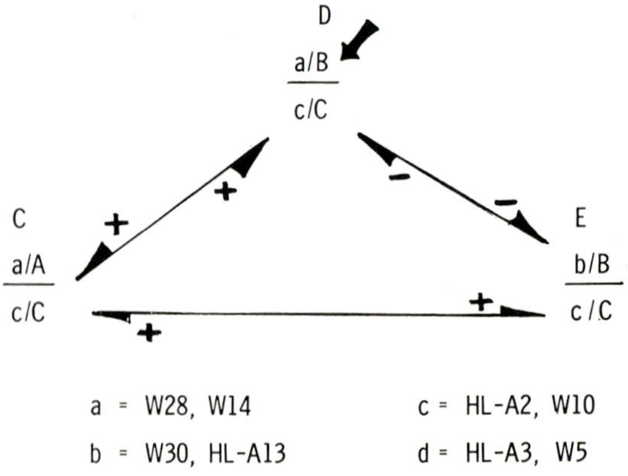

Fig. 2. Family Ba. An LD2 recombinant outside SD1 and SD2. The capital letter following the haplotype represents the LD2 determinant. The arrows point toward the stimulating cell; if the combination responder–stimulator is MLR-positive, the arrow indicates plus; if negative, the arrow indicates minus.

Table 1. Family Co. CML Testing a^F Versus a^M (and Vice Versa) on the Homozygous Cell a^F/a^M, Through a positive LD2 MLR.

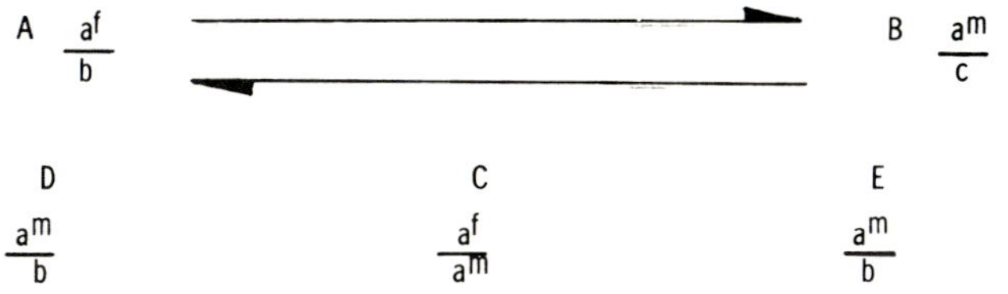

M.L.R. Index	Test Combination	PERCENT CYTOTOXICITY ON TARGETS: A	B	C	D	E	T
42	ABm	−3.7	14.3	16.3	17.5	3.1	N.D.
70	BAm	23.8	−5.0	−19.0	16.7	14.5	14.0
160	TAm	54.7	37.5	22.7	48.9	47.1	6.9
140	TBm	52.2	45.0	46.1	47.7	50.5	7.9

A, father; B, mother; C, homozygous child for the HL-A haplotype 1,8; D and E, phenotypically HL-A-identical to the father A; T, unrelated control. The results are expressed as percentage of specific ^{51}Cr release.

or partly lacking this determinant. The combination BAm, on the contrary, is not cytotoxic to C but is equally cytotoxic to D and E, when the b haplotype is the target of the effector cells. There is, therefore, no abnormal resistance to lysis of the E target cell. In summary, the maternal cells have a determinant that appears to segregate independently of the a^M haplotype (ABm/D vs. ABm/E); this determinant elicits cytotoxic effectors only when A is the responding cell but not when E is the responding cell. This determinant may or may not be located on the HL-A chromosome. In the combination ABm, the MLR activation is secondary to a LD2 incompatibility.

Table 2 demonstrates that the unexpected MLR response of A to the homozygous child C is capable of generating cytotoxic effectors to the maternal determinant present on target cells B, C, and D but not on E. In this combination, although the MLR is probably not due to a LD2 gene activation, cytotoxic effectors are nevertheless generated. The meaning of such findings will be discussed below, as will the absence of cytotoxic effectors in the combination ECm.

Although both D and E have received the HL-A haplotype a^M from their mother and are therefore phenotypically identical to the father, they behave differently in the CML test, both as target and stimulating cells (Table 3). The combination ADm (borderline positive in MLR) generates highly cytotoxic effectors toward the maternal determinant present on cells B, C, and D, while only a slight cytotoxicity can be seen on target E. AEm, however (MLR-negative), does not generate cytotoxic cells against any of the family-member cells.

These last data, combined with the preceding results, demonstrate clearly that D possesses a maternal determinant that segregates with the a^M haplotype in D and C but not in E. This determinant does not seem to have a MLR ability by itself (ECm is MLR-negative, as is EDm) but is highly efficient as target for cytotoxic effectors. The determinant may be or may not be linked to the HL-A haplotype. In this family, cytotoxic effectors are generated independently of the level of MLR activation.

Family Le (No. 0225). As can be seen in Tables 4 and 5, combinations ABm,

Table 2. Family Co. CML Testing a^F Versus a^M (As Well as a^M Versus a^F) on the Homozygous Cell a^F/a^M, Through a Negative LD2 MLR

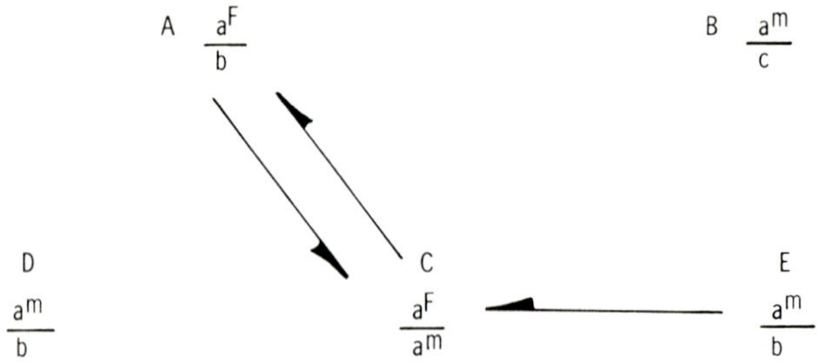

M.L.R. Index	Test Combination	A	B	C	D	E	T
		PERCENT CYTOTOXICITY ON TARGETS:					
10	ACm	2.0	21.0	15.1	26.3	4.8	2.6
2.6	ECm	N.D.	-6.5	-10.8	1.7	-0.1	2.8
115	CAm	15.2	5.2	1.2	17.0	15.0	N.D.

Table 3. Family Co. CML Testing a^F Versus a^M (and Vice Versa) Through a Negative LD2 MLR.

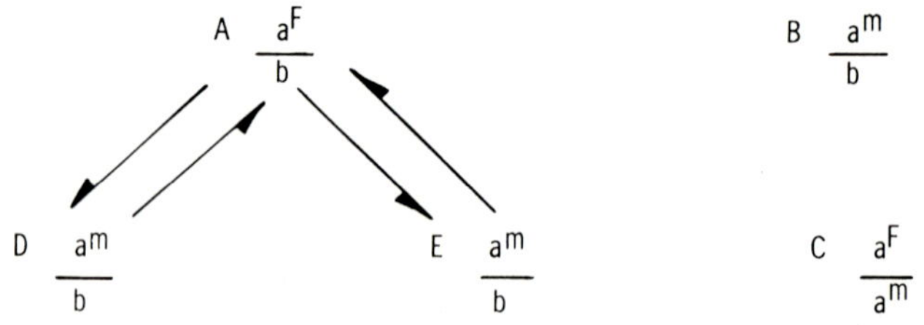

M.L.R. Index	Test Combination	A	B	C	D	E	T
		PERCENT CYTOTOXICITY ON TARGETS:					
3.0	ADm	-5.0	14.7	12.6	21.3	8.7	3.3
4.3	AEm	0.7	-4.2	-12.3	6.1	3.4	1.8
42	ABm	-3.7	14.3	16.3	17.5	3.1	N.D.
10	ACm	2.0	21.0	15.1	26.3	4.8	2.6
2.4	DAm	1.0	-1.5	-3.2	3.0	0.8	2.1
0.9	EAm	2.5	-1.7	-10.6	1.3	0.8	5.5
70	BAm	23.8	-5.0	-19.0	16.7	14.5	14.0

Summary for the evidences that D expresses a maternal determinant absent (or greatly reduced) on E. The boxes show the strikingly different immune lysis of D as compared to E, when the father A cells are sensitized by the mother B or sibs C and D. In contrast, sibs E and D have an identical immune lysis when the effector cells are sensitized toward the haplotype b.

Table 4. Family Le. CML Testing a^F Versus a^M (and Vice Versa) through a Positive LD2 and a Negative LD2 MLR

Test Combination	MLR Index	Targets: A a/A^F / b/B	B a/A^M / d/D	C a/A^F / a/A^M	D a/A^F / a/A^M	E a/A^M / b/B	F d/A^M / a/A^F
ABm	21.2	0.2	23	4.7	0.6	2.7	38.5
ACm	1.2	0.4	−1.9	1.3	0.6	0.6	1.2
ADm	10.0	−0.9	−6.8	1.9	1.6	1.0	−1.7
AEm	1.0	−2.2	−9.1	0	−6.2	−2.0	−2.3
AFm	1.6	−1.8	3.6	0.5	−1.5	−0.9	4.1
TCm	107	11.6	4.2	36.0	44.7	9.0	16.1
TDm	96.6	13.1	6.0	28.2	28.0	20.9	6.9

A, father; B, mother; C and D, HL-A-homozygous sibs; E, HL-A phenotypically identical to mother B, but LD2-recombinant; therefore sibs C, D, and F are LD2-identical and -homozygous; T, unrelated control. A capital letter beside the HL-A haplotype stands for the LD2 locus. Results are expressed as percentage of specific ^{51}Cr release.

BAm, ACm, ADm, AEm, and AFm do not generate cytotoxic effectors to the homozygous cells C and D, despite a MLR activation in combination ABm and ADm.

Because of the LD2 recombinant in sib F, who is therefore LD2-identical to sibs C and D but SD-different, a third-man experiment was performed. The activation of C was provided by the cells from sib E, thus permitting the bypassing of the absence of MLR activation of C by F. As can be seen, neither CEm (MLR-positive) nor CFm (MLR-negative) is cytotoxic toward F; however, in combination, CFm Em becomes cytotoxic to F; C therefore has become able to generate cytotoxic effectors to F through the MLR activation provided by Em. An allogeneic cell combination, TCm or TDm, much more efficiently kills the homozygous cells C and D than the heterozygous cells for the haplotype shared by A and B.

Family Ba (No. 0168). As can be seen in Table 6, DEm (MLR-negative) does not generate cytotoxic effectors to target E, although D and E are SD-different. However, in the combination DCm Em, where Cm provides a MLR activation of D, D generates cytotoxic effectors to the haplotype b present on E (bc). In two experiments, the combination DCm was found cytotoxic for itself. As in family Le, it was possible to bypass, by a third-party cell, the absence of MLR between D and E, thus

Table 5. Family Le. CML With a Third-Party Cell E Allowing Sensitization Despite Absence of LD2 Activation Between Responding Cell C and Sensitizing Cell F, SD-different From C

MLR Index	Test Combination	Targets: A a/A^F / b/B	B a/A^M / d/D	C a/A^F / a/A^M	D a/A^F / a/A^M	E a/A^M / b/B	F d/A^M / a/A^F
4	CDm	3.5	−6.1	0	0.9	3.6	2.8
1.64	DCm	0.7	−7.1	1.7	0.3	3.0	−1.7
12	CEm	4.35	−1.9	−0.8	−0.6	8.9	−0.4
1.4	CFm	−4.3	−11.8	0	−6.3	3.0	−5.6
	CFm Em	6.0	−1.6	2.1	4.9	9.2	4.4
	CDm Em	9.7	−6.1	1.3	3.7	9.7	5.8
23.52	FBm	2.9	−4.5	4.8	5.0	7.4	6.9
107	TCm	11.6	4.2	36.0	44.7	9.0	16.1
96.6	TDm	13.1	6.0	28.2	28.0	20.9	6.9

Neither combination CEm (MLR-positive and SD-identical) nor CFm (MLR-negative but SD-different) is cytotoxic to target F. However, CFm Em becomes cytotoxic toward target F.

Table 6. Family Ba. Another Example of Sensitization of a Responding Cell Toward a Stimulating Cell, SD-different but LD2-identical to the Responding Cell, by an LD2 Recombinant Through a Third-Party Cell Providing LD2 Activation

M.L.R. Index #1	M.L.R. Index #2	Test Combination		A a/A / b/B	B c/C / d/D	C a/A / c/C	D a/B / c/C	E b/B / c/C	T x/X / y/Y
91	80	CDm	#1	-8.5	-2.1	-2.1	-3.7	1.8	-0.6
			#2	-9.2	2.3	2.2	5.8	5.0	-5.1
90	34	DCm	#1	1.1	13.9	8.6	9.3	7.2	2.3
			#2	4.6	8.3	13.4	7.8	13.4	-0.2
4.4	1.6	DEm	#1	-6.8	N.D.	-6.6	-4.1	-2.3	-0.3
			#2	-2.7	0	5.2	0.9	8.3	0.3
106	42	DCm Em	#1	24.8	19.4	9.9	9.4	30.1	8.3
			#2	45.4	23.5	22.1	16.7	54.0	0.3

(Columns A–T are TARGETS.)

Nos. 1 and 2 stand for two successive experiments. The capital letter beside the haplotype represents the LD2 locus. A, father; B, mother; C, D, and E are the children; D is the paternal LD2 recombinant; D and E are, therefore, LD2-identical but SD-different; C and D are LD2-different but SE-identical; T, unrelated control. In the boxes it can be seen that D becomes sensitized to the haplotype b of the cell E only when co-cultivated with both Cm and Em.

allowing D to generate cytotoxic effectors toward the SD-different cell E, SD2-identical to D.

DISCUSSION

Neither MLR nor HL-A typing is entirely predictive of the fate of a given graft in man. Phenotypically identical HL-A sibs who are MLR-negative do reject skin grafts, although less rapidly than unrelated grafts.[2] HL-A-identical sibs who are MLR-negative can develop GvH reaction after bone marrow grafting.[7] So far, in humans it has been shown that CML can develop only when there is a positive MLR and a difference of the SD antigens between the responding and the stimulating cells.[4] It is also apparent that SD-different but LD2-identical cells cannot generate cytotoxic effectors in vitro;[3] however, a third-party cell accurately chosen to activate the MLR but not to allow sensitization to SD determinants present on the SD MLR-negative target cell allows the bypassing of the absence of MLR between two cells, SD-different but LD2-identical.[3,8]

The data on family Col provide the first evidence that a specificity coded for by the HL-A chromosome or another chromosome may be the target of CML effectors (Fig. 1). If linked to HL-A, this specificity is entirely included in the HL-A1,8 haplotype of the father (BAm is not cytotoxic for the homozygous cell); it may therefore be an additional specificity located outside SD1 or SD2 at a recombinant distance on the maternal chromosome. If not linked to HL-A, this specificity is present in the mother B and has segregated only in sibs C and D but not in sib E. This antigen may well be serologically definable. As stated in Materials and Method, during the immunization of A by D a leukoagglutinin as well as a weak cytotoxic antibody appeared in the serum of the father A. This leukoagglutinin was positive against 89 unrelated cells out of 108 tested with apparently no HL-A correlation.[2] Family studies are underway to further clarify this specificity.

Data in family Co provide nuances to the generally accepted rules in regard to the CML test, as defined both in mouse[3] and man.[4,8] Cytotoxic effectors in this family were generated apparently independently of the level of MLR activation. No difference can be seen in the lysis of the target C with combination ABm (MLR index 42.0), ACm (MLR index 10.0), or ADm (MLR index 3.0). Furthermore, if the ABm activation is clearly provided through an LD2 incompatibility, this is not the case for ACm nor for ADm. Apparently only A generates cytotoxic effectors to the additional maternal specificity, while combinations ECm and EDm are not cytotoxic for the targets C and B. The only difference between A and E (who should not both express this maternal determinant) is essentially due to the status of immunization of A toward D. The combination of an extensive preimmunization of A by D and the presence of an additional specificity on D made possible the generation of cytotoxic cells toward the maternal determinant in the absence of an in vitro MLR. This suggests that in a secondary response, provided there is an additional specificity on the sensitizing cell, a positive MLR is no longer a prerequisite for a positive CML test. To clearly demonstrate or exclude this possibility, we intend to immunize E by C, D, or B, and to follow the behavior of ECm or EDm in CML, E should became cytotoxic to D without a positive MLR if our hypothesis should stand valid.

In family Le, the negativity of the various combinations testing a^F vs. a^M (and vice versa) on the homozygous cells may be related either to the absence of an additional specificity between the shared haplotype or to the less extensive immunization of A.

In families Le and Ba, the LD2 recombinant allows the testing, in the CML assay, of the two following combinations: SD identity with LD2 differences and SD differences with LD2 identity. In each family, no cytotoxic effectors are generated by these combinations. However, an additional family cell, LD2-different to the responding cell, allows the responding cell to become sensitized to a SD-different but LD2-identical cell. These data are identical to those already found in mouse[3] and man.[8]

From the data discussed here, it appears that the CML assay in immunized families provides biologic informations far beyond that collected from the MLR or CML in unimmunized families. Specificities that may be relevant to transplantation but to date are not definable by serotyping or by CML in the absence of preimmunization can be detected by an in vitro test and parallel in vivo data where skin grafts between HL-A phenotypically identical related individuals are rejected, although less quickly than between nonidentical sibs. In the future, a valuable in vitro test should be developed to allow the detection of such specificities, even in the absence of an LD2 activation.

SUMMARY

The data herein presented provide mainly three types of evidence: (1) a positive MLR may not be a prerequisite for the generation of cytotoxic effectors, and types of activation other than LD2 may be as efficient for a positive CML; (2) specificities different from SD1 or SD2 may provide an efficient target to CML effectors; (3) MLR activation is not required to be specific to allow sensitization toward SD antigens.

REFERENCES

1. Sasportes M, Mawas C, Bernard A, et al: Transplant Proc 5:1517, 1973

2. Sasportes M, Lebrun A, Rapaport FT, Dausset J: Transplant Proc 4:209, 1972

3. Alter BJ, Schendel DJ, Bach ML, et al: J Exp Med 137:1303, 1973

4. Eijsvoogel VP, Dubois MJGJ, Melief CH, et al: in: Histocompatibility Testing 1972, p 501

5. Lightbody JJ, Bernoco O, Miggiano VC, Ceppellini R: J Bacteriol Virol Immunol 64:243, 1971

6. Hartzman RJ, Segall M, Bach ML, Bach FM: Transplantation 2:268, 1971

7. Graw RG Jr, Leventhal BG, Yankee RA, et al: Transplant Proc 3:405, 1971

8. Eijsvoogel VP, Dubois MJGJ, Melief CH, et al: Transplant Proc 5:1301, 1973

Cell-mediated Cytotoxicity Toward Human Lymphocytes: Comparison Between In Vivo Immunization and In Vitro Sensitization

By C. Mawas, Y. Christen, L. Legrand, and J. Dausset

SINCE Eijsvoogel et al.[1] have shown that after skin grafting and/or subcutaneous human leukocyte injections, cytotoxic effectors appear in the peripheral blood of the human recipient, a methodology has been available to follow planned immunization in human volunteers, both in terms of humoral immunity and cellular immunity. Furthermore, it is possible (1) to study the specificity of the effector cells in relation to SD determinants; (2) to check if humoral cross-reactivities could also be found at the cellular level; (3) to compare the spectrum of the cullular vs. the humoral killing; and finally (4) to compare whether or not in vivo immunization and in vitro sensitization through the CML assay would generate cytotoxic effectors to the same determinants. This report deals with our preliminary results.

MATERIALS AND METHOD

Recipient A and donor B were two healthy brothers of known HL-A genotype. A was W24, W18/W26, HL-A5, and B was W32, W27/W26, HL-A5. A received 150×10^6 lymphocytes from B on March 12, 1973, according to a previously described technique.[2] Three control donors from our panel were used; they were T1 = HL-A1, 3, 8, W18; T2 = HL-A3, 7; T3 = W31, HL-A8, HL-A2, W10. Following these initial results, a second set of unrelated targets were chosen according to their positivity or negativity toward the recipient serum. The following cells were used: (A) Cells killed by the recipient serum: X1 = B = W32, W27/W26, HL-A5; X2 = HL-A1, W32, HL-A12; X3 = W28, W30, W18, W22; X4 = T1 = HL-A1, 8, 3, W18; X5 = W23, W28, HL-A12, W27; X6 = HL-A1,W32,HL-A7; (B) Cells not killed by the recipient serum: X7 = HL-A3,W24,HL-A12,W22. It should be noticed that cells X3 and X4 (T1) gave an unexpected positivity according to present knowledge in HL-A cross-reactivities.

The technique used for the direct cytotoxic assay of the peripheral blood lymphocytes has been described by Eijsvoogel et al.[1] In short, the lymphocytes were separated through a Ficoll Hypaque gradient. Effector cells were washed and adjusted to a concentration of 2×10^7 cells per milliliter. Target cells were prepared as follows: 3 days prior to the test, 10×10^6 cells in 10 ml of medium were cocultivated with PHA M (Difco No. RIS057) at a final concentration of 1:100. The PHA-transformed cells are collected on the test day, washed, and labeled with 100 μCi of ^{51}Cr (C.E.A., France, 1 mCi per ml; specific activity between 150 and 400) in a total volume of 1 ml for 1 hr at 37°C with occasional shaking. After two washes the cells were resuspended at a concentration of 2×10^5 per milliliter.

Each test was performed in triplicate (or duplicate). In a plastic hemolysis tube, 0.5 ml of effector cells (1×10^7) were mixed with 0.5 ml of target cells (1×10^5). Before incubation they were spun down for 2 min at 800 g. Incubation was then allowed for 4 hr at 37°C. The reaction was ended by a 10-min centrifugation at 800 g; 0.5 ml of the supernatant was collected in another plastic tube and each pellet and supernatant were counted in a gamma counter (Intertechnique, France, CG 30). The maximum release was determined by freeze-thawing three times with distilled water. Control release was always calculated both as spontaneous release of the target cell alone and release in the presence of the autologous effector cell. Whenever a discrepancy was present between these two controls, the release in the presence of the autologous control was used. Results were expressed as percentage specific release:

$$\left(\frac{\text{c.p.m. test supernatant}}{\text{c.p.m. test (pellet + supernatant)}} - \frac{\text{c.p.m. control supernatant}}{\text{c.p.m. control (pellet + supernatant)}}\right) \times 100$$

MEM Gibco F14 buffered with Tris containing 20% AB plasma was used throughout all the experiments.

Serologic studies of the recipient serum were performed by one of us (L.L.) according to techniques

From the Laboratoire d'Immuno-Hématologie, INSERM U93, Institut de Recherches sur les Maladies du Sang, Hôpital Saint-Louis, Paris, France.

Supported in part by grant A1-CA-9293, National Institutes of Health, Bethesda, Md.

© 1973 by Grune & Stratton, Inc.

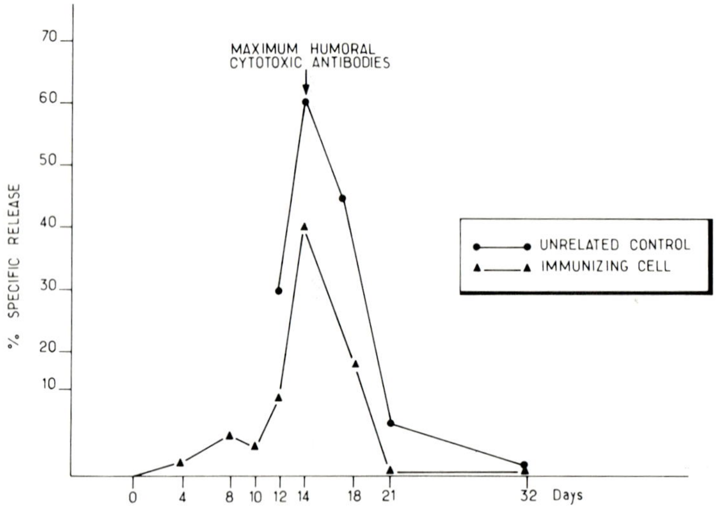

Fig. 1. Kinetics of cellular response of recipient A to his brother B. Immunization between HL-A-haploidentical sibs W32, W27/W26, 5 → W24, W18/W26, 5. Fresh recipient cells (1 × 10^7 in 0.5 ml) were incubated 4 hr at 37°C with either 1 × 10^5 in 0.5 ml donor cells or control cells, both of them labeled with ^{51}Cr. Results are expressed as percentage of specific release, i.e., test release minus release from an unimmunized control (the same for each day tested) corrected for the maximum release.

previously described.[2] Detailed data will be the object of a specific paper (L.L., manuscript in preparation). The CML assay was performed according to the technique of Lightbody and Bach,[3] modified by Alter et al.,[4] with an in vitro sensitization done using the technique of Hartzmann et al.[5] The technique used has already been described in the preceding paper.[6]

RESULTS

Figure 1 describes the kinetics of the response of recipient A to his brother B. The spike of this primary response was found on day 14, and cytotoxic effectors were not more detectable against B target cells 3 wk following immunization. An unexpected result was found with the unrelated control T1 who shares no HL-A specificities and who has no known cross-reactivity antigens with the B haplotype. Cytotoxic effectors from A were not cytotoxic to T1 before the immunization, and after 3 wk no cytotoxic effectors could be found against T1. Therefore the cytotoxicity of A to T1 was in relation to the immunization of A by B, and its knietics were parallel to the cytotoxicity of A toward B.

Table 1 further studies the specificity of the killing induced by A following immunization of B. There is no autologous kill; only the cell T2 (HL-A3, 7) seems to be unaffected by the A effector cells. T1 (unimmunized control) is negative toward all five target cells.

Table 1. Specificity of Effector Cells on Day 18

EFFECTORS	TARGETS				
	A	B	T_1	T_2	T_3
	W24, W18, / W26, HL-A5	W32, W27, / W26, HL-A5	HL-A1, 3, / HL-A8, W18	HL-A3, 7	W31, HL-A8 / HL-A2, W10
A	- 2	17	45	6	10
T_1	- 4.5	2.5	2	- 1	- 9

A, recipient; B, donor; T1, T2, T3, unrelated controls unimmunized. T_1 genotype should be read HL-A1,8/3,W18

Results are expressed as percentage of specific ^{51}Cr release.

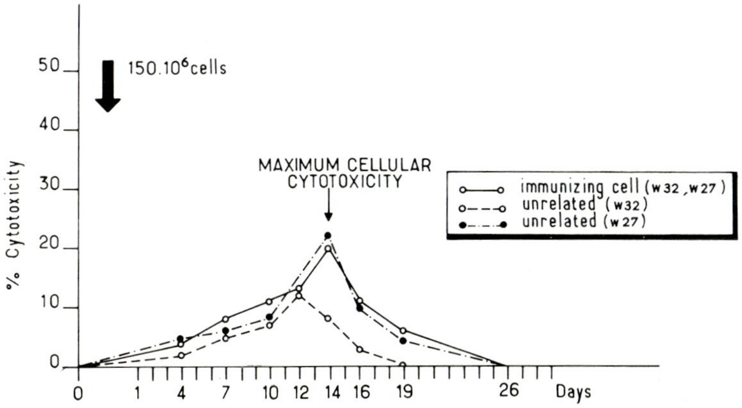

Fig. 2. Kinetics of humoral response of recipient A to his brother B. Immunization between HL-A-haploidentical sibs W32, W27/W26, 5 → W24, W18/W26, 5. Humoral response. The results are expressed as percentage of 2,000 cells in 1 μl killed by 5 μl of the immune serum undiluted; 5 μl undiluted rabbit C was used. Viability was assessed by the absorbed trypan blue vital dye.

Figure 2 describes the kinetics of the appearance of the humoral response against both W32 and W27. The spike of the humoral response is parallel to the cellular response but very weak (less than 20% of 2,000 cells/μl are killed by 5 μl of undiluted serum from A). It can therefore be concluded that T1 possesses a specificity that is a good target for the A cytotoxic effectors and that this specificity (or specificities) was not serologically predictable from the HL-A typing. It may be a cross-reactive antigen to W32 or W27 or a shared factor or a specificity different from SD1 and SD2, either linked or not linked to HL-A; only further studies will demonstrate this fact.

Table 2 further confirms the weakness of this antiserum, which by day 14 is unable to block the cytotoxicity of A for B or T1. Furthermore, this serum does not induce an antibody-mediated lymphocytotoxicity in 4 hr (nor in 15 hr—data not shown).

Table 3 summarizes CML data where the test combination was ABm and compares the data obtained on a panel of target cells by in vivo immunization (both at the humoral and cellular level) to the in vitro sensitization. As can be seen, the HL-A typing was predictive only of the CML data; both the day-14 effector cells from A and the recipient serum are cytotoxic for targets X3 and X4 (which should be neutral according to the HL-A typing); on the contrary, the CML results totally parallel the HL-A typing. Only one cell, X7, remains entirely negative for the three different immune effectors. SD1 and SD2 antigens are good targets for direct cytotoxicity or CML effectors.

Table 2. Day-14 Cytotoxicity of Recipient Peripheral Blood Lymphocytes in Presence of Day-14 Immune Serum

EFFECTORS			TARGETS B	TARGETS T_1
		Medium only	40	59
A	+	Serum A day 14	36	57
		Medium only	7	5
T_1	+	Serum day 14	2	6

Target cells were incubated with the day-14 immune serum at a final dilution of 1:10 or with medium, 1 hr at 37°C, followed by three washes. Effector cells were then added for 4 hr to the preincubated target cells.

Results are expressed as percentage of ^{51}Cr release corrected for the maximum release.

DISCUSSION

These results are confirmatory of the work of Eijsvoogel et al.[1] showing the feasibility of measuring the recipient cellular cytotoxicity against the donor cells after a skin graft and/or lymphocyte injection. Three additional facts can be seen in this work:

(1) To date, HL-A typing is not sufficient to predict whether a given target cell will be negative in regard to effectors cells drawn from a recipient peripheral blood after in

Table 3. Comparison of Specificity of Immune Killing Between In Vivo Effectors (Humoral and Cellular) and In Vitro CML Effectors

HL-A Typing	W32, W27 W26,HL-A5	HL-A1, W32 HL-A12	W28, W30 W18, W22	HL-A1,HL-A8 HL-A3,W18	W23, W28 HL-A12, W27	HL-A1, W32 HL-A7	HL-A3, W24 HL-A12, W22
Target cells	X1 (B)	X2	X3	X4 (T1)	X5	X6	X7
Cytotoxicity: Predicted from HL-A typing	+	+	−	−	+	+	−
Observed with immune serum A*	22%	12%	21%	18%	22%	14%	2%
Observed with direct cytotoxicity†	40%	technical failure	3%	32%	18%	17%	−4%
Observed with CML effectors	24%	10%	0%	−7%	16%	8%	−3%

X2 to X7 are unrelated controls. X1 is the donor B and X4 is the T1 control.

*Results are expressed as the percentage of 2,000 cells in 1 μl killed by 5 μl of undiluted day-14 immune serum in presence of rabbit C.

†Results are expressed as percentage of ^{51}Cr released either by day-14 fresh frozen lymphocytes or by CML effectors.

vivo immunization. The cells of donor T1, especially chosen as control in our experiment on the basis of HL-A typing, were very efficiently killed by recipient A, and the kinetics of this killing was entirely parallel to the specific killing of the target B.

(2) The specificity (or specificities) through which effectors A were able to kill T1, although not definable by present HL-A typing, may be serologically definable; immune serum from A was cytotoxic toward T1. Further studies are underway to elucidate this point and should allow us to determine whether we are in the presence of a cross-reactivity or antigen sharing between SD antigens, so far undescribed, or whether this specificity (or specificities) belongs to another system. The fact that such an overlap of the effector cells outside the HL-A system can be found only through the in vivo immunization may be an argument against a cross-reactivity or an antigen sharing inside the HL-A system.

(3) Finally, in vivo immunization generates immune effectors, both humoral and cellular, that kill targets beyond the HL-A system as it is defined to date; the specificities of the CML effectors are entirely included in the present HL-A typing. Obviously, the in vivo system is much more complicated than the in vitro one. However, it remains to be demonstrated whether the observed difference is secondary to the different nature of the effector cells collected in vivo or in vitro, or to the different mode of sensitization in vivo, with more than one pathway of activation, versus the in vitro one, where the only prerequisite is a positive MLR as starter of the sensitization. It could very well be that such specificities outside LD1 and LD2 necessitate another pathway of sensitization that is not provided in the test tube.

In conclusion, it appears from this work that the CML assay is probably not a completely satisfactory in vitro correlate of the in vivo immunization.

SUMMARY

A comparison between in vivo immunization and in vitro sensitization against a known HL-A haplotype provides evidence that the in vivo effectors, both humoral and cellular, have become sensitized against HL-A specificities, as well as specificities different from the main HL-A determinants, in contrast to the CML cytotoxic effectors, which follow the HL-A typing. The implications of these results are discussed.

REFERENCES

1. Eijsvoogel VP et al: Transplant Proc, 5:1301, 1973

2. Legrand L, Dausset J, Rapaport FT: Transfusion 11:233, 1971

3. Lightbody JJ, Bach FM: Transplant Proc 4: 307, 1972

4. Alter B, Bach FM, Segall M: personal communication

5. Hartzmann RJ, Segall M, Bach MC, Bach FM: Transplantation 2:268, 1971

6. Mawas C, Sasportes M, Christen Y, et al: Transplant Proc, 5:1683, 1973

T Cells In Mixed-Lymphocyte-Culture-Induced Cytolysis (MLC–CML)

By Pekka Häyry and Leif C. Andersson

LYMPHOCYTES sensitized in one-way mixed lymphocyte culture (MLC) specifically kill allogeneic target cells (CML).[1-3] This method has become a useful technique to study allograft response in vitro.[4-6] Moreover, provided that the MLC–CML interaction is a B-independent T-autonomous function, the response may be used as a probe to investigate T-cell physiology. This paper summarizes the preliminary results of the recent unpublished work done in our laboratory in this respect. Detailed reports will be given elsewhere.

T AUTONOMY OF MLC–CML INTERACTION

Several reports demonstrate that the MLC response in the mouse is a T-dependent function.[7-9] Moreover, the CML of MLC-sensitized cells is largely abolished in the mouse by treating the cultured cells with relatively T-cell-specific anti-θ serum[10] plus complement.[11] The killer cells also behave in electrophoresis as T cells do.[5,12] The possibility remains, however, that T cells may recruit B cells to proliferate (although B cells in these conditions may not be performing any substantial amount of target-cell lysis). This possibility was excluded by using the following in vitro chimeric technique.

Responder cells in one-way CBA + DBA/2m MLC were electrophoretically fractionated[13,14] T cells of CBA/H-T6T6 strain and/or B cells of karyotypically distinguishable histocompatible CBA/Ca strain, or vice versa. Adequate controls were performed to ensure the viability of each separated cell type in functional (PHA or LPS) tests and to exclude the proliferation of mitomycin-C-blocked stimulator cells. Karyotype analyses were performed on the fourth through ninth culture days to examine the origin of dividing cells. The result (Table 1) demonstrates that 91 to 97% of mitoses in these cultures were of T origin.[15]

This result, which is at variance with the observation of Piquet and Vassalli,[16] who used (CBA/Ca × CBA/H-T6T6) thymus–bone marrow cell chimeric mice as responders, demonstrates that at least under our culture conditions[5] the proliferative phase of the MLC interaction is nearly completely a T-cell phenomenon. To investigate only T-cell responses in the MLC, however, highly standardized conditions must be used, since, for example, removal of serum from MLC culture medium has been shown to activate B cells to antibody production.[17,18]

T VS. B CELLS AS STIMULATORS IN THE MLC

DBA/2 spleen lymphocytes, probably representing mature T plus B cells, were purified by two incubations in glass plus cotton-wool filtration and were fractionated in preparative cell electrophoresis. The T and B cells (blocked with mitomycin C) were separately tested for their ability to stimulate CBA spleen lymphocytes in the MLC. The results (to be published), analyzed at a very low level of background proliferation, demonstrate that B cells alone induce only a very weak blast response, whereas T cells alone stimulated strongly, even better than nonfractionated (T + B)

From the Third Department of Pathology, University of Helsinki, Helsinki, Finland, and the Fourth Department of Surgery, University of Helsinki Central Hospital, Helsinki, Finland.

Supported by grants from the National Research Council for Medical Sciences, Helsinki, Finland; Association of Finnish Life Insurance Companies, Helsinki, Finland; and the Délégation Générale à la Recherche Scientifique et Technique, Paris, France.

© *1973 by Grune & Stratton, Inc.*

Table 1. Blast Responses and Results of Karyotype Analyses of Proliferating Cells in One-Way MLC of CBA + DBA/2m With Electrophoretically Fractionated Histocompatible CBA/Ca T and CBA/H-T6T6 B Responder Cells

Responder Cells* 1.5 × 10^6		Stimulating Cell† 3.0 × 10^6	Response‡ Days in Culture							
T Cell	B Cell		2	3	4	5	6	7	8	9
CBA/Ca	—	DBA/2m			190			480		
—	CBA/H-T6T6	DBA/2m			0			0		
CBA/Ca	CBA/H-T6T6	DBA/2m	10	50	93	115	150	230	195	160
% ToTo (T-cell derived) mitoses: §										
CBA/Ca	CBA/H-T6T6	DBA/2m			91	95	95	96	96	97

*T and B cells were obtained by fractionation in free-flow cell electrophoresis. In cultures with recombined mixtures of T plus B responders, 0.75 × 10^6 cells of each type were used.

†Blocked with mitomycin C.

‡Blasts per culture × 10^3.

§The Ca karyotype is designated as ToTo and the T6 karyotype (carrying the marker chromosomes) as T6T6.

spleen lymphocytes. Since B cells in control cultures die faster than do T cells, it is difficult to judge with certainty whether T cells are superior to mature B cells in inducing the MLC response. This finding, however, would not be contradictory to the results of von Boehmer et al.[19] in the mouse system, where partially purified T vs. B cells were compared as stimulators in allogeneic MLC. The result is also compatible with the result of Eijsvoogel et al.[20] in the human system, where the authors demonstrated that lymphocytes from a patient with thymic aplasia, which carried a normal set of HL-A antigens, were unable to stimulate allogeneic lymphocytes in vitro.

NECESSITY OF BLAST TRANSFORMATION (AND PROLIFERATION) FOR CML TO OCCUR

If the MLC response is carried out in the presence of a 2.5 × 10^{-6} M concentration of BUdR, and the cultures are illuminated prior to CML testing, the CML is negative.[5,21] Similarly, nontoxic mitosis-inhibiting concentrations (1.0 μg/ml) of Colcemid (Ciba) abolish both the blast response and the CML.[22] This shows that the removal of proliferating cells abolishes the CML response, although it leaves open the possibility that blast transformation (vide infra) without proliferation could be sufficient to trigger the T-autonomous killing function.

MORPHOLOGY OF KILLER CELLS

The question of whether the killing function is performed in the MLC culture by blast cells or by lymphocytes was examined as follows. The cells in one-way CBH + DBA/2m MLC were fractionated on the sixth culture day in 1-g velocity sedimentation of Miller and Phillips, and the cells in the resulting fractions were separately tested for CML to DBA/2 P-815 mastocytoma cells. The results[22] demonstrate that at this stage of the MLC all killer cells are >8.5 μm in diameter, and morphologically they are blasts. No cytotoxicity was observed in fractions with an average diameter of <8 μm (lymphocytes).

If the fractionation and subsequent CML are performed at day 10 in the MLC, the majority of the killer cells are no longer blasts (diameter >8.5 μm) but are smaller cells, morphologically resembling large lymphocytes (unpublished data).

A similar change in the size distribution of killer cells has also been observed in vivo in the Brunner[23] type of system.[24] Five and 10 days after in vivo immunization with allogeneic cells, the killer cells are >8 μm in diameter, whereas later, during the course of the immune response, it is mostly small cells that perform target-cell lysis.

The result demonstrates that the morphology of killer cells varies characteristically during the course of immunization both in vitro and in vivo. Moreover, the results indicate that all activated cells at a certain stage of the MLC response are blast cells, and the method also provides a possibility for their selective recovery and the study of their subsequent behavior.

THE BLAST-DERIVED LYMPHOCYTES (BDL)

The subsequent functions of blast cells primed in one-way MLC were studied as follows: either (1) they were transferred to macrophage or fibroblast feeder layers syngeneic to responder cells,[25] (2) the (primary) MLC culture was carried on up to 3 wk, or (3) they were injected intravenously into B mice (adult thymectomized, 800-R irradiated, and anti-θ-plus-complement-treated bone marrow reconstituted animals) syngeneic to responders. In all these conditions the blast cells reverted to lymphocytes (BDL).[26]

BDL were tested for secondary blast responses in secondary one-way MLC (2-MLC) and also for their ability to respond to the T mitogens Con-A and PHA. Characteristic blast responses of BDL recovered from syngeneic recipient spleens are given in Fig. 1. The BDL responded promptly to the original (and H-2-cross-reactive) stimulator cells (not shown). The peak of the response was observed on the second to third day of culture (instead of on the sixth to seventh day of 1-MLC). The BDL did not respond to PHA and responded very weakly to Con-A (Fig. 1). Nontransferred B mice did not give any MLC, Con-A, or PHA responses. B mice transferred with similar amounts of nonprimed spleen and lymph node cells gave weak responses of 1-MLC pattern. More than 90% of blast cells recovered from 2-MLC cultures were lysed by anti-θ serum plus complement.

Thus blast cells primed in one-way MLC revert back to lymphocytes and are both primed (since they respond in an accelerated manner in 2-MLC) and restricted (since although they are T cells, they no longer respond to PHA, and very weakly to Con-A). Essentially similar proliferative responses in 2-MLC, after transfer of 1-MLC-sensitized cells to B rats, have been obtained by Wilson and Howard (personal communication and reference 27).

The BDL, primed in CBA + DBA/2m MLC and reverted by any of the three methods, were also tested for their ability

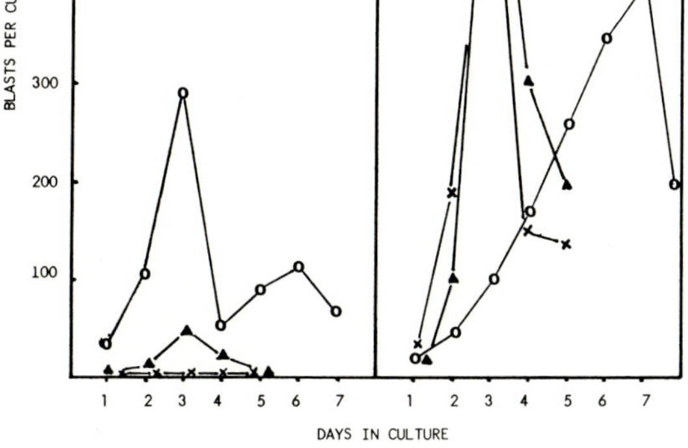

Fig. 1. Blast responses of CBA spleen lymphocytes to DBA/2m (○), PHA (×), and Con-A (▲). (A) Lymphocytes from B mouse transferred with 5 × 10^6 MLC-primed CBA + DBA/2m blasts 4.5 wk earlier. (B) Lymphocytes from normal CBA mouse.

Table 2. Target-Cell Lysis by MLC Blasts (CML) and by Spleen Lymphocytes of B Mice Transferred With Blast Cells

Effector Cell	Effector/Target Ratio	Specific ^{51}Cr* Release
CBA + DBA/2m MLC blasts	5:1	65%
CBA B-mouse spleen lymphocytes after transfer of CBA + DBA/2m blasts†	100:1 50:1 25:1	33% 18% 8%
CBA B-mouse spleen lymphocytes after transfer of nonprimed CBA spleen and lymph node cells	100:1 50:1 25:1	3% −1% 1%
CBA B-mouse spleen lymphocytes	100:1	−3%
CBA normal spleen lymphocytes	100:1	−2%

*Target cell: P-815 (DBA/2); exposure time 16 hr.

†5 × 10⁶ MLC-primed blasts or nonprimed spleen plus lymph node lymphocytes injected intravenously to recipient B mice 4.5 wk prior to test.

to lyse P-815 mastocytoma (DBA/2) target cells. Regardless of the method used, the BDL were cytotoxic to target cells. Table 2 demonstrates the persistence of tne effector function in BDL produced by transfer of blasts to B mice.

When 1-MLC was initiated in BALB/c + DBA/2m combination differing in respect to the M locus but identical in H-2,[28] both blast cells and BDL were incapable of lysing PHA or LPS blasts of DBA/2 origin, did lyse P-815 (DBA/2) mastocytoma and were able to respond to DBA/2 in 2-MLC in approximately the 1-MLC pattern (Festenstein and Häyry, unpublished results).

T-CELL SYNERGY IN MLC–CML

When mixtures of CBA thymus plus lymph node cells were tested for their ability to respond to DBA/2m spleen cells, the blast responses in certain combinations were higher than expected (Fig. 2); 0.9×10^6 thymus plus 0.1×10^6 lymph node cells

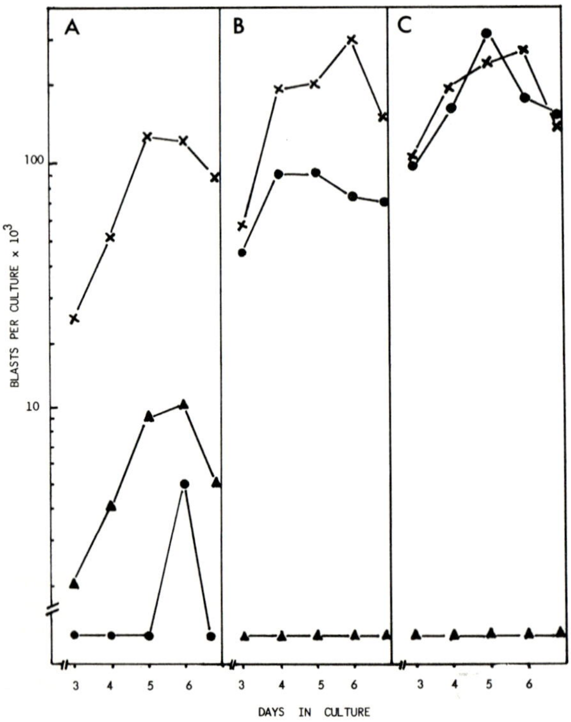

Fig. 2. Superadditive blast responses in CBA + DBA/2m MLC with thymus (ThC) plus lymph node (LNC) responder cells. ●, LNC; ▲, ThC; ×, LNC plus ThC. (A) 0.9×10^6 ThC and 0.1×10^6 LNC. (B) 0.5×10^6 ThC and 0.5×10^6 LNC. (C) 0.1×10^6 ThC and 0.9×10^6 LNC.

responded approximately ten times better than expected on the basis of responses when stimulated separately. When mixed in equal proportions the responses were still superadditive, but no superadditive response was obtained when 0.9×10^6 lymph node cells plus 0.1×10^6 thymus cells were used as responders. The results suggest[29] that the lymph node cell population contains cells capable of amplifying thymus cell response; this organ, on the other hand, may contain extra responders. Amplifying cells were also found in the blood, and to a lesser extent in the spleen, whereas both thymus and spleen contained extra responders (Häyry and Andersson, article in preparation). The responses have so far been quantitated in terms of blast per culture,[5] and it is not known which cell type responds to what extent by proliferation.

Tigelaar and Feldmann (this issue) have tested the CML responses when an excess of thymus cells and small numbers of blood lymphocytes are primed in one-way MLC with allogeneic cells. The CML, when both types of cells are primed together, is synergistic, as compared to when they are primed separately. We have made a similar observation in those MLC–CML experiments where an excess of thymus cells and small numbers of lymph node cells are used as responders.*

THE ABILITY OF BDL TO SYNERGIZE

The BDL that are derived after in vivo transfer of CBA + DBA/2m blast cells to B mice have also been examined for their ability to amplify CBA thymus cells to blast transformation. Spleens of B mice transferred by primed cells contained amplifiers, and the amplifying effect was several times higher than with spleen lymphocytes of B mice transferred with similar amounts of nonprimed cells. Nontransferred B-mouse lymphocytes were unable to amplify.

DISCUSSION

The MLC–CML interaction, at least in certain culture conditions, is a T-autonomous B-independent phenomenon. Since all cytotoxic cells (and possibly all activated cells) can be recovered from the blast fraction at a certain stage of the MLC response, their subsequent behavior may thus be studied, and the MLC–CML response may be used as a probe to investigate T-cell physiology.

When both thymus and lymph node cells are used as responders in one-way MLC, blast responses higher than expected (synergistic responses) may be obtained. This is the case when the majority of responders come from the thymus and the minority from the lymph node. The blast response of large numbers of lymph node cells cannot be further enhanced by adding a small number of thymus cells to the responder population. In the former case also the capacity of in vitro primed cells to perform CML is similarly superadditive, as it is in the case when large numbers of thymus cells and small numbers of blood cells are similarly primed (Tigelaar and Feldmann, this issue).

The results indicate that lymph node tissue contains cells capable of amplifying thymus cells (responders) to blast transformation and to cytotoxicity. Cells capable of amplifying normal thymus cells to blast transformation were also found in the blood and to a lesser degree in the spleen, and preliminary experiments indicate that small numbers of amplifying cells are also present in the thymus of mice that have received a high dose (5 mg intraperitoneally) of hydrocortisone 2 days prior to sacrifice. Responder cells in terms of superadditive blast responses were also found in the spleen in addition to the normal thymus.

This phenomenon closely resembles the synergistic GvH responses observed by Asofsky et al.[29] when a combination of large

*Note added in proof: Comparable results on in vitro synergism by T cells in MLC–CML have recently been published by L. Cohen and M. L. Howe, *Proc Natl Acad Sci* 70:2707, 1973.

numbers of thymus cells and small numbers of blood lymphocytes were used to elicit the response. Studies by Stobo et al.[30] indicate that the cooperating cells may represent two functionally distinct subsets of T cells, although it is not yet certain whether they belong to the same or to different lineages of T cells.[31]

Several studies indicate that passenger leukocytes trapped in the graft parenchyma are important immunogens in the triggering of the host's response.[32,33] Although macrophages[34] or even skin cells[35] are able to induce a proliferative response under certain conditions in vitro, T cells may be somewhat more important than B cells in the stimulation of the T cell response in the MLC.

The blast cells of one-way MLC cultures revert to lymphocytes. Similar reversion has been observed by Ginsburg et al.[25] in lymphocyte populations stimulated by other means. We call these secondary lymphocytes blast-derived lymphocytes (BDL), since these experiments demonstrate that they really are derived from the blast cells. At least four peculiar properties have so far been assigned to the BDL: (1) they are prompt responders in 2-MLC to the original (or H-2-cross-reactive) stimulator cells, (2) they do not respond to the T mitogens PHA and Con-A at optimal concentrations, (3) they act as killer cells to allogeneic target cells in the CML, and (4) they act as amplifying cells with thymus cells. When the 1-MLC is induced in an M-locus-unidentical, H-2-identical combination, at least the third property (CML) is lacking. Experiments to test the lifetime of the BDL in B mice, as correlated to these four properties, are currently under way.

Alter et al.[36] and others[28] have found that incompatibility in the Ir region of the major histocompatibility complex of the mouse is necessary and is alone capable of inducing proliferative response in the MLC. It has also been demonstrated that CML does not usually occur unless (1) the proliferative response takes place and (2) there is an H-2 (serologic) incompatibility between the responder cell and the target cell.[28,36]

Our data may be discussed in terms of the two-cell hypothesis of the MLC–CML interaction.[37-39] A modified version of the hypothesis is summarized in Fig. 3. This also includes the experimentally proven fact that T blasts revert back to lymphocytes.

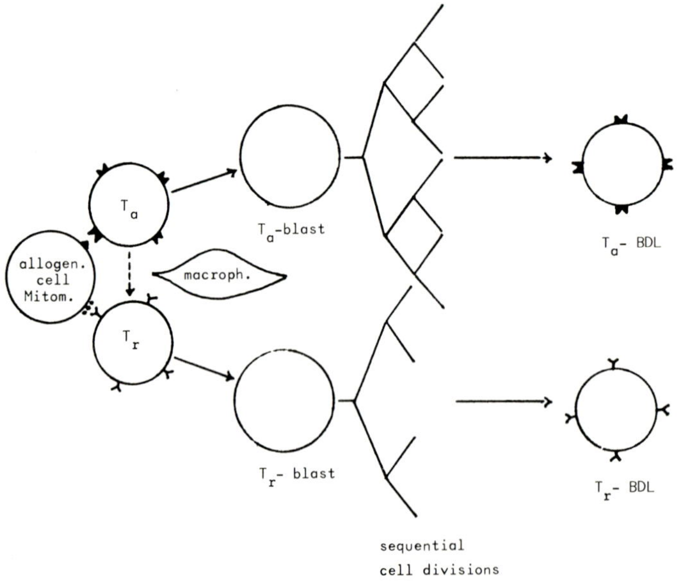

Fig. 3. Modified two-cell hypothesis of MLC–CML interaction. T_a (amplifier) and T_r (responder) carry different receptors and recognize different antigenic determinants on stimulating cell surface. The presence of macrophages is necessary for the interaction. Both T_a and T_r transform to blasts, divide and revert to lymphocytes carrying the original receptors. T_a BDL is possibly a long-lived cell, able to reamplify and unable to mediate target lysis, whereas T_r BDL may be a relatively short lived cell, able to lyse the target cell and able to respond promptly by second exposure to the original and H-2-cross-reactive SD antigens.

Since it is disturbing that the progeny of a single-cell clone might have receptors for antigens other than those initiating its proliferation, we suggest that a MLC interaction taking place both across H-2 and Ir barriers may result in two types of BDL, each carrying receptor sites of its own. This naturally means that there are two subsets of T cells, each one carrying specialized receptors and functions.

REFERENCES

1. Häyry P, Defendi V: Science 168:133, 1970
2. Solliday S, Bach FH: Science 170:406, 1970
3. Lightbody J, Bernoco D, Miggiano VC, Ceppellini R: J Bact Virol Immunol 67:243, 1971
4. Wagner H: J Immunol 109:630, 1972
5. Häyry P, Andersson LC, Nordling S, Virolainen M: Transplant Rev 12:91, 1972
6. Bach FH, Bach HL, Sondel PM, Sundharadas G: Transplant Rev 12:30, 1972
7. Tyan ML, Ness DB: Transplantation 13:198, 1972
8. Mosier D, Cantor H: Eur J Immunol 1:459, 1971
9. Wagner H: Eur J Immunol 1:498, 1971
10. Greaves MF, Raff MC: Nature [New Biol] 233:239, 1971
11. Wagner H, Harrish AW, Feldmann M: Cell Immunol 4:39, 1972
12. Andersson LC, Nordling S, Häyry P: Scand J Immunol 2:107, 1973
13. Häyry P, Andersson LC, Nordling S: Transplant Proc 5:87, 1973
14. Nordling S, Andersson LC, Häyry P: Eur J Immunol 2:405, 1972
15. Andersson LC, Nordling S, Häyry P: J Exp Med 138:324, 1973
16. Piquet PF, Vassalli P: J Exp Med 136:962, 1972
17. Mann PL, Falk JA, Fald RE: Transplant Proc 5:349, 1973
18. Coutinho A, Möller G: Eur J Immunol, (in press)
19. Boehmer H, Shortman K, Adams P: J Exp Med 136:1648, 1972
20. Eijsvoogel VP, Schellekens PTA, Breur-Vriesendorp B, et al: Transplant Proc 3:85, 1971
21. Bach ML, Alter BJ, Lightbody JJ, Bach FH: Transplant Proc 4:169, 1972
22. Andersson LC, Häyry P: Cell Immunol 8:470, 1973
23. Brunner KT, Mauel J, Cerottini JC, Immunology 14:181, 1968
24. Andersson LC: Scand J Immunol 2:75, 1973
25. Ginsburg H, Hollander N, Feldman M: J Exp Med 134:1062, 1971
26. Andersson LC, Häyry P: Eur J Immunol (in press)
27. Wilson DB, Howard JC, Nowell PC: Transplant Rev 12:3, 1972
28. Festenstein H, Démant P: Transplant Proc (in press)
29. Asofsky R, Cantor H, Tigelaar RE: in Amos DB (ed): Progress in Immunology. New York, Academic, 1971, p 369
30. Paul WE, Stobo JD: J Immunol 110:362, 1973
31. Raff MC, Cantor H: in Amos DB (ed): Proggress in Immunology. New York, Academic, 1971, p 83
32. Steinmuller D: Science 158:127, 1967
33. Guttmann RD, Lindquist RR: in McIntyre OR ed: Proceedings of the Fourth Leucocyte Culture Conference. New York, Appleton-Century-Crofts, 1971, p 29
34. Bain B, Lovenstein L: in Rieke W (ed): Proceedings of the Third Leucocyte Culture Conference. New York, Appleton-Century-Crofts, 1969, p 87
35. Thibault PM, Main RK, Kountz SL: Transplant Proc 5:397, 1973
36. Alter BJ, Schendel DJ, Bach ML, et al: J Exp Med 137: 1303, 1973
37. Eijsvoogel VṖ, de Bois R, Melief CJM, et al: Transplant Proc 5:1301, 1973
38. Bach FH: Transplant Proc 5:23, 1973
39. Thorsby E: Research in Immunochemistry and Immunobiology (in press)

Virus Plaque Assay and Enumeration of Effector Cells in Mixed Lymphocyte Cultures

By B. R. Bloom, S. Kano, and M. L. Howe

PERHAPS the major obstacle to our understanding of the mechanism of cell-mediated immune reactions has been the lack of a quantitative assay for enumerating sensitized or effector T lymphocytes analogous to the Jerne plaque assay for antibody-forming cells. Measurement of blast-cell transformation usually correlates with cell-mediated immunity, but thymidine incorporation is seen also in secondary antibody responsiveness and, as this paper will indicate, may occur in the absence of effector function. Lymphocyte–target-cell cytotoxicity is a very important assay of effector function, yet it yields results primarily in terms of percentage of target cells destroyed and probably depends as much on the nature of the target cell as on the number of sensitized cells in the immune population. Mediators or products of activated lymphocytes (PALs) are found only in minute amounts, and their quantitation has been extremely difficult to date; in no case is it possible to extrapolate to the number of sensitized lymphocytes.

A virus plaque assay has been introduced as a method of enumerating antigen- and mitogen-activated lymphoid cells.[1,2] The assay is based on the observation that while resting lymphocytes are incapable of supporting the replication of a variety of viruses, antigen- or mitogen-stimulated lymphocytes rapidly acquire the ability to do so. Increases in the number of lymphocytes replicating virus, i.e., increased virus plaque-forming cells (VPFC) have been observed in cultures of human or guinea pig lymphocytes obtained from delayed hypersensitive donors stimulated in vitro by specific antigens[1,3] or mixed lymphocyte cultures.[4] In contrast to the kinetics of thymidine incorporation, the increase in VPFC in cultures of sensitized lymphocytes stimulated with antigen over a 4-day period was found to be linear and unaffected by the mitotic inhibitor vinblastine.[3] This suggested the existence of a nondividing antigen-sensitive lymphocyte that had properties of the effector cell in cell-mediated immune reactions.[5]

The present work explores the nature of virus plaque-forming cells, specifically whether they are activated T or B lymphocytes or both. Second, the virus plaque assay was applied to mixed lymphocyte cultures, and results were compared in systems generating cytotoxic lymphocytes. The latter were limited solely to a proliferative response without development of effector cells.

NATURE OF THE VIRUS PLAQUE-FORMING CELL

The basic experimental design for elucidating the nature of the virus plaque-forming cell was to explore the enhancement of VPFC in mouse spleens by mitogens known selectively to stimulate T lymphocytes (concanavalin-A and phytohemagglutinin), B lymphocytes (lipopolysaccharide), and both T and B lymphocytes (pokeweed mitogen). At various times after stimulation the lymphocytes were harvested and infected with vesicular stomatitis virus; free virus was neutralized and the infected lymphocytes were plated in a thin layer of agar above an indicator L-cell monolayer.[2] When a lymphocyte is activated it becomes

From the Departments of Microbiology and Cell Biology, Albert Einstein College of Medicine, Bronx, N.Y., and the Department of Microbiology and Immunology, State University of New York, Brooklyn, N.Y.

Supported by NIH grants AI 09807, AI 10702, and AI 10158.

© 1973 by Grune & Stratton, Inc.

Table 1. Stimulation of Virus Plaque-forming Cells by Mitogens

Mitogen	VPFC ± SE*	ΔVPFC†
—	1,811 ± 369	—
Con-A	59,561 ± 5,137	57,750
PWM	31,420 ± 4,604	29,609
LPS	3,889 ± 377	2,078

*VPFC, virus plaque-forming cells/10^6 plated.

†ΔVPFC = VPFC mitogen-stimulated spleen − VPFC unstimulated spleen.

capable of producing and releasing virus, which diffuses through the agar, infects the indicator layer, and produces a visible plaque. There is a background of virus-forming cells in all lymphoid populations comprised predominantly of glass-adherent cells, probably macrophages. However, when lymphocytes are stimulated by mitogens or antigens, there is an increase in VPFC above this background, and this represents the number of activatable lymphocytes or ΔVPFC. As seen in Table 1, stimulation of mouse spleen with concanavalin-A produced a 33-fold increase in VPFC above background, pokeweed mitogen (PWM) produced a 17-fold increase, and *Escherichia coli* lipopolysaccharide (LPS), known to activate B lymphocytes, produced only a slight, though statistically significant, increase. In order to assess the contribution of T lymphocytes to the production of VPFC, two types of T-lymphocyte-depleted spleen were studied. As shown in Table 2, treatment of mouse spleen with anti-thy.1^b (AKR anti-θ C3H) serum plus complement prior to stimulation decreased the VPFC response to Con-A or PWM by greater than 99%. In additional experiments,[6] generation of VPFC by Con-A in athymic nude-mouse spleen was totally absent. These experiments clearly demonstrate the thymus-dependence of the virus plaque-forming response. In order to prove that the VPFC were in fact T lymphocytes, normal spleens stimulated for 2 days in culture by Con-A were treated just before infection with VSV with high doses of congenic anti-thy.1^b sera* (Table 2). Under these conditions there was a reduction of 97% in the number of VPFC, unambiguously demonstrating that the virus plaque assay measures activated T lymphocytes. While never greater than 10% of the response to Con-A, the small VPFC response in LPS-stimulated cultures requires some comment. The fact that LPS and PWM produced the same degree of thymidine incorporation, and yet the VPFC responses differed widely, suggested either that there was a very low efficiency of virus replication in activated B lymphocytes or that virus was capable of replicating in only a small subpopulation of B cells. We have previously found that VSV is capable of replicating in an IgM-producing murine plasmacytoma, MOPC-104, and we were able to demonstrate[6] that the small increase in VPFC stimulated by LPS could be reduced by at least 50% by treatment of the activated spleens with an anti-PC.1 serum, a serum that selectively reacts with plasma cells but not B lymphocytes. Thus it seems clear that the VPFC measures activated T lymphocytes and that activated B lymphocytes or plasma cells, or possibly macrophages, account for less than 10% of the virus plaque-forming cells in these experiments. This contribution

Table 2. Virus Plaque Formation by T Lymphocytes in Con-A-stimulated Mouse Spleens*

	ΔVPFC†	% reduction
(A) Treatment on day 0 with		
NMoS (1/32) + C	49,000	
anti-thy.1^b‡ (1/32) + C	4,600	90.6
(B) Treatment on day 2 with		
NMoS (1/8) + C	161,000	
congenic anti-thy.1^b (1/8) + C	4,700	97.0

*Conditions for the treatments can be found in reference 6.

†ΔVPFC/10^6 viable cells plated.

‡Anti-thy.1^b = AKR anti-θ C3H.

*The congenic anti-thy.1^b serum was donated for these experiments by Dr. Edward Boyse, Sloan-Kettering Institute for Cancer Research, New York, N.Y.

would undoubtedly be diminished further by use of cell sources containing fewer B lymphocytes than macrophages, e.g., peripheral blood, lymph node, or spleen treated with immunoadsorbants.

VIRUS PLAQUE ASSAY AND MIXED LYMPHOCYTE CULTURES

Mixed lymphocytic reactions occur generally when T lymphocytes are stimulated by lymphoid cells that differ across a major histocompatibility complex. Recently a dissociation between serologically determined loci and those controlling the mixed lymphocyte reaction has been found in both human[7] and murine systems.[8] Festenstein has previously described another gene, not linked to H-2, the M locus, that is responsible for stimulation of a mixed lymphocyte reaction by cells that do not differ serologically in their major histocompatibility complex. In this system, BALB/c ($H\text{-}2^d$) spleen or thymus cells proliferate when stimulated by mitomycin-C-treated DBA/2 ($H\text{-}2^d$) spleen cells. Most interesting, however, was the observation that BALB/c lymphocytes activated in MLC by DBA/2 cells are quite incapable of exerting cytolysis of DBA/2 target cells, either P-815 mastocytoma cells or Con-A-activated spleen cells.[9] In contrast, CBA ($H\text{-}2^k$) spleen cells, when stimulated by DBA/2 ($H\text{-}2^d$), proliferate to a somewhat lesser degree but are nevertheless highly effective at lysing DBA/2 target cells. When the virus plaque assay was performed on the lymphocytes arising from the mixed lymphocyte cultures between these strains, an increase in VPFC was obtained only in CBA spleens stimulated by DBA/2 cells (Table 3), although the BALB/c vs. DBA combination caused greater proliferation. These experiments clearly demonstrate that lymphocyte proliferation in MLC is not a sufficient condition for generating either cytotoxic lymphocytes or virus plaque-forming cells. They further suggest the parallelism between cytotoxic effector cells and the virus plaque-forming cells.

DISCUSSION

The virus plaque assay was designed to provide a quantitative method for enumerating antigen-sensitive lymphocytes in cell-mediated immune responses. Previous correlations between the virus plaque assay and cell-mediated immunity were: (1) increased VPFC were observed when cells obtained from delayed hypersensitive donors were stimulated in vitro with specific antigens;[1,3] (2) the virus-producing cell in this situation was observed by electron microscopy to be generally an enlarged small lymphocyte;[10] and (3) the kinetics of activation of antigen-sensitive cells was linear over a 4-day period and not affected by mitotic inhibitors. It seemed that the virus plaque assay detected a nondividing antigen-sensitive cell, and it was proposed that this cell had many of the characteristics of differentiated effector cells in cell-mediated immunity.[11] For example, cells obtained from sensitized animals are capable of transferring delayed hypersensitivity or graft rejection in vivo following treatment with mitomycin C[12] or x-irradiation,[13] demonstrating that sensitized effector cells need not divide in order to produce re-

Table 3. Generation of VPFC and Cytotoxic Lymphocytes in MRL

	DNA Synthesis (c.p.m.)	In Vitro Cytotoxicity	Virus Plaque Assay ΔVPFC/10^6
CBA × $DBA/2_m$	24,292 ± 2,413	78.0 ± 11.6%	59,128 ± 2,828
CBA	6,277 ± 2,468		
BALB/c × $DBA/2_m$	31,963 ± 8,253	2.2 ± 1.4%	3,183 ± 715
BALB/c	4,341 ± 807		

Adapted from *Proc Natl Acad Sci* 70:2299, 1973.

actions in vivo. This cell seemed similar to cells producing migration-inhibitory factor[14,15] and to immune T lymphocytes exerting target-cell cytotoxicity in vitro.[16] The experiments described here extend these observations and demonstrate that mitogens known to activate T lymphocytes produce a large increase in virus plaque-forming cells; in contrast, only a very slight increase above background in VPFC results from stimulation of B lymphocytes by LPS. Second, the failure of anti-θ-treated spleens or spleens from nu/nu mice to generate VPFC following stimulation with Con-A demonstrates a thymic dependence of this response. Further, the abrogation of VPFC in already stimulated spleen cells (Table 2) by treatment with anti-θ sera unambiguously establishes the VPFC as an activated T lymphocyte.

A dissociation between the proliferative response and production of VPFC or mediators in vitro has been observed previously.[3,14] It was of interest to learn whether, in a MLC across an M locus, which generates a strong proliferative response in cells that are identical at the major histocompatibility complex, there was a correlation between VPFC and proliferating cells or effector cells. In the system described, with only an M-locus difference, while there was a sevenfold increase in thymidine incorporation, there was no generation of cytotoxic lymphocytes in vitro. Similarly, there was no VPFC response. In contrast, control MLC with cells that differed across the major histocompatibility complex, produced a marked cytotoxic activity and parallel increase in virus plaque-forming cells. The conclusion is inescapable that these MLC generate at least two functionally different populations of T cells, proliferating cells that lack effector capacity and cells that have effector capacity and are also biologically altered so that they are capable of replicating viruses. It has been argued that in other systems in which dissociation between proliferation and cytotoxic activity has been described, the dissociation may be largely a function of complexities in the assays for cytotoxicity, e.g., high rates of spontaneous chromium release, relatively short times in which lysis can be studied, or failure of commonly used target cells such as non-lymphoid tumors or mitogen-activated lymphocytes to express certain surface antigens, e.g., MLC gene products. The salient fact is that the virus plaque assay detects a striking difference in lymphocytes as they are harvested from the MLC, and it must be emphasized that these results must reflect a fundamental difference in the biology of the different populations of lymphocytes activated in the MLC, since target-cell effects are excluded in our system. These results are consistent with those of Bach et al.[18,19]

There are two general models that can be invoked to explain these results. One would hold that there are two distinct subpopulations of T lymphocytes, one of which is capable of becoming activated by antigen to proliferate but lacks cytotoxic activity, the other of which is capable of activation, perhaps without proliferation, and effector function. The obvious difficulties of this view are that it adds additional complexity to the immune system by postulating an additional T-cell class, it fails to explain the apparent requirement of cell proliferation for the generation of the effector cell, and it is not easily amenable to direct experimental test. An alternative view would argue, in analogy to the generation of fully differentiated terminal plasma cells from precursor cells of the B-lymphocyte system,[17] that there is only a single population of T lymphocytes but that T cells vary in their biologic capabilities at different stages in their differentiation. For example, at early stages they may be capable of antigen recognition and clonal expansion but not effector function; in a more differentiated state, after much proliferation, they may have acquired the capacity to exert cytotoxicity, produce mediators, and replicate viruses, but may possibly be incapable of further proliferation. This view, because it adds no additional complexities, is the one most easily amenable to experimental tests: for example, by interruption of proliferation at early stages in the response or by destruction of one or more cell types, as by continuous viral infection. A variant of the one-cell hypothesis would hold that each T cell has two separate receptors, one for MLC and one for H-2 gene products. Because of the potential self-destructive capacity of the system, using an analogy with the common requirement for two keys to open a bank safe, it could be argued that stimulation of only the MLC receptor will result only in proliferation; two signals would be required for generation of cytotoxic effector cells. The difficulty with this argument is the cell biologic problem: how does one control the process of differentiation in two populations in which there may be equal numbers of cell divisions and yet where one population acquires no effector function and the other has differentiated with a high degree of such function? In any case, it is hoped that the virus plaque assay will prove to be useful in approaching such questions and testing these hypotheses.

REFERENCES

1. Bloom BR, Jimenez L, Marcus PI: J Exp Med 132:16, 1970
2. Jimenez L, Bloom BR: in Bloom BR, Glade PR (eds): In Vitro Methods in Cell-Mediated Immunity. New York, Academic, 1971, p 553
3. Jimenez L, Bloom BR, Blume MR, Oettgen HF: J Exp Med 133:740, 1971
4. Jimenez L, Bloom BR: in Harris JE (ed): Proceedings of the Fifth Leukocyte Culture Conference. New York, Academic, 1970, p 467
5. Bloom BR, Maillard J, Gaffney J, et al: Transplant Proc 4:329, 1972
6. Kano S, Bloom BR, Howe ML: Proc Natl Acad Sci USA (in press)
7. Yunis E, Amos DB: Proc Natl Acad Sci USA 68:3031, 1971
8. Bach FH, Widmer MB, Segall M, et al: Science 176:1024, 1972
9. Howe ML, Berman L: J Immunol (in press)
10. Nowakowski M, Feldman JD, Kano S, et al: J Exp Med 137:1042, 1973
11. Bloom BR: Adv Immunol 13:101, 1971
12. Bloom BR, Hamilton LD, Chase MW: Nature 201:689, 1964
13. Salvin SB, Smith RF: J Exp Med 109:325, 1959
14. Bloom BR, Gaffney J, Jimenez L: J Immunol 109:1395, 1972
15. Rocklin RE: J Immunol 110:674, 1973
16. Mauel J, Rudolf B, Chapuis B, Brunner KT: Immunology 18:517, 1970
17. Williamson AR, Askonas BA: Nature [New Biol] 238:337, 1972
18. Bach FH, Segall M, Zier K, et al: Science, 180:403, 1973
19. Bach FH, et al: Transplant Proc 5:1717, 1973

Synergy Among Thymocytes and Peripheral Lymph Node Cells in the In Vitro Generation of Lymphocytes Cytotoxic to Alloantigens

By Robert E. Tigelaar and Marc Feldmann

RECENT studies have detailed the phenomenon of synergy among subpopulations of parental-strain thymus-derived (T) lymphocytes in initiating the graft-vs.-host (GvH) reaction in neonatal F_1 recipients.[1-6] Mixtures of thymocytes and small numbers of either peripheral blood or peripheral lymph node (PLN) cells regularly gave reactions significantly greater than would be expected by summation of the reactivities of the components of the mixture measured separately. This synergy has been observed when the reactions were quantitated either by a spleen weight assay or a mortality assay in sublethally irradiated recipients. Experiments utilizing cells from neonatally thymectomized donors or cells pretreated with anti-θ serum and complement demonstrated that both subpopulations were thymus-derived. Most recently, the existence of two subpopulations of T cells within a single peripheral lymphoid tissue, both of which appear to be necessary for expression of the GvH reactivity characteristic of that tissue, has been demonstrated on the basis of differential migratory patterns of these subpopulations in intermediate syngeneic recipients.

The difficulties in elucidating the actual mechanism or mechanisms of this synergy in an in vivo model as complex as the GvH reaction are obvious. In addition, one may legitimately inquire as to the potential relevance of this synergy to other models of cell-mediated immunity. For these reasons we decided to explore the possibility that a similar type of synergy could be demonstrated in another cell-mediated immune response, such as the in vitro generation of cytotoxic lymphocytes to allogeneic cells. The preliminary studies reported here suggest that synergy also occurs in this model.

Approximately 5 × 10^6 CBA (H-2^k) cells from thymus and/or PLN were cultured in the presence of 5 × 10^6 irradiated (1500 R) DBA/2 (H-2^d) spleen cells in flat-bottom tubes (12 mm in diameter) in 4 ml of Dulbecco's fortified Eagle's medium containing 10% heat-inactiviated fetal calf serum (DF_{10}) and 3 × 10^{-5}-M 2-mercaptoethanol (J. C. Cerottini, personal communication). After 5 days incubation at 37°C in 10% CO_2, the cells were harvested, washed, and tested for their capacity to lyse ^{51}Cr-labeled target cells. The target cell used was the DBA/2 mastocytoma P-815X2. Conditions for labeling have been described.[7] Various numbers of viable in vitro-sensitized cells in 1 ml DF_{10} were then mixed with 5 × 10^4 labeled target cells (0.1 ml) in 16-mm tissue-culture wells. After incubation on a rocking platform for 4 hr in an atmosphere of 10% CO_2, the contents of the wells were harvested, centrifuged at 600 g for 10 min, and the supernatant fluid counted in a well-type gamma counter. Controls included ^{51}Cr-labeled targets incubated with either medium alone (background) or with 5% detergent (maximum releasable ^{51}Cr). Specific ^{51}Cr release was calculated according to the formula: specific ^{51}Cr release (%) = 100 × (experimental − background)/(maximum releasable ^{51}Cr −

From the Tumor Immunology Unit, Imperial Cancer Research Fund, Department of Zoology, University College, London, England.

Dr. Tigelaar is on working assignment from the Laboratory of Microbial Immunity, NIAID, National Institutes of Health, Bethesda, Md.

Supported by C. J. Martin Fellowship of the National Health and Medical Research Council of Australia.

© 1973 by Grune & Stratton, Inc.

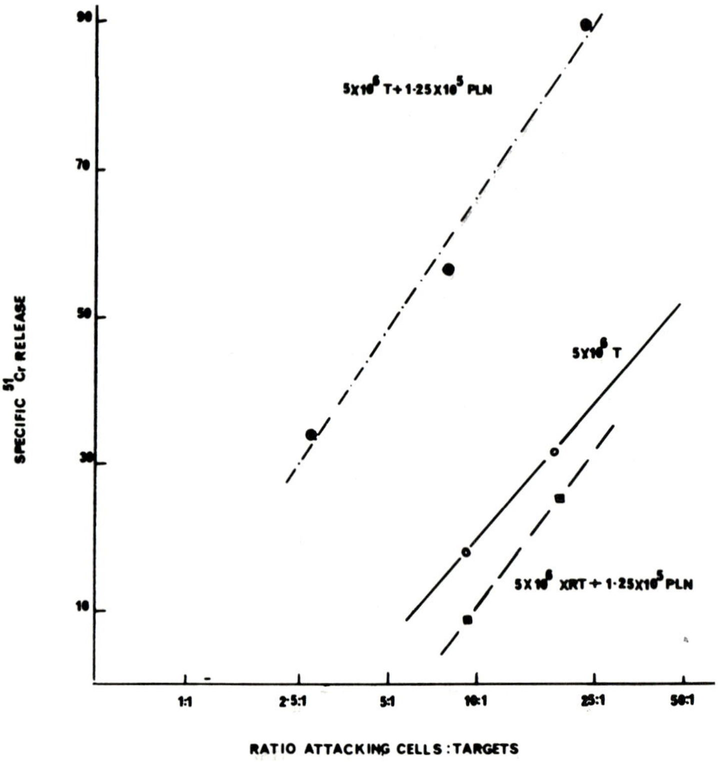

Fig. 1. Activity profiles of various populations of CBA cells sensitized in vitro to irradiated DBA spleen cells. Cultures were initiated 5 days before testing, each tube containing 5 × 10^6 irradiated DBA spleen cells and either 5 × 10^6 normal CBA thymocytes (open circles), 5 × 10^6 irradiated CBA thymocytes + 1.25 × 10^5 CBA PLN cells (squares), or 5 × 10^6 normal CBA thymocytes + 1.25 × 10^5 CBA PLN cells (black circles). Assay performed as described in text using 5 × 10^4 ^{51}Cr-labeled P-815X2 cells as targets. Number of viable attacking cells per well was estimated by trypan blue dye exclusion of harvested cultures. Each point represents the mean of triplicate determination.

background). All data points are the means of triplicate determinations.

Figure 1 illustrates the dramatic increase in cytotoxic activity that occurs when CBA thymocytes were sensitized against irradiated DBA spleen cells in the presence of a very small number of CBA PLN cells, compared with the activity generated by either thymocytes in the absence of these PLN cells or by small numbers of PLN cells alone. Sensitized thymocytes alone caused about 30% specific lysis at an attacking cell: target cell ratio of 20:1. Similarly, cultures containing 1.25 × 10^5 CBA PLN cells sensitized to alloantigen either alone (data not shown) or in the presence of 5 × 10^6 irradiated (1500 R) CBA thymocytes generated low levels of cytotoxicity, i.e., about 20% specific lysis at a ratio of 20:1. On the other hand, cells harvested from cultures containing 5 × 10^6 thymocytes + 1.25 × 10^5 PLN cells were approximately 8 times as active as the other groups; 30% specific lysis was seen at an attacking cell:target cell ratio of only about 2.5:1. The fact that PLN cells sensitized to alloantigen either alone or in the presence of irradiated syngeneic thymocytes generated similar levels of cytotoxic activity argues that the mechanism of enhanced reactivity observed when thymocytes are cultured together with PLN cells does not involve a radioresistant cell in the thymocyte population augmenting the reactivity of the PLN cells.

Although the enhanced cytotoxic potential of mixtures of thymocytes and PLN cells is obvious, the data presented in Fig. 1 alone do not permit a quantitative analysis of this heightened reactivity; i.e., how much more lytic activity is obtained from cultures containing mixtures of thymocytes and PLN cells than is accounted for by summing the activities obtained from the separate cultures of these two populations? This data can be obtained by first establishing activity profiles for the sensitized

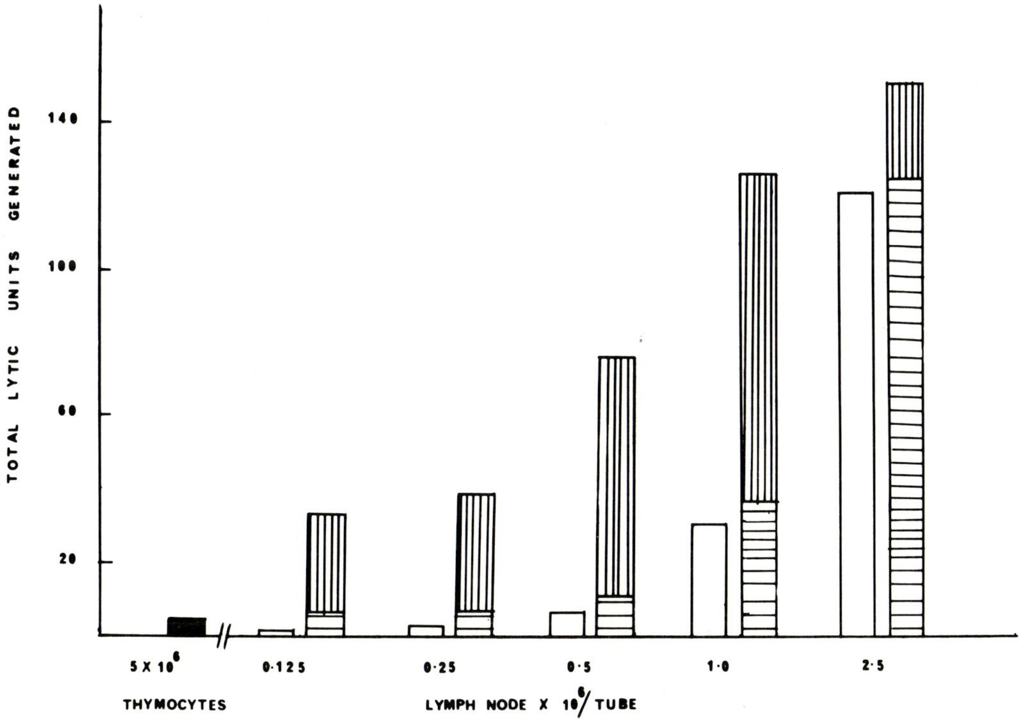

Fig. 2. Total lytic activity generated in 5-day in vitro alloantigen-stimulated cultures. Five cultures/group were initiated with 5×10^6 irradiated DBA spleen cells and the indicated number of normal CBA PLN cells + either 5×10^6 irradiated CBA thymocytes (plain bars) or 5×10^6 normal CBA thymocytes (bars with vertical and horizontal lines). Total activity generated by five cultures each containing 5×10^6 irradiated DBA spleen cells and 5×10^6 normal CBA thymocytes is shown by solid bar. Number of total lytic units generated calculated as described in text. Bars with vertical lines represent the number of LU generated by mixtures of thymocytes + PLN cells in excess of the sum of activities generated by the components of the mixture measured separately (solid bar + plain bar = horizontally hatched bar*).

populations as has been done in Fig. 1. If one then arbitrarily defines 1 lytic unit (LU) as the number of viable sensitized cells required to produce 30% specific lysis of a fixed number (5×10^4) of target cells, then the total lytic activity (in LU) of any population is simply the quotient of the total number of viable cells recovered from the cultures divided by this number. One can now sum the numbers of LU generated by cultures of thymocytes alone and PLN cells alone and compare this to the number of LU generated by cultures containing the mixture of these two populations.

Figure 2 is a graphic presentation of data calculated in this way and shows the results of culturing a fixed number of normal or irradiated thymocytes (5×10^6) with various numbers of PLN cells (five cultures/group). Thymocytes alone sensitized to alloantigen generated a total of 4 LU of cytotoxic activity (solid bar). Cultures of, for example, 5×10^5 PLN cells + 5×10^6 irradiated thymocytes generated a total of 6 LU (open bar). The expected (i.e., assuming no synergy) reactivity of cultures initiated with 5×10^6 normal thymocytes + 5×10^5 PLN cells would be 4 + 6 = 10 LU (horizontally hatched bar). However, the observed reactivity of these mixed cultures of 75 LU was 7.5 times more, or 65 LU more (vertically hatched bar), then expected by simple addition.

Figure 2 also shows that the observed

synergy tended to increase with increasing numbers of PLN cells. The greatest increase above simple addition in total LU generated was seen with 10^6 PLN cells, i.e., 91 LU. Mixtures of thymocytes and 2.5×10^6 PLN cells, however, only showed an increment of 25 LU above that expected by addition of the activities of these populations cultured separately.

Having established the requirement for a radiosensitive cell within the thymocyte population in order for synergy to be observed, it was of interest to see whether the active cell in the PLN population was also radiosensitive. Accordingly, cultures were initiated with either 5×10^6 thymocytes alone, 5×10^6 thymocytes + 2.5×10^5 normal PLN cells, or 5×10^6 thymocytes + 2.5×10^5 irradiated (1500 R) PLN cells (all cultures contained 5×10^6 irradiated DBA spleen cells as antigen). Both the sensitized thymocytes alone and sensitized thymocytes + irradiated PLN cells caused about 20% specific lysis at attacking cell:target cell ratios of 12:1, whereas the cells obtained from cultures set up with thymocytes and normal PLN cells caused nearly 60% lysis at this same ratio of 12:1.

These studies have clearly demonstrated that the cytolytic capacity of in vitro alloantigen-stimulated thymocytes is markedly augmented by the addition of very small numbers of syngeneic PLN cells. To this extent, these in vitro observations correlate well with the previously described synergy seen with these populations in eliciting in vivo GvH reactions in neonatal mice. Other observations of both increased cytolytic activity (Wagner, manuscript submitted) and increased blastogenesis (Häyry, this issue) in in vitro alloantigen-stimulated mixtures of thymocytes and PLN cells similar to the present model have recently been reported. On the other hand, the present studies have yet to answer a number of important questions. In the synergy observed in GvH reactions, it has been shown that both of the populations involved are T cells.[3,5,6] Preliminary studies in the present model would indicate that pretreatment of PLN cells with anti-θ serum and complement significantly decreases the synergy otherwise seen with thymocytes, but additional studies are in progress to see to what extent the augmented cytolytic activity of these cell mixtures may be due to the immunologically nonspecific enhancement of thymocyte survival in vitro. All of the data from the GvH model were consistent with the hypothesis that thymocytes were providing precursors of the cells that inflicted the immunologically specific injury, while the PLN cells were acting as amplifiers of this reactivity.[3,4] It remains to be seen in the present model to what extent the enhanced cytolytic activity of mixtures of thymocytes and PLN cells is due to augmentation of the reactivity of the thymocyte population.

There are many possible explanations for the decreased synergy observed when the number of PLN cells in the mixture was increased to 2.5×10^6 (Fig. 2). While deterioration of culture conditions secondary to cell crowding, etc., must certainly be considered, an intriguing alternative is that an excess of PLN cells physiologically inhibits a cell in the thymocyte population that in the presence of fewer PLN cells can be activated. If PLN cells are indeed amplifying thymocyte reactivity in this model, then perhaps excess amplifying activity has a negative effect similar to that observed in the humoral antibody response to thymus-dependent antigens.[8]

Finally, in the synergy observed in GvH reactions, both populations had to have the capacity to recognize foreign antigens in the F_1 recipient.[2-4,6] Recent experiments have shown that substitution of the CBA PLN cells in the mixtures with either DBA or CBA/DBA F_1 PLN cells results in cytolytic activity similar to that seen with the thymocytes alone. However, the important question as to whether the synergizing populations in either the in vivo or the in vitro model are recognizing the same antigenic determinant(s) on the sensitizing cell remains to be answered. Nevertheless, it is tempting to speculate that there is a relationship between the synergizing populations in this model and the apparently separable populations involved in the recognitive and destructive phases of cell-mediated immunity described by Bach et al. (reference 9 and also this issue).

ACKNOWLEDGMENT

The helpful comments and collaboration of Dr. R. Gorczynski in pursuing these studies are gratefully acknowledged.

REFERENCES

1. Cantor H, Asofsky R: J Exp Med 131:235, 1970
2. Asofsky R, Tigelaar R, Cantor H: in Amos B (ed): Progress in Immunology. New York, Academic, 1971, 369
3. Cantor H, Asofsky R: J Exp Med 135:764, 1972
4. Tigelaar R, Asofsky R: J Exp Med 135:1059, 1972
5. Cantor H: Cell Immunol 3:461, 1972
6. Tigelaar R, Asofsky R: J Exp Med 137:239, 1973
7. Wagner H, Harris AW, Feldmann M: Cell Immunol 4:39, 1972
8. Feldmann M: Nature [New Biol] 240:282, 1973
9. Bach FH, Segall M, Zier KS, et al: Science 180:403, 1973

The Nature of Cells Responding in Mixed Leukocyte Cultures and Cell-mediated Lympholysis

By Fritz H. Bach, Karen Stouber Zier, and Paul M. Sondel

THE duality of genetic control over lymphocyte activation in mixed leukocyte cultures (MLC) and target cell destruction in cell-mediated lympholysis (CML) has been documented in both man[1,2] and mouse.[3] The lymphocyte-defined (LD) regions of the major histocompatibility complex (MHC) that are important for MLC activation are genetically separable from the loci determining the serologically defined (SD) antigens. Whereas the LD differences play the primary role in causing lymphocyte proliferation in MLC, the SD loci or alleles of loci very closely linked to the SD loci determine the targets for CML, or factors necessary to obtain lysis.

One question concerning the findings stated above concerns the nature of the cellular response to the LD and SD components of the MHC. One might think of a single lymphocyte as recognizing both the LD and SD differences on an allogeneic target cell. Such a hypothesis would require that a given cell have specificity for both the LD and SD antigens, each presumably on a clonal basis, since both the response in MLC[4] and the cells mediating cytotoxicity show specificity prior to sensitization. An alternative suggestion by one of us (F.H.B.), based on the above findings as well as on the suggestions of several authors that there may be more than one type of T cell,[5] was that the cell population responding to the LD differences was not then and would not differentiate into a cytotoxic lymphocyte, but rather was simply a proliferating helper cell (PHC). The hypothesis was advanced that proliferation of the PHC in response to the LD stimulus would allow a second population of cells, the cytotoxic lymphocytes, to react to the specific SD difference on the target cell. Collaboration between the PHC and the cytotoxic lymphocyte would, therefore, lead to increased cytotoxicity. At the time, there was no evidence concerning which cell was responsible for cytotoxicity in CML; the recent work by Häyry et al.[6] suggests this is a T lymphocyte. Based on this data we will call the killer cell in CML a cytotoxic T lymphocyte (CTL).

This paper summarizes the data we recently presented[2] supporting the two-cell model for the LD–SD response and discusses the alternative explanations of the data presently available.

It is known that lymphocytes which mediate cytotoxicity adhere to monolayers in vitro either prior to[7] or following sensitization.[8] Experiments were designed to test whether cells activated in MLC could be separated into two populations by adsorption on monolayers. To summarize we will refer all experiments to a general model in which cells for MLC, for CML, or for monolayer preparation are obtained from individual B, the stimulating (sensitizing) cell in MLC; from individual A, the responding (effector) cell in MLC; or from a third donor C. Likewise, CML was tested against target cells from the same three sources. The two protocols followed are illustrated in Fig. 1. In Fig. 1A, cells sensitized in MLC for 6 days are incubated at 37°C for 1 hr on a fresh monolayer. In some experiments these cells are incubated with tritiated thymidine for the last hours of culture prior to adsorption on the monolayer;

From the Departments of Medical Genetics and Surgery, University of Wisconsin, Madison, Wisc.

Supported by NIH grants GM-15422, AI-08439, and AI-06525; NF-MOD grant CRBS 246; and ONR grant N00014-67-A-128-0003.

This is Paper No. 1698 from the Laboratory of Genetics, University of Wisconsin, Madison, Wisc.

©1973 by Grune & Stratton, Inc.

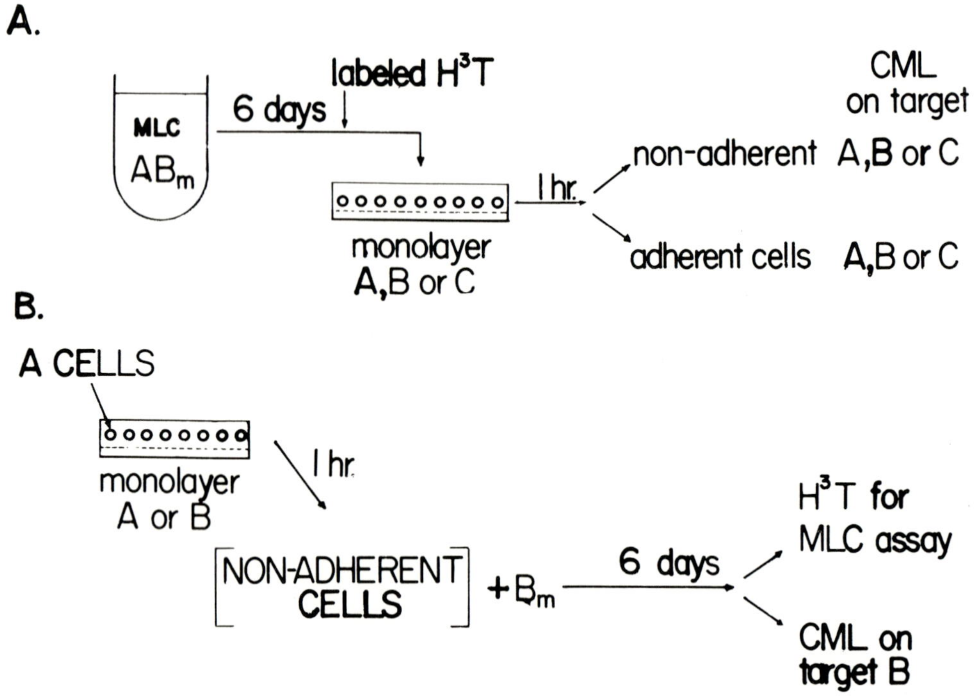

Fig. 1.

alternatively, the nonadherent cells are labeled with tritiated thymidine after removal from the monolayer. Nonadherent cells are removed by gently pipetting the supernatant medium over the adherent cells and removing the medium. Cells adhering to the monolayer are collected by scraping with a rubber policeman; these preparations serve as adherent cell effectors in CML. The protocol given in Fig. 1B attempts to separate the MLC and CML active cell populations prior to sensitization in MLC. In a prototype experiment, cells of an individual A are placed on a monolayer of either A or B and incubated for 1 hr at 37°C. The nonadherent cells are removed as described above and serve as responding cells in MLC to mitomycin-treated cells of either A, B, or C. After incubation for 6 days the cultures are assayed not only for MLC activation by studying the incorporation of tritiated thymidine, but also for CML activity by assaying for cytotoxicity on target cells of A, B, or C.

The data we have obtained since the publication of results[2] using these protocols represents a further confirmation of the conclusions presented at that time. The only addition to the protocols has been that we have preliminarily tested for and found specificity using the second protocol described in Fig. 1B by including cells of a third-party individual C. We will thus simply describe the general conclusions from these experiments here and refer the reader to the published paper for experimental details.

The results obtained by the two protocols are in accord. These general results are summarized in Table 1. In contrast to the general lack of adsorption of the proliferating cells, a highly significant percentage, and in some cases all, of the CML potential was removed by adsorption on the specific B monolayer. This was demonstrated both by the reduction in the nonadherent cells, sometimes to background levels, of CML potential after adsorption on B monolayers

Table 1. Qualitative Summary of Adsorption Experiments*

Adsorption of MLC Sensitized Cells

Responding (Effector) Cell	Stimulating (Sensitizing) Cell	Adsorbing Monolayer	Nonadherent cells: MLC (^{3}H-TdR) Incorporation	Nonadherent cells: CML on Target Cell B	Nonadherent cells: CML on Target Cell C
A	Bm	A	+++	+++	+
A	Bm	B	+++	−/+†	−
A	Bm	C	+++	+++	−

Adsorption of Nonsensitized Cells

Responding (Effector) Cell	Adsorbing Monolayer	Stimulating Cell	Nonadherent Cells: MLC (^{3}H-TdR) Incorporation	Nonadherent Cells: CML on Target Cell B
A	A	Bm	+++	+++
A	B	Bm	+++	−/+†

*This table is meant to serve as a strictly qualitative synopsis of the results we have obtained. The reader is referred to the previous publication[2] for the actual data.

†CML is always significantly reduced when effectors are adsorbed on the specific monolayer B, sometimes to background levels.

and by the recovery from the monolayers of CML effector cells for the specific target cells. Yet of the total tritiated thymidine present in the adherent plus nonadherent cells, less than 10%, on the average, stuck to the B monolayer. When ABm cells adsorbed on A monolayers gave significant CML on C target cells, the CML potential toward C was removed in every experiment by adsorption on either the B or the C monolayers, compared with adsorption on the A monolayers. Similarly, preadsorption of A cells on a B monolayer prior to MLC activation removed the capability for the nonadherent cells to develop CML potential following stimulation with Bm, but did not significantly reduce the tritiated thymidine incorporated following specific adsorption.

It is possible to interpret these results as supporting the existence of two separate cell populations involved in MLC–CML. The great majority of cells incorporating radioactive thymidine in MLC are included in the nonadherent population; a highly significant percentage and in some cases the entire CML capability is removed by adsorption on the specific monolayer. It is possible that there is a minority population of dividing cells in MLC that are CML effector cells. This finding is consistent with the somewhat higher number of counts per minute found on the B monolayer in some experiments. Our previous findings that early treatment of MLCs with bromodeoxyuridine and light, which kills dividing cells, abrogates CML[9] can be explained either if the CML effector cells divide or if the dividing nonadherent cells (PHCs) are needed to collaborate with the effector cells. The genetic evidence mentioned at the beginning of this article regarding the LD–SD cooperation suggests that the two cell populations would be collaborating ones.[3,10]

A two-cell model consistent with the above discussion would favor a series of LD-responsive clones; those clones that recognize LD antigens on the target cell would proliferate in MLC. In addition, there would be a separate cell population, the clones of which would be responsive to the SD antigens on the target cell.

The data are also interpretable on a one-cell population model. In such a model each responsive cell would have receptors for both LD and SD. As such there would be some cells having a specific receptor for an LD difference as well as a specific receptor for the SD difference. This population, the only one in this model that can mediate CML, would be removed by the protocols in Fig. 1. As such, CML potential would be removed. One would hypothesize, however, that there are many other clones of cells that have LD receptors for the LD differences on the target cell but that do not have the specific SD receptor. Such cells would proliferate without being specifically cytotoxic. The ratio of such cells to those carrying both a specific LD receptor for the target cell and a specific SD receptor would be large, thus explaining why the great majority of tritiated thymidine remains in the nonadherent cells. Such a model would require each cell to have specific receptors for LD and SD, each presumably distributed on a clonal basis.

At the present time the data presented by the adsorption experiments are thus interpretable to suggest that there are at least some LD-responsive cells in a given individual that can, either before or after sensitization, be separated from a second cell population that mediates cytotoxicity in CML. Whether the cells in the second population can themselves respond to the LD differences on the target cell is the subject of further investigation.

REFERENCES

1. Eijsvoogel VP, du Bois R, Melief CJM, et al: Transplant Proc 5:1301, 1973

2. Bach FH, Segall M, Zier KS, et al: Science 180:403, 1973

3. Alter BJ, Schendel DJ, Bach ML, et al: J Exp Med 137:1303, 1973

4. Zoschke DC, Bach FH: Science 172:1350, 1971

5. Bach FH: Transplant Proc 5:23, 1973

6. Hayry P: Transplant Proc 5:1697, 1973

7. Lonai P, Wekerle H, Feldman M: Nature [New Biol] 235:235, 1972

8. Brondz BD, Goldberg NE: Folia Biol (Praha) 16:20, 1970; Golstein P, Svedmyr E, Wigzell H: J Exp Med 134:1385, 1971

9. Bach ML, Alter BJ, Lightbody JJ, Bach FH: Transplant Proc 4:169, 1972

10. Schendel DJ, Alter BJ, Bach FH: Transplant Proc 5:1651, 1973

Nude Mice and the Mixed Leukocyte Reaction

By B. Anne Croy and David Osoba

MICE of the genotype nu/nu are hairless and fail to develop a normal thymus, whereas their +/nu littermates are phenotypically normal in these respects.[1,2] In the immunologic system of nu/nu mice, the major deficiency is in T cells (θ-positive cells),[3] but the numbers and functions of B cells and A cells appear to be normal.[4] The deficiency of T cells is most apparent in those immune responses where helper T cells are required, e.g., the response to sheep erythrocytes. Despite the T-cell deficiency, spleen cells of nu/nu mice can both respond[5] and stimulate[6] in the mixed leukocyte reaction (MLR). However, they do not give rise to effector cells cytotoxic for target cells carrying the H-2 antigens to which they have been exposed during the MLR.[5,7] Thus mice bearing this genetic mutation are a useful model for studying the cellular requirements in immune reactions and for dissecting the various stages of immune responses that culminate in effector function.

The results we present in this brief communication confirm and extend the above results. Further experiments indicate that T cells are required in the MLR, but they need not be present in the responding population of cells, i.e., a response in the MLR will occur if T cells are present only in the stimulating population of allogeneic spleen cells.

Our colony of nu/nu and +/nu mice was originally obtained from R. C. Roberts, Edinburgh, and the mice used in the experiments reported here were in the 11th to 13th generations of brother–sister matings. As yet, our colony cannot be regarded as being an inbred line, but preliminary skin graft data suggest that the major histocompatibility region of these mice is H-2^k.

The method used for the one-way MLR has been described in detail elsewhere.[8] Both the responding and stimulating populations of cells are obtained from the spleen, and the suspension of stimulating cells is heavily irradiated with 2500 rad of gamma radiation. In mixtures of allogeneic cells, the peak of tritiated-thymidine (^{3}H-TdR) incorporation is on the third or fourth day of incubation.

Neither nu/nu nor +/nu spleen cells respond to each other in culture. However, both nu/nu and +/nu spleen cells regularly respond to stimulating cells from BALB/cJ, DBA/2J, DBA/1J, C57BL/6J, C3H/HeJ, and CBA/J mice. The magnitude of the response is in the order given above, being greatest to BALB/cJ spleen cells and least to CBA/J spleen cells. There is no response above control levels to AKR/J spleen cells, nor do spleen cells from nu/nu and +/nu mice stimulate a response by AKR/J spleen cells. However, both nu/nu and +/nu spleen cells stimulate responses by BALB/cJ, DBA/2J, and C57B1/6J spleen cells. From the pattern of responses seen in these allogeneic combinations, we suspect that these mice bear the M1 allele of the M locus described by Festenstein.[9] Further testing on the appropriate F_1 backcrosses is required before a definite assignment can be made.

In all of the above experiments the magnitude of the response by nu/nu spleen cells to stimulating cells from a particular strain of mice is similar to the response produced by equal numbers of +/nu spleen cells.

From the Institute of Medical Science and the Department of Medicine, Ontario Cancer Institute, University of Toronto, Toronto, Ontario, Canada.

Supported by the Medical Research Council of Canada (grant MA-1609).

Dr. Croy is a Fellow of the Medical Research Council of Canada and Dr. Osoba is an Associate of the Medical Research Council of Canada.

©1973 by Grune & Stratton, Inc.

Thus, nu/nu spleen cells appear to be as capable as +/nu spleen cells of incorporating ^{3}H-TdR when incubated with appropriate allogeneic stimulating cells.

We have attempted to characterize the nature of the responding cell in the spleens of nu/nu and +/nu mice. Treatment of either nu/nu or +/nu spleen cells with cytotoxic anti-θ C3H antibody (in the presence of complement) before incubating them in the MLR does not significantly alter the magnitude of the response even though this antibody is cytotoxic for more than 95% to +/nu thymus cells and about 25% of +/nu spleen cells. Yet the same batch of anti-θ C3H antibody significantly depresses the response of C57BL/6J spleen cells to DBA/2J stimulating cells. Thus the response of nu/nu and +/nu spleen cells appears to be by cells other than T cells.

The nature of the responding cells is still uncertain. Separation of nu/nu and +/nu spleen cells by the velocity sedimentation[10] and density centrifugation procedures[11,12] indicates that the responding cells in the MLR possess sedimentation and density characteristics similar to those of B cells that give rise to plaque-forming cells in the Marbrook culture system. However, without more direct evidence, these results cannot be interpreted to mean that the responding cells in nu/nu and +/nu spleen are B cells. For the moment we prefer to state that the response in the MLR is by a non-T-cell population of cells.

When mixtures of either nu/nu or +/nu spleen cells and DBA/2J stimulating cells are cultured in the one-way MLR for 6 days and then assayed for their capacity to lyse ^{51}Cr-labeled DBA/2J mastocytoma cells, only the cells from mixtures containing +/nu spleen cells produce a significant release of ^{51}Cr. The degree of ^{51}Cr release produced by cells from mixtures of +/nu spleen cells appears not to be affected by the possible presence of antibody in the supernatant fluid, since the amount of ^{51}Cr released is the same regardless of whether or not the effector cells are washed prior to being mixed with the target cells. Thus although nu/nu spleen cells incorporate ^{3}H-TdR in the MLR, they do not give rise to cytotoxic effector cells in the ^{51}Cr-release assay. Since cytotoxic effector cells are not produced when the responding cells are deficient in T cells, this implies that T cells are either the direct precursors of cytotoxic effector cells or that they have a helper function necessary for another class of cells to express cytotoxicity. It is also possible that the nu gene in the homozygous state results in an impairment in the capacity of a non-T-cell precursor to differentiate into a cytotoxic effector cell.

The above results confirm the reports of other workers.[5–7] Thus far our experiments were designed to characterize the cellular populations in the immune system of nu/nu and +/nu mice. The experiments that follow are of a different nature. Here we have used the effects of the nu mutation as a tool to investigate the cellular requirements in the MLR itself. It has been suggested that the responding cell, which proliferates in the MLR, is a T cell,[13,14] and thus the MLR is often thought of as an assay for the presence of T cells. The experiments reported above indicate that a non-T-cell population is capable of incorporating ^{3}H-TdR when nu/nu spleen cells are incubated with allogeneic cells. Thus responses in the MLR need not be entirely due to T-cell proliferation. It can be asked, then, whether T cells are required in the MLR at all.

Mixtures of nu/nu spleen cells (T-cell-deficient) were incubated with BALB/cJ stimulating cells that had been pretreated with anti-θ C3H antibody and complement before irradiation. Therefore the stimulating-cell suspensions were also T-cell-deficient. In these cultures, incorporation of ^{3}H-TdR did not occur above the control levels found in cultures containing nu/nu cells mixed with irradiated nu/nu spleen cells. In further experiments, when both the

+/nu responding cells and the BALB/cJ stimulating cells were pretreated with anti-θ C3H antibody and complement, the response was also abolished. It is unlikely that pretreatment with anti-θ C3H antibody was toxic to all the spleen cells treated in this way, since pretreatment of only the responding +/nu cells or only the stimulating BALB/cJ cells did not abolish the response. Thus we conclude that T cells are required for a response in the MLR, but it seems not to matter whether the T cells are present in the responding population or in the stimulating population of cells. This conclusion does not contradict previous results indicating that under some conditions T cells in the responding population do proliferate in response to allogeneic cells.[13,14] However, under the conditions we have described it is evident that the T cells need be provided only by either the responding or the stimulating population of cells. Since the T-cell function in the stimulating population persists after treatment with 2500 rad of irradiation, continued T-cell proliferation would appear to be unnecessary for the expression of this function.

Our results suggest two possibilities. Either the responding cells in the MLR are responding to the presence of T cells in the stimulating population or the T cells in the stimulating population supply a function that allows a non-T class of cells in the responding population to incorporate ^{3}H-TdR. We can exclude that the irradiated T cells in the stimulating population are themselves incorporating significant amounts of ^{3}H-TdR, since mixtures of allogeneic cells in which both populations contain T cells and both have been irradiated with 2500 rad do not incorporate significant amounts of ^{3}H-TdR. Of the two possibilities presented above, we think that the first is unlikely because untreated +/nu spleen cells do respond to stimulating BALB/cJ spleen cells that have been treated with anti-θC3H antibody and complement. Since the T cells in this latter population have been removed, they obviously cannot act as stimulators for the responding cells. Therefore we favor the second possibility, that T cells supply a function enabling a non-T class of cells to recognize and respond to allogeneic cells in the MLR. The exact nature of this function is unknown, but it may be to produce a cell-free factor that affects the function of non-T cells. Studies are underway to test this possibility.

In this brief communication we have presented a summary of experiments on the nature of the responding cells and on the function of T cells in the MLR. A detailed presentation will be published elsewhere.

REFERENCES

1. Flanagan SP: Genet Res Camb 8:295, 1966
2. Pantelouris EM: Nature (Lond) 217:370, 1968
3. Raff MC, Wortis HH: Immunology 18:931, 1970
4. Croy BA, Osoba D: Cell Immunol (in press)
5. Wagner H: J Immunol 109: 630, 1972
6. Cheers C, Sprent J: J Immunol 15: 336, 1973
7. Feldman M, Wagner H, Basten A, Holmes M: Aust J Exp Biol Med Sci 50:651, 1972
8. El-Arini MO, Osoba D: J Immunol 110:926, 1973
9. Festenstein H, Abbasi K, Sachs JA, Oliver RTD: Transplant Proc 4:219, 1972
10. Miller RG, Phillips RA: J Cell Physiol 73:191, 1969
11. Gorczynski RM, Miller RG, Phillips RA: Immunology 5: 817, 1970
12. Messner H, Till JE, McCulloch EA: Ser Haemat 5:22,1972
13. Festenstein H, Davies AJS, Leuchars E, et al: in Fiore-Donati L, Hanna MG Jr (eds): Lymphatic Tissue and Germinal Centers in Immune Response. New York, Plenum, 1969, p 121
14. Johnston JM: in McIntyre OR (ed): Proceedings of the Fourth Leukocyte Culture Conference. New York, Appleton-Century-Crofts, 1971, p 14

The Proliferative Response of T Lymphocytes to Alloantigens in Irradiated Mice: A Mixed Lymphocyte Reaction In Vivo

By Jonathan Sprent

THE FIRST unequivocal demonstration that small lymphocytes were immunologically competent was the demonstration by Gowans that thoracic duct lymphocytes (TDL) from parental-strain rats underwent extensive blast transformation and proliferation in the spleens of irradiated F_1 rats.[1] Since this phenomenon was not observed when the host and donor were syngeneic, Gowans concluded that blast-cell transformation was a manifestation of antigenic recognition. The subsequent development and widespread use of the mixed lymphocyte reaction (MLR) in vitro[2] has fully confirmed this view.

Although the MLR has yielded valuable information on various aspects of cellular immunity, as a technique it has two distinct disadvantages. First, it is only semiqualitative. Second, by its nature it cannot take into consideration the importance of cell migration during the immune response. The aim of this article is to draw attention to the feasibility of studying the MLR in vivo. Most of the data presented here were derived from studies on the response of lymphocytes from CBA/J (H-2^k) mice to antigens present in [CBA/J × C57BL/6 (H-2^b)] F_1 hybrid mice; these studies have been published in detail elsewhere.[3-5] The system described here with these two strains is offered as a prototype for studying responses between a variety of other strain combinations.

KINETICS OF T-CELL PROLIFERATION IN VIVO

When parental-strain T cells, either thymus or TDL, were injected into heavily irradiated F_1 mice, the cells homed predominantly to the spleen and lymph nodes and there responded against the alloantigens of the host by blast transformation and proliferation.[3] The spleens of the hosts, although initially small as the result of extensive host-cell necrosis following irradiation, became enlarged after 3 to 4 days, the enlargement being proportional to the number of parental T cells injected. Histologic examination of the spleens at this time showed massive accumulation of blast cells around the central arterioles. The vast majority of these cells were shown to be of donor T-cell origin. Large numbers of blast cells were also found in the paracortical regions of the lymph nodes. No evidence of cell proliferation was found in irradiated F_1 recipients of F_1 T cells.

When tritiated thymidine (^{3}H-TdR) was injected intravenously every 8 hr into irradiated F_1 recipients of parental T cells, autoradiographs prepared from the spleen and lymph nodes showed that virtually all of the blast cells present in these organs were heavily labeled; very few labeled cells were seen in recipients of syngeneic (F_1) T cells.[3] Further studies showed that the extent of cell proliferation in the spleen and lymph nodes could be quantitated by measuring uptake of ^{3}H-TdR soon after an intravenous pulse. This approach is illustrated in Fig. 1. Irradiated F_1 mice were injected with various sources of T cells. At daily intervals, groups of the mice were pulsed intravenously with 25 μCi ^{3}H-TdR, and their spleens were removed 30 min later for estimation of radioactivity levels. When 2×10^5 TDL or mesenteric lymph node (MLN) cells were used as sources of T cells, ^{3}H-TdR incorporation increased progressively between 3 and 6 days after cell injection; in other experiments, radioactivity

From the Basel Institute for Immunology, Basel, Switzerland.
© 1973 by Grune & Stratton, Inc.

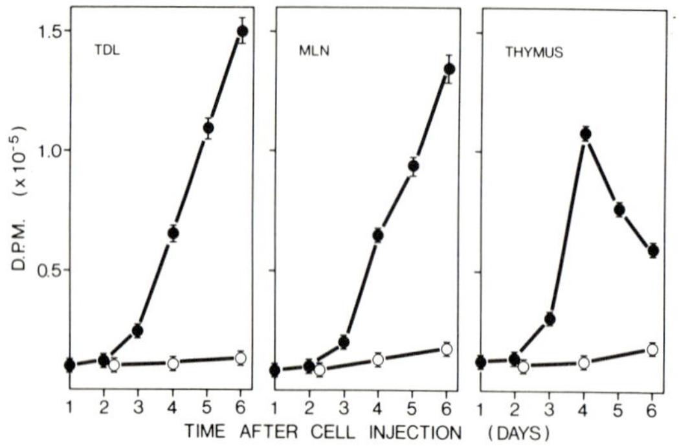

Fig. 1. Incorporation of ^{3}H-TdR in spleens of irradiated (CBA/J × C57BL/6) F_1 mice given 25 μCi ^{3}H-TdR intravenously 30 min before killing. Spleens were removed at various times after intravenous injection of 2 × 10^5 TDL, 2 × 10^5 MLN cells, or 10^7 thymus cells. Black circle indicates recipients of CBA/J lymphocytes; open circle indicates recipients of (CBA/J × C57BL/6) F_1 lymphocytes. Arithmetic means of results obtained from four mice per point are shown, and vertical bars indicate magnitude of SE.

levels were found to fall rapidly at later stages. With recipients of syngeneic T cells, only low levels of radioactivity were found; these levels increased only slightly during the term of the experiment and, unless large numbers of cells were injected, were not significantly higher than the background levels found in irradiated mice not given lymphocytes.

Parental thymus cells also proliferated extensively in irradiated F_1 mice, but only when large numbers were injected. By calculating the numbers of cells required to produce a certain level of ^{3}H-TdR incorporation in the spleen of the recipients, the proliferative capacity of thymus cells was assessed to be 50 to 100 times less than that of peripheral T cells, e.g., TDL. This is consistent with evidence that the immunocompetent cells in thymus are represented by only 1 to 2% of the total population, namely, the cortisone-resistant TL-negative cells of the medulla.[6,7] The proliferative response of thymus cells characteristically reached a peak at 3 or 4 days after cell injection and then declined rapidly (Fig. 1), i.e., much earlier than the peak reached at about 6 days with TDL or MLN.

Within certain cell dose ranges, ^{3}H-TdR incorporation was found to be directly proportional to the number of parental T cells injected. This is exemplified in Fig. 2 where a direct relationship is apparent with doses up to 5 × 10^5 TDL and 6 × 10^7 thymus cells. A plateau was eventually reached when higher doses of these cells were injected.

The above technique provides a simple and reproducible method for measuring cell proliferation in vivo. Some index of its sensitivity is evident in Fig. 2 where ^{3}H-TdR incorporation in recipients of as few as 5 × 10^4 parental TDL was twice that found in recipients of syngeneic cells. A similar method for estimating lymphocyte prolifer-

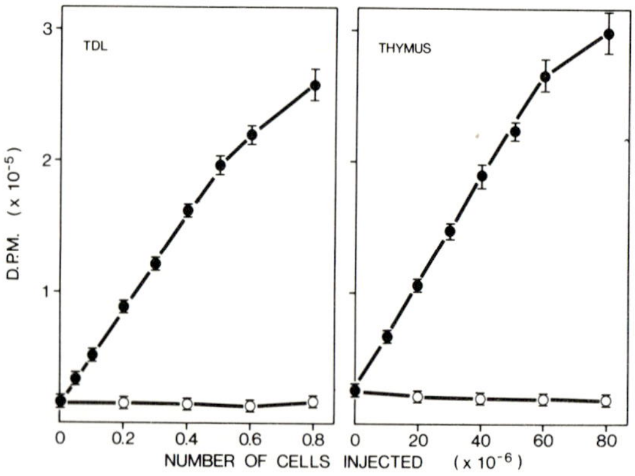

Fig. 2. Incorporation of ^{3}H-TdR in spleens of irradiated (CBA/J × C57BL/6) F_1 recipients of various numbers of CBA/J (●) or (CBA/J × C57BL/6) F_1 (○) TDL or thymus cells. Measurements were at 4 days after cell injection in the case of TDL and 3.5 days with thymus cells. Arithmetic means of results obtained from four mice per point are shown, and vertical bars indicate magnitude of SE.

ation in irradiated allogeneic mice has been described by Bennett.[8] His method involves injecting 5-iodo-2′-deoxyuridine-^{125}I intraperitoneally and then measuring radioactivity in the spleen 1 day later.

Most of the cells that proliferate after injection into irradiated F_1 mice appear to be T cells. Thus treatment of parental TDL (which contain 15 to 20% B cells[9]) with anti-θ serum and complement before injection completely abolished the proliferative capacity of the cells when measured after 4 days by ^{3}H-TdR incorporation.[10] Recent evidence has suggested, however, that B cells may also proliferate in response to alloantigens in vivo.[11] The response of B cells is weaker than that of T cells and reaches a peak within 2 to 3 days of cell injection; it is not detectable at 4 days postinjection, i.e., when the response of T cells becomes prominent.

Lymphocytes are rich in histocompatibility antigens[12] and are highly radiosensitive.[13] Since T cells are activated in the thymus-dependent areas of irradiated semiallogeneic mice, the question arises of whether the main immunogenic stimulus in these areas is provided by the host T cells. Two lines of evidence suggest that this is probably not the case. First, if T-cell-depleted F_1 mice, i.e., thymectomized, irradiated, and marrow-protected mice, were used as the irradiated recipients of parental T cells, the stimulus for proliferation offered by these mice was actually greater than that given by normal irradiated F_1 mice.[3] Second, the immunogenicity of various cell types was tested by injecting T cells of parental strain into syngeneic irradiated mice that, 18 hr before irradiation, had been injected with F_1 lymphoid cells. With this approach, preinjection of F_1 bone marrow provided the most effective stimulus (Table 1); TDL, which consist largely of immunocompetent T cells, were poorly immunogenic. These findings are at variance with the report of McLaurin[14] that in the MLR in vitro, cell populations depleted of T cells provided a poor stimulus. In our hands, TDL from nu/nu mice, i.e., a population containing no detectable T cells and consisting almost entirely of B cells, proved as immunogenic to allogeneic lymphocytes in vitro as TDL from nu/+ mice, which contain 80% T cells.[15] It would seem likely that a variety of cell types can stimulate allogeneic lymphocytes, cells of bone marrow origin being particularly effective. Since macrophages are required for the MLR, at least

Table 1. ^{3}H-TdR Incorporation in Spleens of CBA/J Mice Injected With Either (CBA/J × C57BL/6) F_1 or CBA/J Cells, Irradiated 18 Hr Later, and Then Given 5 × 10^7 CBA/J Thymus Cells

		Disintegrations per Minute per Spleen ($\times 10^{-3}$) ± SE*	
Source of Cells Injected	Number of Cells Injected	CBA/J Recipients of (CBA/J × C57BL/6) F_1 Cells	CBA/J Recipients of CBA/J Cells
Thoracic duct	1 × 10^7	62 ± 2	28 ± 3
	5 × 10^7	71 ± 2	23 ± 1
Thymus	1 × 10^7	63 ± 6	22 ± 1
	5 × 10^7	112 ± 8	28 ± 4
Spleen	1 × 10^7	85 ± 15	25 ± 4
	5 × 10^7	160 ± 20	25 ± 3
Bone marrow	1 × 10^7	105 ± 11	21 ± 5
	5 × 10^7	260 ± 15†	34 ± 4

*25 μCi ^{3}H-TdR given 3 days after injection of thymus cells; mice killed 30 min later; four to six mice per group.
†Compared to 287 ± 40 for irradiated (CBA/J × C57Bl/6) F_1 recipients of 5 × 10^7 CBA/J thymus cells.

in vitro,[16] it is probable that the immunogenic stimulus is not provided by intact cells per se but by antigen released from the cells following degradation by macrophages; this might not necessarily apply for generation of effector cells.

FATE AND FUNCTION OF ACTIVATED T CELLS

Donor cells proliferating in irradiated semiallogeneic mice did not remain confined to the lymphoid organs, but after 4 days appeared in large numbers in thoracic duct lymph. More than 95% of the cells collected at this time were recently divided cells of donor thymus origin.[4] These thymus-derived thoracic duct lymphocytes (T.TDL) had the following properties:

(1) As a population, T.TDL were highly immunocompetent, but only toward the antigens that provoked their formation (the host antigens). This applied to the capacity of the cells to reject skin grafts on adoptive transfer, to lyse target cells in vitro, and to prevent growth of tumor cells in vivo.[5]

(2) T.TDL, unlike normal T cells, failed to elicit splenomegaly when transferred to appropriate neonatal mice.[5]

(3) In an MLR in vitro, approximately 25% of T.TDL synthesized DNA when reexposed to the host antigens, but not to other antigens. Significantly, DNA synthesis was not accompanied by cell division. This suggested that the proliferative potential of the cells had been exhausted. In view of the restricted functional specificity of T.TDL (see above), it was therefore considered likely that the failure of the remaining 75% of the cells to synthesize DNA in culture reflected complete exhuastion of this fraction of the population, rather than that these cells were reactive to other antigens.[17]

(4) When T.TDL were transferred to syngeneic mice, they homed largely to the spleen and intestines. Most of the cells were able to recirculate, i.e., they appeared in thoracic duct lymph after intravenous injection. Very few T.TDL, however, remained in the recirculating pool for more than a few days.[4,10]

The above findings can be interpreted as follows: shortly after injection of T cells into irradiated semiallogeneic mice, the cells are recruited from the circulation to the spleen and lymph nodes and there proliferate extensively in response to the alloantigens of the host; the work of Ford and Atkins[18] indicates that the cells do in fact leave the circulation at this time. After 4 days the progeny of the responding cells rejoin the recirculating pool and can be collected in large numbers in thoracic duct lymph. These cells, a virtually pure population of specifically reactive lymphocytes, appear to represent the effector cells generated against the host antigens. Most of the cells are short-lived and probably die soon after mediating their functions. They may thus be considered as the T-cell analogue of the plasma cell, the effector end cell of the B-cell line.

ACKNOWLEDGMENT

The author is indebted to his colleague Dr. J.F.A.P. Miller for publishing in this article data obtained with his collaboration.

REFERENCES

1. Gowans JL: Ann NY Acad Sci 99:432, 1962
2. Bain B, Vas M, Lowenstein L: Fed Proc 22:428, 1963
3. Sprent J, Miller JFAP: Cell Immunol 3:361, 1972
4. Sprent J, Miller JFAP: Cell Immunol 3:385, 1972
5. Sprent J, Miller JFAP: Cell Immunol 3:213, 1972
6. Blomgren H, Andersson B: Cell Immunol 1:545, 1970
7. Lance EM, Cooper S, Boyse EA: Cell Immunol 1:536, 1970
8. Bennett M: Transplantation 11:158, 1971
9. Sprent J: Cell Immunol 7:10, 1973

10. Sprent J: unpublished data

11. Sprent J, Wagner H: unpublished data

12. Aoki T, Hammerling U, de Harven E, et al: J Exp Med 130:979, 1969

13. Trowell OA: J Pathol Bacteriol 64:687, 1952

14. McLaurin BP: Clin Exp Immunol 10:649, 1972

15. Cheers C, Sprent J: Transplantation 15:336, 1973

16. Gordon J: Proc Soc Exp Biol Med 127:30, 1968

17. Cheers C, Sprent J, Miller JFAP: Cell Immunol (in press)

18. Ford WL, Atkins RC: Nature [New Biol] 234: 178, 1971

Surface Immunoglobulin on H-2-activated T Lymphocytes

By Jonathan Sprent and Leslie Hudson

THE controversy on the nature of the antigen-specific receptors on T cells[1-4] inevitably centers around the question of whether these cells, like B cells, express membrane-bound immunoglobulin (Ig). Opinion on this point is strongly divided. Thus while some groups have been unable to demonstrate Ig on T cells,[5] others claim to have found as much Ig on T cells as on B cells.[6]

In previous studies it was shown that cells collected from thoracic duct lymph of (H-2^k × H-2^b) F_1 mice given 800 R irradiation and injected 4 days before with H-2^k thymus cells were almost entirely of donor thymus origin.[7] Sixty to eighty percent of these thymus-derived thoracic duct lymphocytes (T.TDL) were blast cells with reactivity only to the antigens that provoked their formation.[8] Since the cells are usually 100% viable and contain 0.3% or less B cells, T.TDL offer distinct advantages for studying T-cell functions.

By a variety of approaches, T.TDL have been shown to carry surface Ig.[9-12] Two lines of evidence now suggest that at least a proportion of Ig on activated T cells is passively adsorbed antibody of B-cell origin. First, recent work has shown that the helper activity of thymus cells activated in vivo to heterologous erythrocytes can be reduced by passing the thymus cells through a rabbit anti-mouse Ig-coated column before injection, i.e., to remove B cells;[13] injection of appropriate antiserum raised against the erythrocyte antigens partially restored the helper activity of the passaged cells. Second, surface Ig on T.TDL could no longer be detected if these cells were first cultured in vitro for 20 hr at 37°C.[12]

The effect on cell surface Ig of preparing T.TDL from thymus-cell suspensions depleted of B cells was investigated as follows: T.TDL were prepared from thymus cells passed through high-capacity immunoadsorbent columns containing Sephadex G-100 covalently linked either to purified rabbit anti-mouse Ig antibody or to normal rabbit IgG.[14] A high proportion of T.TDL showed surface Ig when they were derived from thymus cells passaged through the control (normal rabbit IgG) columns (Table 1). With thymus cells passed through rabbit anti-mouse Ig-coated columns, however, a much lower proportion of T.TDL derived from these cells were Ig-positive. T.TDL generated under these conditions were unimpaired in their capacity to lyse appropriate ^{51}Cr-labeled target cells in vitro (Table 2). The continuous presence of purified rabbit anti-mouse Ig (1 mg/ml) in the cultures did not impair target-cell lysis by either population of T.TDL.

The above experiments are consistent with the concept that Ig detected on T.TDL represented cytophilic alloantibody derived from B cells in the thymus-cell inocula. As suggested elsewhere,[12] cytophilic antibody might be attached in two ways. First, it might be absorbed nonspecifically onto antibody Fc receptors expressed by the cells as the result of their activated state; this would conform to claims that activated T cells do indeed display Fc receptors.[17,18] Second, the immunoglobulin could be alloantibody attached to T.TDL via the Fab region, i.e., to soluble host antigens held to antigen-specific receptors on the cells. In preliminary experiments, T.TDL derived from B-cell-depleted thymus cells were found to bind mouse myeloma proteins after incubation with these proteins in vitro

From the Basel Institute for Immunology, Basel, Switzerland, and the Department of Immunology, Middlesex Hospital Medical School, London, England.
© 1973 by Grune & Stratton, Inc.

Table 1. Reduction of Surface Ig on T.TDL Derived From Thymus Cells Passed Through Rabbit Anti-Mouse Ig Immunoadsorbent Columns*

T.TDL Incubated With†	% T.TDL Stained With Sheep Anti-Rabbit Ig-rhod‡: T.TDL From Thymus Passed Through Normal Rabbit IgG-coated Column§	% T.TDL Stained With Sheep Anti-Rabbit Ig-rhod‡: T.TDL From Thymus Passed Through Purified Anti-Ig-coated Column
Normal rabbit IgG	6	17
Purified anti-Ig	76	24
Anti-μ	89	26

*T.TDL were collected from irradiated (750 R) (CBA × C57BL) F_1 mice between 4 and 5 days after injection of 2×10^8 CBA thymus cells. Before injection, the thymus cells were passed through Sephadex G-100 immunoadsorbent columns.[14] Under the conditions used, B cells were selectively retained on columns coated with purified antibody of a polyvalent rabbit anti-mouse Ig antiserum (purified anti-Ig) but not on normal rabbit IgG-coated columns.

†T.TDL were incubated on ice with 1 mg/ml of IgG fractions of normal rabbit serum (NRS), rabbit anti-mouse μ antiserum (anti-μ), or 1 mg/ml of rabbit anti-mouse Ig purified antibody (purified anti-Ig). The preparation and specificity of these reagents will be described elsewhere;[15] 90% of the purified anti-Ig was specific antibody.

‡After incubation with unconjugated rabbit IgG, the cells were washed thoroughly and then incubated with a rhodamine-conjugated Ig fraction of sheep anti-rabbit IgG antiserum (sheep anti-rabbit Ig-rhod, provided by Dr. F. Loor) as described elsewhere[16] and then examined by fluorescent microscopy. This technique did not stain T-cell populations other than T.TDL. The results are from a single experiment; two other experiments gave similar results.

§Similar results were obtained with T.TDL derived from unfractionated thymus cells.

(data not shown). In a previous study, however, it was concluded that T.TDL did not express Fc receptors, since these cells, unlike B cells, failed to bind immune complexes in vitro.[20] Since T.TDL in this study were generated from normal (B-cell-contaminated) thymus cells, it now seems possible in view of the present data that immune complexes were not bound because of presaturation of the receptors with antibody in vivo. This explanation is currently being explored.

Recent work has indicated that when surface Ig on T.TDL is detected with an anti-mouse Ig serum raised in chickens rather than rabbits, the Ig demonstrable on the cells is not reduced when they are generated from B-cell-depleted thymus cells (unpublished data of L. Hudson, J. Sprent, and F. Loor). Thus the present data cannot be taken as firm evidence against the concept that antigen-specific receptors on T cells are immunoglobulin in nature.

Table 2. Cytotoxicity of T.TDL Depleted of Surface Ig*

Treatment of Thymus-Cell Progenitors of T.TDL	% Fluorescent T.TDL After Incubation With		% Lysis of ^{51}Cr-Labeled DBA/2 Mastocytoma Cells Incubated With†		
	NRS	Purified Anti-Ig	T.TDL Alone	T.TDL + Purified Anti-Ig	T.TDL + Normal Rabbit IgG
Filtered through normal rabbit IgG column	9	69	94	85	88
Filtered through purified anti-Ig column	24	16	94	87	93

*T.TDL prepared as in Table 1 except that the irradiated recipients of the CBA thymus cells were (CBA × DBA/2) F_1 mice; T.TDL were collected between 5 and 6 days after thymus cell injection.

†Cytotoxicity was determined by the method of Brunner et al.[19] using a killer cell:target cell ratio of 20:1, Ig was added to the cultures at a concentration of 1 mg/ml; spontaneous lysis of mastocytoma cells alone was 19%.

REFERENCES

1. McDevitt HO, Benacerraf B: Adv Immunol 11: 31, 1969

2. Feldmann M, Nossal GJV: Transplant Rev 13:3 1972

3. Crone M, Koch C, Simonsen M: Transplant Rev 10:36, 1972

4. Miller JFAP: Int Rev Cytol 33:77, 1972

5. Vitetta ES, Bianco C, Nussenzweig JW, Uhr JW: J Exp Med 136:81, 1972

6. Marchalonis JJ, Cone RE, Atwell JL: J Exp Med 135:956, 1972

7. Sprent J, Miller JFAP: Cell Immunol 3:385, 1972

8. Sprent J, Miller JFAP: Cell Immunol 3:213, 1972

9. Bankhurst AD, Warner NL, Sprent J: J Exp Med 134:1005, 1971

10. Nossal GJV, Warner NL, Lewis H, Sprent J: J Exp Med 135:405, 1972

11. Cone RE, Sprent J, Marchalonis JJ: Proc Natl Acad Sci USA 69:2556, 1972

12. Pernis B, Miller JFAP, Forni L, Sprent J: Cell Immunol (in press)

13. Playfair JHL, Marshal-Clark S, Hudson L: submitted for publication

14. Modified from Schlossman SF, Hudson L: J Immunol 110:313, 1973

15. Hudson L, Sprent J, Miller JFAP, Playfair JHL: manuscript in preparation

16. Hudson L, Roitt IM: Eur J Immunol 3:63, 1973

17. Yoshida TO, Andersson B: Scand J Immunol 1:401, 1972

18. Lee ST, Paraskevas G: J Immunol 109:1262, 1972

19. Brunner KT, Mauel J, Cerottini JC, Chapuis B: Immunology 14:181, 1968

20. Basten A, Miller JFAP, Sprent J, Pye J: J Exp Med 135:610, 1972

Significance of Antigen Binding by T Cells

By Jeannine Charreire and Jean-François Bach

DIRECT demonstration of antigen binding by T cells has been a matter of controversy in the last few years. Whereas antigen binding by B cells is easily demonstrated by the rosette test and radioautography using labeled soluble antigens, these two techniques have often been found inoperative for T cells. Technical reasons probably explain these failures,[1-4] such as the use of weakly labeled antigens for the radioautography studies[5] or techniques not delicate enough for rosettes.[6] The latter include turbulent resuspension and omission of detection of rosettes with few red cells, which have been shown to include the majority of T rosettes.[6] Respecting all necessary technical requirements, many authors[5-17] have now reported the existence of T-antigen-binding cells (ABC) in spleen cells using anti-θ serum (AθS), sometimes made fluorescent,[12] in thymus cells[17] or in educated thymocytes[6,11,14] either detected by the rosette test[7-14] or by radioautography.[5,15,16] Now that the controversy is somewhat settled, one may wonder what is the significance of these T-ABC, or more precisely what is the nature of their receptors and whether these receptors are produced by the ABC itself or secondarily fixed on its surface as cytophilic antibodies. We have approached these problems by studying rosette-forming cells (RFC) in pure T-cell preparations, paying particular attention to their antigenic specificity and looking at the possibility of their passive formation in vitro and in vivo. Before describing these studies, we shall report experiments confirming directly the thymic origin of θ-positive RFC.

From INSERM U25, Clinique Nêphrologique, Hôpital Necker, Paris, France.

©1973 by Grune & Stratton, Inc.

MATERIALS AND METHOD

Animals. Mice were of CBA-Lac Harwell, CBA-T6T6 Harwell, and C57BL/6 strains. (C57BL/6 × CBA-Lac) F_1 were also used in some experiments. Chimeras with T6-labeled T cells were prepared as described by Davies:[18] adult CBA-Lac mice were thymectomized, irradiated (850 R) and reconstituted intravenously with 50×10^6 thymus cells from CBA-T6T6 mice and 35×10^6 bone marrow cells from CBA-Lac H mice. They were simultaneously injected i.v. with 6×10^8 sheep red blood cells (SRBC) or 3×10^8 pigeon red blood cells (PRBC). Other chimeras with T cells bearing an allogeneic marker were prepared by reconstituting thymectomized irradiated CBA-Lac mice with 60×10^6 thymus cells intraperitoneally from (C57BL/6 × CBA-Lac) F_1 mice and 15×10^6 syngeneic bone marrow cells.[13] Such chimeras were used 4 wk later for rosette inhibition studies.

Educated thymocytes. Educated thymocytes were obtained from CBA-Lac mice irradiated (850 R) and reconstituted with 50×10^6 syngeneic thymus cells and stimulated simultaneously with 5×10^8 SRBC or 3×10^8 PRBC.

Rosette test. The rosette test was performed as previously described.[6] Particular attention was given to gentle resuspension and to evaluation of rosettes with few RBC.

Karyotypes. The rosette technique was adapted to the karyotype technique using formalin-treated RBC. Formalin treatment was performed as previously reported.[19] PRBC were used without formalin treatment since their nuclei resist the hypotonic shock and still bear PRBC antigenicity. The karyotype technique was that of Ford.[20]

Immunizations. Immunizations were generally obtained by i.v. injection of 5×10^8 SRBC and 3×10^8 PRBC. Cytophilic antibodies were obtained by injection of 5×10^8 SRBC i.v. or 3×10^8 PRBC into normal mice and collecting their sera 5 days later.

Cytotoxicity tests. Cytotoxicity tests were performed as already described.[8] CBA anti-C57BL/6 serum was prepared by the repeated weekly injection of 2×10^8 thymus lymph nodes and spleen cells i.p. into normal CBA-Lac mice for 6 wk and bleeding 1 wk after the last injection.[13]

RESULTS

T6 and Allogeneic Markers

Chimeric mice bearing T6-labeled T cells showed a significant rosette formation and

T6 mitosis response to SRBC or PRBC as early as 3 days after immunization. More than 92% of mitotic RFC bear the T6 chromosome on day 3, both for PRBC and SRBC stimulation, and 80% anti-PRBC RFC and 20% anti-SRBC RFC still bear the T6 chromosome on day 4. The specificity of the technique was verified by showing that rosettes were only formed against the immunizing antigens.

Chimeric mice bearing T cells with the allogeneic C57BL/6 antigens were studied for spontaneous rosette formation, since the chromosome technique does not apply for spontaneous RFC that do not divide. Rosette formation by spleen cells was inhibited by low anti-C57BL/6 serum concentration (1:500) in the presence of complement (60% inhibition). Conversely, no inhibition was obtained with the same antiserum using CBA spleen cells. AθS and azathioprine (AZ) tested under similar conditions[8] inhibited 55 to 65% RFC in both strains of mice at identical concentrations.

Educated Thymocytes

Significant numbers of anti-SRBC rosettes were observed in educated thymocytes (3300 RFC/10^6 cells on day 7). Rosettes in thymocyte-reconstituted mice remained lower than 900/10^6 without immunization with SRBC or in mice immunized with SRBC but not reconstituted with thymocytes. Absence of hemagglutinin production was verified in all instances. The specificity of the rosette response was furthermore examined by immunizing thymocyte-reconstituted mice with both SRBC and PRBC. The majority (85%) of RFC formed in the presence of SRBC and PRBC proved to be specific for one red blood cell species.

Passive Rosette Formation

Cytophilic serum was injected intraperitoneally into normal CBA-Lac mice (0.5 ml) or incubated in vitro with normal CBA-Lac spleen cells for 30 min at 37°C. In both cases a significant increase[2-4] of rosette number was obtained when rosettes were read immediately after collecting spleen cells for in vivo experiments or at the end of the incubation time for in vitro experiments. However, no significant increase in rosette number was noted when spleen cells were incubated 90 min at 37°C before rosettes were read, as was the case in rosette-inhibition experiments performed with AθS in order to eliminate macrophages from the cell suspension.

Specificity of T Rosettes

Antigen specificity of educated thymocytes has already been mentioned. The absence of double rosette formation was always observed in normal thymus and spleen cells. A few double RFC were observed after double immunization with SRBC and PRBC,[21] particularly 5 to 7 days after immunization, and these double RFC proved to be sensitive to inhibition by AθS[22] but always represented a minority of RFC (<15%).

DISCUSSION

The existence of T rosettes in the mouse as has been previously discussed, seems now well established and is confirmed here using a chromosomal marker for immunized mice and an allogeneic marker for unimmunized mice. Similar results had already been obtained with allogeneic markers in immunized mice.[9,13]

The antigen specificity of T rosettes is also shown here, although it is probably less strict than that of antibody-producing cells. Such specificity argues very much against passive fixation of cytophilic receptors, which should lead to a much higher incidence of double rosette formation. The absence of passive rosette formation in vitro or in vivo using the adequate rosette technique after elimination of macrophages by in vitro incubation with sera shown to contain cytophilic antibodies is another result on the same line. Rosette formation in educated thymocytes when no antibody is produced is also against the cytophilic hypothesis. Different results obtained by Kapp and Benacerraf[23] are probably explained by the use of a different rosette technique not including the incubation time at 37°C referred to above. Lastly, rosette inhibition by antimetabolites such as AZ[8] is also against a passive receptor fixation.

Another problem is the nature of the T-ABC receptor. It has been reported that T-ABC were inhibited by anti-light-chain antibodies.[5,24] Conversely, McDevitt[16] did not observe such inhibition. Both the fact that columns coated with anti-light-chain antibody let pass θ-positive RFC[25] and that the inactivation of T-antigen-sensitive cells by antigen (in the suicide experiment) is prevented by anti-light-chain antibodies,[15] as well as the recent demonstration of antigen capping of T-ABC induced by anti-light-chain serum,[5] all support the relationship between T-ABC receptors and immunoglobulins, which, however, obviously deserves much more investigation.

SUMMARY

Rosette-forming cells (RFC) include T cells, as shown directly using chromosomal or allogeneic markers. T-RFC are antigen-specific and are found in educated thymocytes when no antibody is produced. They do not seem to be due to cytophilic antibodies because of their high specificity and the impossibility of producing them passively in vivo and in vitro.

ACKNOWLEDGMENT

We would like to thank Bernadette Bertin for competent technical assistance.

REFERENCES

1. Crone M, Koch C, Simonsen M: Transplant Rev 10:36 1972

2. Hemmingson EJ, Alm GV: Eur J Immunol 2:379, 1972

3. Hunter P, Munro A, McConnell I: Nature [New Biol] 236:52, 1972

4. Takahashi T, Old LJ, McIntyre KR, Boyse EA: J Exp Med 134:815, 1971

5. Roelants G, Forni L, Pernis B: J Exp Med 137:1060, 1973

6. Charreire J, Dardenne M, Bach JF: Cell Immunol 9:32, 1973

7. Bach JF, Muller JY, Dardenne M: Nature 227:1251, 1970

8. Bach JF, Dardenne M: Cell Immunol 3:11, 1972

9. Greaves MF, Moller E: Cell Immunol 1:372, 1970

10. Schlesinger M: Nature 226:1254, 1970

11. Haskill JS, Elliott BE, Kerbel R, et al: J Exp Med 35:1410, 1972

12. Ashman RF, Raff MC: J Exp Med 137:69, 1973

13. Wilson JD, Miller JFAP: Eur J Immunol 1:501, 1971

14. Argyris BF, Haritou A, Cooney A: Cell Immunol 3:101, 1972

15. Basten A, Miller JFAP, Warner NL, Pye J: Nature [New Biol] 231:104, 1971

16. McDevitt H: Transpant Proc 5:1799, 1973

17. Bach JF, Dardenne M: Cell Immunol 3:1, 1972

18. Davies AJS: Transplant Rev 1:43, 1969

19. Bach JF: Transplant Rev (in press)

20. Ford CE: in Micklem HS, Loutit JF (eds): Tissue Grafting and Radiation. New York, Academic, 197

21. Liacopoulos P, Amstutz M, Gille F: Immunology 20:57, 1971

22. Taieb C, Liacopoulos P, Bach JF: submitted for publication

23. Kapp J, Benacerraf B: Eur J Immunol 2:467, 1972

24. Greaves MF, Transplant Rev 5:45, 1970

25. Hudson L, Greenberg AH, Roitt J, Bach JF: Scand J Immunol 2:425, 1973

Antibody-induced Cytotoxicity by Nonsensitized Lymphocytes in Humans

By T. Kovithavongs and J. B. Dossetor

IN VITRO cytotoxicity by nonsensitized lymphocytes can be produced in several ways:[1] (1) by stimulation with PHA or ALS, (2) upon contact with histoincompatible lymphocytes, (3) upon contact with membrane-bound antigen–antibody complex. Our experience in humans has been with the last category. We have found that when an antibody specific for a tissue antigen on a cell binds with the cell, this cell-bound antibody can activate nonsensitized lymphocytes to kill that cell. This phenomenon was first described by E. Möller[2] and has been extensively studied by Perlmann[3] and MacLennan.[4] The mechanism, we believe, is as postulated by G. Möller:[5] as the $F(ab')_2$ of the antibody molecule specifically binds to the target, the Fc portion becomes activated and can trigger normal lymphocytes to exert cytotoxicity by binding to the Fc receptors present on the surface of lymphocytes. The exact mechanism of how the target cell is killed remains unknown at present, although close contact between the effector cells and the target cells is required, and the effector cells must be viable and capable of active metabolism.

We call this phenomenon antibody-mediated cell-dependent immune lympholysis, or ABCIL, and we have studied this phenomenon in multiparous women[6,7] as well as in hemodialysis patients and renal transplants[8] using peripheral blood lymphocytes as target cells labeled with ^{51}Cr. We have found that this system is indeed extremely sensitive for the detection of histoincompatible antigen sensitization, as compared to the conventional complement-dependent cytotoxicity test. Serum diluted down to $1{:}10^6$ can still detect the presence of this ABCIL antibody, whereas the highest titer for the cytotoxic antibody is about 1:5000. We have performed some comparative studies of these two systems and found that the ABCIL antibody can be detected with a higher frequency than the cytotoxic antibody. However, this is not due to the degree of sensitivity of the two systems, for in certain sera that were negative for ABCIL antibody, cytotoxic antibody was present (Table 1). So far we have found ABCIL activity only in the IgG fraction. Neutralization with rabbit anti-human gamma globulin indicates that this ABCIL activity is due to an immunoglobulin. Removal of the Fc portion by pepsin digestion decreases the ABCIL activity. This would support the view that an intact Fc is necessary for the cytotoxicity to be manifested.

The specificity of this system has not been fully delineated. In some instances it appears to be HL-A-specific; in others it has clearly extended beyond the present serologically defined HL-A system. In one multiparous woman that we studied, ABCIL antibody was detected in her serum against a panel of 13 cells in addition to her husband's. In fact, the only instance in which ABCIL was negative was when her serum

Table 1. ABCIL and Lymphocytotoxicity Tests on the Same Cell as Measured by Percentage ^{51}Cr Release

	% ^{51}Cr Release
S1	3.45
S1 + C′	4.62
S1 + lymphocytes	20.52
S2	3.44
S2 + C′	30.70
S2 + lymphocytes	5.17

The first serum (S1) is positive for ABCIL, negative for lymphocytotoxicity. In contrast, the second serum (S2) was positive for lymphocytotoxicity but negative for ABCIL.

From the MRC Transplantation Group, University of Alberta, Edmonton, Alberta, Canada.
©1973 by Grune & Stratton, Inc.

Table 2. Correlative Study in the L. Family

	WIFE	HUSBAND	PANEL												
HL-A	2 3 50 14	3 →11 →7 →12	→11 W32 →12 50	2 →11 →12	1 →11 →7 8	1 →11 →7 W15	2 →7 27	2 W30 8 →12	2 10 W22 14	9 5	2 28 5 50	28 W32 W22 14	1 W30 8 60	2 W29 60	2 W30 60 W22
CYT		(+) -	(+) -	(+) -	-	-	-	(+) -	-	-	-	-	-	-	-
CAT		+	+	+	-	+	-	+	-	-	-	-	-	-	-
AGG		-	-	+	-	-	-	-	-	-	-	-	-	-	-
ABCIL	-	+	+	+	+	+	+	+	+	+	+	+	+	+	+
UMLC		↓	↓	↓	-	↓	↓	↓	↓	↓	↓	↓	↓	↓	↓
MIF-Sw		+	+	N. D.	+	+	-	-	-	+	-	-	-	-	-
MIF+Sw		-	-	N. D.	+	+				+					

Arrow toward right indicates HL-A antigen similar to husband's; (+) = previously + ve; CYT, cytotoxicity test; CAT, capillary agglutinating test; AGG, leukoagglutination test; ABCIL, antibody-mediated cell-dependent immune lympholysis; UMLC, unidirectional mixed lymphocyte culture; vertical arrow indicates inhibition by serum; MIF − Sw = MIF in the absence of wife's serum; MIF + Sw = MIF in the presence of wife's serum; N.D., not done. Positive reactions in CYT, CAT, AGG are strictly confined to the husband and panel sharing husband's incompatible HL-A antigens. Positive reactions in ABCIL and UMLC inhibition are widespread and not confined by HL-A.

was reacted against her own lymphocytes as target (Table 2). It is interesting to note that her serum was also inhibitory in unidirectional mixed lymphocyte cultures in which her lymphocytes were the responding cells. In this woman, however, a limited absorption study was able to identify that the major ABCIL activity was directed against an HL-A antigen, namely HL-A12 (Fig. 1). In another study performed on an Eskimo family in which the parents and 11 children were all serologically HL-A-identical, ABCIL antibody was detected in the mother's serum against the father and three of the children tested (Tables 3 and 4). In this instance, then, the ABCIL antibody was clearly directed against a non-HL-A antigen. In this family it is also remarkable

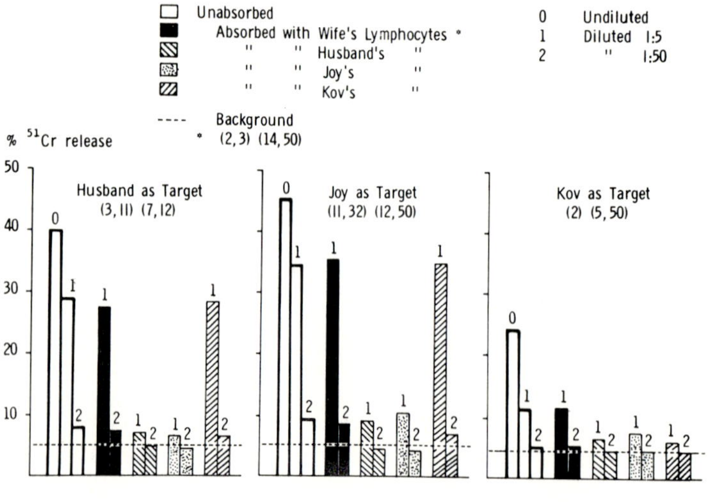

Fig. 1. ABCIL absorption study. Wife's serum absorbed with husband's and panel cells, then reacted in ABCIL with husband's and panel cells.

Table 3. HL-A-identical Eskimo Family* T.

	Rufus	Sarah
HL-A	9	9
W	10	10
ABO	A	AB

	Winnifred	Trudy	Ray	Nadia	Merlin	Pat	Glen	Lorna	Mary Lou	Abel	Rhoda
HL-A	9	9	9	9	9	9	9	9	9	9	9
W	10	10	10	10	10	10	10	10	10	10	10
ABO	B	AB	A	A	A	A	AB	B	AB	A	A

*HL-A typing sera of Edmonton, Terasaki (621, 781), J. Falk.

Table 4. ABCIL in the T. Family*—Wife vs. Husband and Some Children

Targets	% Background	^{51}Cr Release Specific
Husband	5.42	28.44
Glen	4.53	20.66
Raymond	7.30	17.74
Trudy	4.48	17.15

*Performed 10 yr after her last pregnancy.

that the antibody could be detected after a period of 10 yr since her last pregnancy.

We would like to conclude at this point that this ABCIL phenomenon occurs in man. Its biologic significance in the field of transplantation is unknown. This in vitro system is extremely sensitive for the detection of histoincompatible antigenic sensitization. The specificity of this system is not entirely defined by HL-A.

REFERENCES

1. Lundgren G, Collste L, Möller G: Nature (Lond) 220:298, 1968
2. Möller E: Science 147:873, 1965
3. Perlmann P, Holm G: Adv Immunol 11:117, 1969
4. MacLennen ICM: Transplant Rev 13:67, 1972
5. Möller G: Transplant Proc 3:15, 1971
6. Dossetor JB, Kovithavongs T, Boyd JJ, et al: Proceedings of First International Congress on Immunology in Obstetrics and Gynaecology, 1973. (in press)
7. McConnachie PR, Dossetor JB: Tissue Antigens (in press)
8. Dossetor JB, Kovithavongs T, Lao VSH, et al: Proceedings of the European Dialysis and Transplantation Association, 1973. (in press)

Part III

In Vivo Correlates

Introduction

By Jean Hamburger

TO what extent do recent advances in the knowledge of MLC and other related in vitro data have in vivo implications? The answer is: to a large extent. In fact, the understanding of graft rejection and many other problems has greatly progressed in parallel to and because of progress in the results of in vitro studies.

Indeed, we have some evidence that lymphocyte stimulation and blast transformation occur in the allograft recipient exactly as they do in vitro in the mixed lymphocyte culture. Even in clinically well-tolerated renal grafts in the human, a biopsy will often show some interstitial cell infiltration, and when studied under the electron microscope, some of these cells appear quite similar to immunoblasts. We have described a method of following this in vivo transformation of lymphocytes by collecting renal graft lymph from dog and man.[1] This method is derived from the observations of Pedersen and Morris in sheep.[2] Human graft lymph can be collected for up to 12 days following renal transplantation. In dogs not receiving an immunosuppressive drug, the efferent lymph from renal allografts shows only pure normal lymphocytes during the first days. Transformed cells appear after the fourth day, and their proportion may sometimes reach as much as 60% of the collected cells on the sixth day. In man receiving the usual immunosuppressive treatment, the renal allograft lymph may show only normal lymphocytes during the whole period of observation, but in some cases, despite immunosuppression, transformed lymphocytes with blast and mitotic cells may be seen after the fourth and fifth post-transplantation day, and their proportion may rise to 20% or more and then slowly diminish. The incorporation of tritiated thymidine into the lymph cells increases in a parallel fashion, just as it does in an in vitro mixed lymphocyte culture. In some cases, clinical manifestation of rejection follows the appearance of transformed cells in a transplant lymph.

When comparing the results of mixed lymphocyte cultures performed between donor and recipient cells prior to transplantation to the degree of in vivo lymph transformation, a remarkable correlation can be found. This suggests that mixed lymphocyte culture can be a useful tool for the prediction of the degree of cellular immunologic response that the host will show against the graft. The use of mixed lymphocyte culture and also of cell-mediated lympholysis as tests for the selection of allograft donors will be the first subject of this discussion.

The mixed lymphocyte culture theoretically could also be useful for the follow-up of the allograft immunologic reaction after transplantation. The recipient's cell sensitization against the graft, or contrarily the appearance of a specific unresponsiveness, should be detectable by comparing the in vitro response of the host cells to the donor cells prior to transplantation to the same response after transplantation. This method is, in fact, part of a rapidly growing field, i.e., the use of a series of cell-mediated immunologic in vitro tests for the follow-up of the organ allograft recipient. We will devote the second part of the discussion to this important subject.

Finally, the study of the major histocompatibility complex has recently proved also to be of great importance for many subjects other than organ transplantation. A number of biological problems, as well as the genetic approach to many diseases such as ankylosing spondylitis, myasthenia

From Hôpital Necker, Paris, France.
©1973 by Grune & Stratton, Inc.

gravis, multiple sclerosis, psoriasis, and coeliac disease, are in the process of being enlightened by the study of the chromosomic region bearing histocompatibility antigens.

REFERENCES

1. Hamburger J, Dimitriu A, Bankir L, et al: Nature 232:633, 1971

2. Pedersen NC, Morris B: J Exp Med 131:936, 1970

LD–SD Interaction In Vivo and the Allograft Reaction

By J.J. van Rood

DURING the past year studies by Eysvoogel and Alter have shown the existence of an in vitro interaction between serologically defined (SD) and lymphocyte defined (LD) histocompatibility antigens, notably in the cell-mediated lympholysis (CML) test.[1-3] In brief, these studies indicate that killer-cell activation in the CML test is brought about by a disparity between stimulator and responder cells at the MLC locus, while target-cell destruction takes place only through SD differences and mainly through differences of the Four-series antigens. As was to be expected, these studies have aroused widespread interest, but they suffer from two obvious drawbacks. In the first place, they are performed in vitro, and it is not a priori certain that an extrapolation to the in vivo situation is permissible. In the second place, through limitations inherent in the protocols used, the number of combinations tested is rather limited, and it is for that reason uncertain to what extent the findings obtained thus far can be translated into rules that are valid in general.

In vivo studies of over 50 skin grafts and over 300 kidney grafts led independently to the formulation of exactly the same mechanism for the recognition of foreignness, as was concluded from the in vitro CML work.[4,5] It is our intention to summarize the relevant findings, formulate the different steps by which the homograft reaction might be brought about, and suggest a few topics for further evaluation. In this, we will restrict ourselves mainly to the situation in man.

From the Department of Immunohaematology, University Hospital, Leiden, The Netherlands.

Supported in part by the Dutch Organization for Health Research (TNO), the Dutch Organization for Pure Research (FUNGO), the Whitehall Foundation, the National Institute of Health (contract PH 43-65-992), and the J. A. Cohen Institute for Radiopathology and Radiation Protection.

©1973 by Grune & Stratton, Inc.

EXPERIMENTAL FINDINGS

Effect of Immunization on Graft Survival

Graft survival can be but is not always shortened by the injection of blood or tissue from the graft donor to an unrelated person or persons,[6-8] due to the presence of antibodies. These experiments formed the basis for the postulation of the existence of and the recognition of the transplantation antigens.

Recipients can be divided into responders and nonresponders, because shortening of graft survival is not always observed after injection of blood, etc., even in the face of incompatibility for the transplantation antigens between donor and recipient.[9-12] Generally speaking, this division is based on the presence or absence of cytotoxic antibodies. It is, however, certain that recipients without cytotoxic antibodies can have other antibodies, such as those that can block the MLC test.[13,14] The relative effects of these different types of antibodies and of activated or killer cells in graft survival are uncertain. In our analysis it will thus be necessary to separate graft recipients who have received blood transfusions or who have been pregnant from those who have not. In the latter group, a distinction should be made between those who have formed antibodies and those who have not. Finally, the effect of immunosuppression should be taken into account.

Nonimmunized Recipients Without Immunosuppression

Koch et al.[4] have shown that in SD-identical donor–recipient combinations, skin graft survival is inversely correlated with MLC reactivity, i.e., the stronger the MLC

Table 1. Skin Graft Survival and Matching for LD and SD

	N	Mean Skin Graft Survival	SE	Publication	Significance
LD ≠ SD ≠	24	9.96	17.8	Koch 1973	.02
LD ≠ SD =	14	11.86	0.3	Koch 1973	.01 .04 .001
LD = SD ≠	6	17	12	Sasportes 1973* Ward 1973†[23]	.03
LD = SD =	4	15.25	2.3	Koch 1973	n.s.

≠ indicates non-identity; = indicates identity.

All skin grafts were exchanged between unrelated donor–recipient pairs except the (critical) LD = SD ≠ grafts, which were exchanged between parent and child* and siblings.†

reaction the shorter the skin graft survival. Sasportes et al. have furthermore shown that when donor and recipient are only LD-identical[15] (thus in the face of SD nonidentity), skin graft survival shows approximately the same prolongation (Table 1). In the nonimmunized recipient, matching for LD seems thus to be more important than matching for SD.

Immunized Recipients Without Immunosuppression

Experiments in Rhesus monkeys and in man have shown[16-18] that preimmunization against a specific transplantation antigen will shorten the survival of subsequent grafts carrying that antigen. For instance, after intradermal immunization with buffy coat cells from a donor A who carried the antigen HL-A7, lacking in the recipient, skin grafts from an unrelated HL-A7-positive donor had a mean survival time of 6 days, while skin grafts from an unrelated HL-A7-negative donor had a mean survival time of 11 days (Table 2). Similar findings have been obtained for 4a, 4b, HL-A2, and HL-A8. In the immunized recipient, matching for the SD antigens against which the recipient has been immunized appears to be a most effective way to improve skin graft survival.

Table 2. Skin Graft Survival in HL-A7-negative Recipients After Immunization With HL-A7-positive Leucocytes

Immunizing Dose	Interval (Days)	Survival of Skin Graft HL-A7 pos.	Survival of Skin Graft HL-A7 neg.
1.2×10^8 leuc.	14	0	12
2.2×10^8	18	5	9
2×10^8	16	5½	8½
0.5×10^8	13	7	14
2×10^8	14	9	11
2.1×10^8	14	9½	11½
Mean		6	11

From van Rood et al, 1965.

Nonimmunized Recipients With Immunosuppression

Hamburger[19] has shown that prognosis for kidney grafts exchanged between parent and child correlated best with MLC reactivity, i.e., the lower the MLC reactivity the better the graft prognosis. Although the number of blood transfusions these children had received was not given, it can be assumed that it will have been low. In accordance with those results, van Hooff et al.[9] found in almost 200 kidney graft recipients who had received blood transfusions, but who had no demonstrable leucocyte antibodies, that graft survival appeared to be better only in the SD-identical group. It was argued that in all probability graft survival was superior because in the process of matching for SD, one matches at the same time (through link-

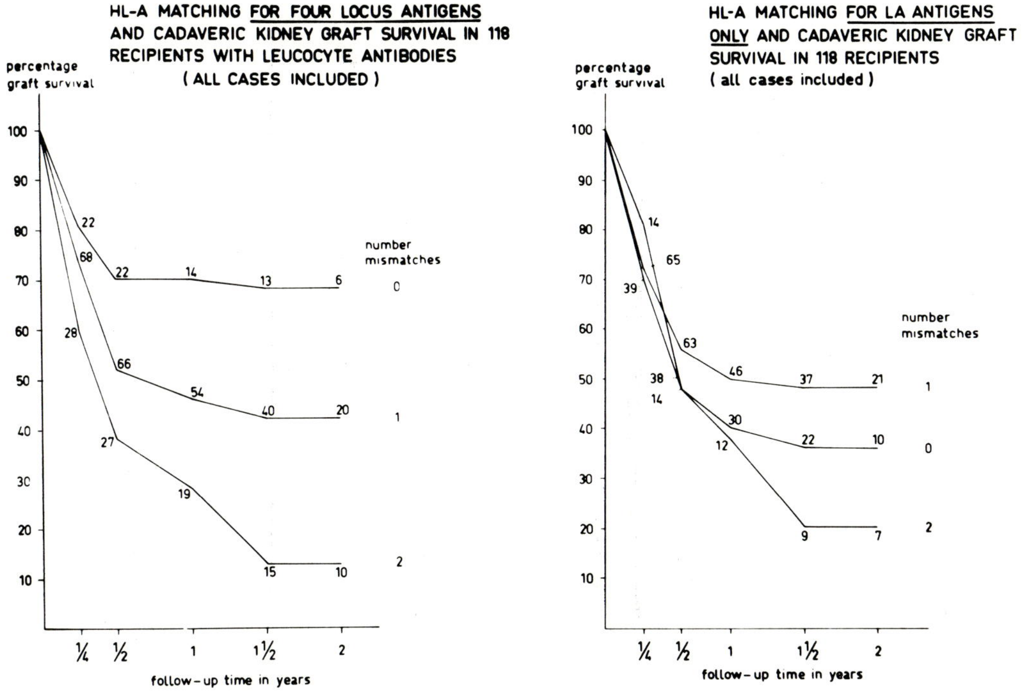

Fig. 1. HL-A matching and kidney graft prognosis. All recipients had formed leucocyte antibodies as a result of previous blood transfusions. Kidney graft prognosis is significantly improved through matching for the Four-locus antigens. Prognosis is not improved through matching for the LA-locus antigens. The (not significant) improved survival of the graft mismatched for one LA antigen might be due to the fact that many of these grafts had zero mismatches for the Four-series antigens.[9]

age disequilibrium) for LD. This received support from the finding that in this group grafts mismatched for four antigens had a prognosis as good as that for grafts mismatched for one antigen. Data by Cochrum et al.[20] also indicate that matching for MLC improves graft survival significantly.

Immunized Recipients With Immunosuppression

Van Hooff et al.[9] have presented significant evidence that in this group, matching especially for the antigens of the Four series improves graft survival (Fig. 1). Especially because of the linear correlation between the number of mismatched antigens of the Four series and graft prognosis, it appears highly likely that one should match for these antigens and not some other product coded for by the MLC chromosomal region. Data by Oliver et al.[12] also indicated that matching for the Four series antigens will improve graft survival significantly.

DISCUSSION

We interpret the in vivo findings as being in almost complete agreement with the in vitro data. In the nonimmunized recipient or in the recipient who has received blood transfusions but has not formed lymphocytotoxic antibodies, graft survival will be improved by matching for LD, which seems even more important than matching for SD. In other words, in the unprimed recipient or in the recipient who has been primed ineffectively (i.e., no cytotoxic antibodies were formed), matching for LD will improve graft survival, probably because the induction of homograft sensitivity develops more slowly or less effectively.

However, after initiation of the homograft reaction the activated immune apparatus of the recipient will attack the donor organ through differences for SD, especially the Four-locus antigens. This is borne out by the finding that if donor and recipient are matched for these antigens, graft survival is significantly improved even if matching is only partial. It could well be, however, that LA-series disparity is easier to suppress by immunosuppressive treatment than Four-series differences. This could explain why presensitization against HL-A2 without immunosuppression seems to make a difference for skin graft survival (without immunosuppression) but not for kidney graft survival (with immunosuppression). This would be in agreement with findings in the mouse.[21] In these considerations, the effects of non-HL-A systems have not been taken into account. It is possible that they form the target through which graft destruction takes place in SD-identical donor–recipient combinations. In this context it will be of interest to assess the role of the only non-HL-A system recognized so far in man, the group Five system.[22]

Some of the skin graft experiments have been interpreted a posteriori. It will be necessary to extend the study with the the critical SD-identical, LD-different and especially SD-different, LD-identical groups and with skin graft experiments in preimmunized recipients.

To unravel the different steps in the homograft reaction (activation through LD differences, development of immunity, role of macrophages, and target-cell destruction through SD differences by killer cells and/or antibody) might be at least partly possible by combining in vitro and in vivo transfer experiments. For instance, it would be of interest to activate lymphocytes in vitro and transfer them to recipients disparate either at LD or at SD with and without simultaneous antibody transfer.

REFERENCES

1. Eijsvoogel VP, du Bois MJGJ, Melief CJM, et al: in Dausset J, Colombani J (eds): Histocompatibility Testing, 1972. Copenhagen, Munksgaard, 1973, p 501

2. Eijsvoogel VP, du Bois R, Melief CJM, et al: Transplant Proc 5:1301, 1973

3. Alter BJ, Schendel DJ, Bach ML, et al: J Exp Med 137:1303, 1973

4. Koch CT, van Hooff JP, van Leeuwen A, et al: in Dausset J, Colombani J (eds): Histocompatibility Testing, 1972. Copenhagen, Munksgaard, 1973, p 521

5. Van Rood JJ, Koch CT, van Hooff JP: Transplant Proc 5:409, 1973

6. Friedman EA, Retan JW, Marshall DC: J Clin Invest 40:2162, 1961

7. Medawar PB: Br J Exp Pathol 27:15, 1946

8. Rapaport FT, Thomas L, Converse JA, et al: Fed Proc 20:36, 1961

9. Van Hooff JP, Schippers HMA, van der Steen GJ, et al: Lancet 1972, ii, 7792:1385

10. Opelz G, Mickey MR, Terasaki PI: Lancet 1972, i, 7756:868

11. Payne R: Arch Intern Med 99:587, 1957

12. Oliver RTD, Sachs JA, Festenstein H, et al: Lancet 1972, ii, 7792:1381

13. Hattler BG, Karesh C, Miller J: Tissue Antigens 1:270, 1971

14. Revillard JP, Robert M, DuPont E, et al: Transplant Proc 5:331, 1973

15. Sasportes M, Lebrun A, Repaport FT, et al: Transplant Proc 5:353, 1973

16. Balner H, Dersjant H, van Rood JJ: Transplantation 3:230, 1965

17. Van Rood JJ, van Leeuwen A, Schippers A, et al: Histocompatibility Testing 1965, Ser Haematol 11:37, 1965

18. Dausset J, Rapaport FT, Iványi P, et al: Histocompatibility Testing 1965, Ser Haematol 11:63, 1965

19. Hamburger JJ, Crosnier JJ, Deschamps B, et al: Transplant Proc 3:260, 1971

20. Cochrum K, Perkins H, Payne R, et al: Transplant Proc 5:391, 1973

21. Démant P: MLC workshop, London, 26 February–2 March 1973 (to be published)

22. Van Leeuwen A, Eernisse JG, Van Rood JJ: Vox Sang 9:431, 1964

23. Ward FE, Seigler HF: Transplant Proc 5:359, 1973

Some Remarks About the Preceding Paper by Prof. J. J. van Rood With Regard to the Interpretation of the Results of Kidney and Skin Allograft Studies in Man

By Jean Dausset

ALTHOUGH the author is in general agreement with the outline presented by Professor van Rood, a number of points raised in his presentation are deserving of more detailed consideration and analysis, with particular reference to differences in the results of kidney transplantation in patients whose sera contain cytotoxic antibodies, as compared to those whose sera do not contain such antibodies. Two additional points of interest worthy of further comment in the light of our own experience refer to the relative role of incompatibility for the two SD HL-A loci, and to a correlation between HL-A identity and the results of transplantation. Statistical studies of the results of kidney transplantation performed under the auspices of the France-Transplant Organization, as well as the results of the 10-yr experience in over 1200 skin allografts performed in collaboration with Dr. Felix T. Rapaport, have provided evidence of a number of rather important points:

(1) The products of the first (LA) and second (Four) HL-A series appear to have about the same weight, in the absence of immunosuppressive therapy, as has been demonstrated with skin allograft studies. Under immunosuppression, there is a trend that the second-series incompatibilities are more detrimental.

(2) The presence or absence of detectable cytotoxic antibodies before cadaver kidney transplantation appears to have no influence on the survival rates observed in the France-Transplant series, as shown in Fig. 1.

(3) The number of transfusions received by the patient before transplantation does, indeed, appear to correlate with kidney allograft prognosis, with a direct proportion between the number of blood transfusions received and the tempo and intensity of renal allograft rejection (Fig. 2).

(4) As noted in Fig. 3, the correlation between HL-A SD incompatibilities and the survival of kidney allografts holds quite well in cadaver kidney recipients, although both groups compared in this figure include subjects with and without cytotoxic serum antibodies, in approximately equivalent numbers.

(5) Figure 4 presents the results of 533 kidney transplants obtained from unrelated (cadaver) donors, and provides clear-cut evidence of the predominant role played by the HL-A SD antigens in conditioning the results of cadaver renal transplantation in man under immunosuppression. A pooling of the data of the France-Transplant Registry with the results of The London Transplant Group, in collaboration with Dr. H. Festenstein, has also provided clear-cut evidence of the tremendous advantages, in terms of long-term renal allograft survival in man, of using full-house phenotypically identical HL-A SD donor–recipient combinations.[1]

From the France-Transplant Registry, Laboratory of Immuno-Hematology, Centre Hayem, Hôpital Saint-Louis, Paris, France.

© *1973 by Grune & Stratton, Inc.*

REFERENCE

1. Dausset J, Festenstein H: Transplant Proc 5:1299, 1973

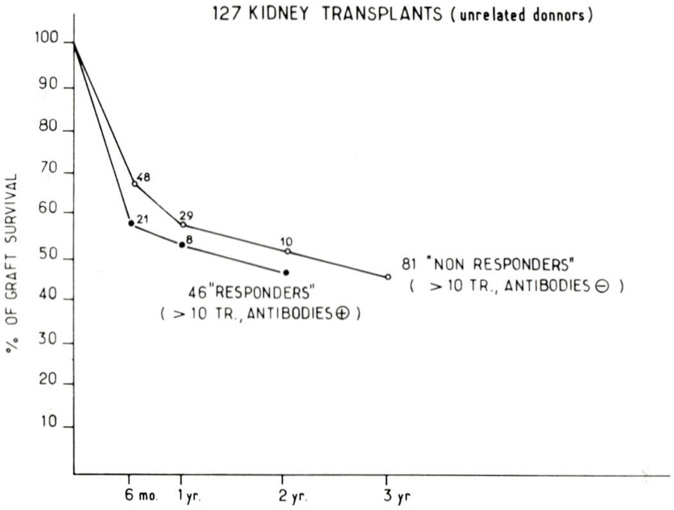

Fig. 1. **Influence of the presence or absence of detectable cytotoxic antibodies in the recipient upon the survival of cadaver-donor renal allografts.**

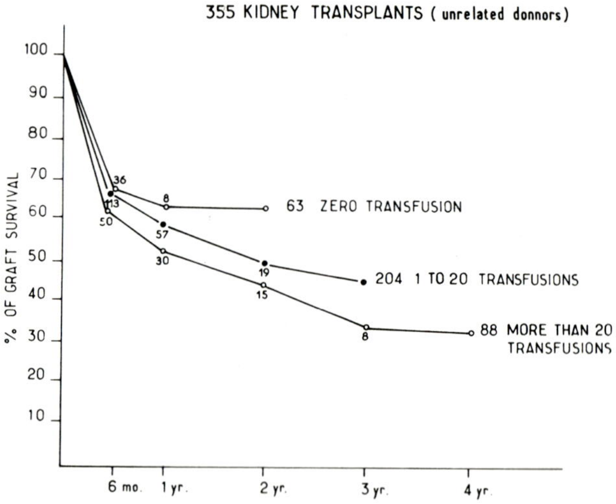

Fig. 2. **Correlation between the prognosis of renal allograft survival and the number of transfusions received by the patient prior to transplantation.**

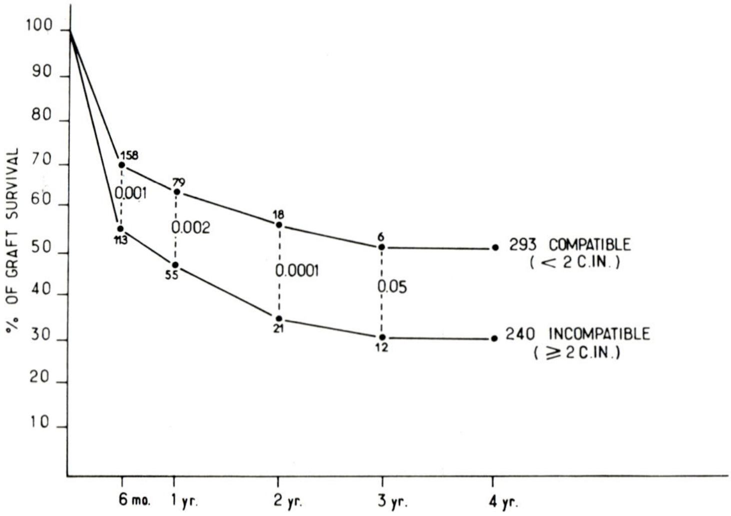

Fig. 3. **Renal allograft survival rates in donor–recipient pairs with two or less HL-A SD incompatibilities, as compared to pairs with two or more incompatibilities, where each patient grouping includes approximately the same number of subjects with detectable cytotoxic antibodies before transplantation.**

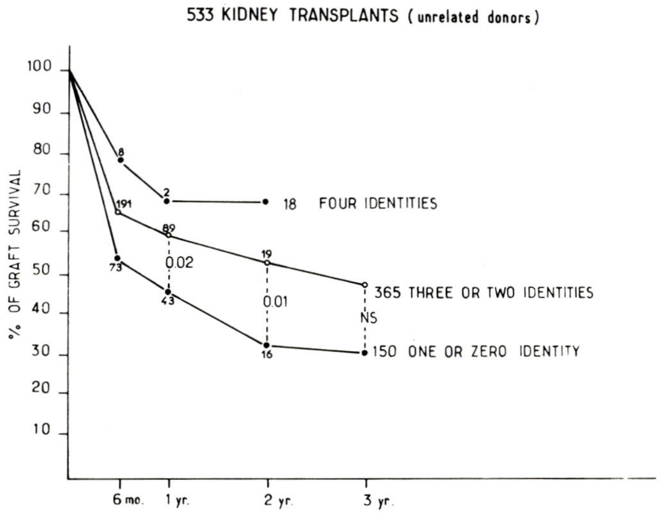

Fig. 4. Evidence of the predominant role played by the HL-A SD antigens in cadaver renal transplantation under immunosuppression.

Proliferating Helper-Cell (PHC) Test: A Possible Addition to the Armamentarium for Histocompatibility Testing

By Marilyn L. Bach and Fritz H. Bach

THE problems of choosing the right donor for a given recipient in allotransplantation has intensely commanded the attention of geneticists and immunologists for more than a decade. Although the evidence suggesting that typing for the HL-A serologically defined (SD) antigens and matching for the lymphocyte-defined (LD) determinants of HL-A with the mixed leukocyte culture (MLC) test has had a highly significant (and salutary) effect within families, the value of these approaches for pairing of unrelated donor and recipient has been put to question.

Recent evidence obtained in bone marrow transplantation in man suggests that even presumed HL-A SD and LD identity is not sufficient in some cases. In approximately 20% of HL-A SD- and LD-identical sibling pairs, a fatal graft-vs.-host reaction ensues following bone marrow transplantation.[1] It would thus appear that histocompatibility factors other than those presently defined may be of importance.

Recent use of the cell-mediated lympholysis (CML) test in man[2,3] may shed some light in this regard. In the CML test, lymphocytes are sensitized in vitro in MLC for 5 to 6 days and then tested for their ability to lyse phytohemagglutinin-stimulated ^{51}Cr-labeled target cells taken from the donor of the sensitizing cells or from another donor; ^{51}Cr release is regarded as an assay of the extent of cytotoxicity, although the test at present can only be used on a semiquantitative basis.

Although it has been demonstrated[4-6] in both man and mouse that the targets for CML killing are at least in part those determined by the SD loci of HL-A and H-2, or the phenotypic product of loci very closely linked to the SD loci, results of recent family investigations in man[7] are consistent with the postulate that in some cases the CML target can be determined by genes segregating independently of HL-A. This would be a possible mechanism to explain the cases of fatal GvH in the HL-A-identical sibling pairs.

The purpose of this article is to suggest a further histocompatibility test that we propose to call the proliferating helper-cell, or PHC, test. It must be noted that at the present time this is based on theoretical considerations only; extensive animal and human testing will be required before its practical usefulness can properly be determined.

The theoretical basis for this test comes from studies in man by Eijsvoogel and his collaborators[5] and from studies in mouse by Schendel and Alter[6] in our laboratory. In both man and mouse there are certain genes of the major histocompatibility complex (HL-A and H-2, respectively) that we have called LD genes—differences at which, between two individuals, lead to proliferation of their lymphocytes in MLC.[8,9] Whereas differences of the LD genes lead to activation of lymphocytes in MLC, the targets for cytotoxicity in CML are (apparently) the phenotypic products of the SD genes, or alternatively the phenotypic products of genes very closely linked to the SD genes. (For purposes of this discussion

From the Departments of Pediatrics, Pharmacology, Medical Genetics, and Surgery, University of Wisconsin, Madison, Wisc.

Supported by NIH grants AI-08439, GM 15422, and AI-06525; NF-MOD grant CRBS 246; and ONR grant N00014-67-A-128-0003.

M.L.B. is a recipient of the American Cancer Society Faculty Research Award.

This paper is No. 1699 from the Laboratory of Genetics, University of Wisconsin, Madison, Wisc.

© 1973 by Grune & Stratton, Inc.

Table 1. The Three-Cell Experiment

Responding (Effector) Cells	Stimulating (Sensitizing) Cells	Difference	MLC Response	Target Cell	CML
A	B_m	LD	+++	B	–
A	C_m	SD	–	C	–
A	$B_m + C_m$	LD + SD	+++	B	–
				C	+++

we will refer to the SD product as being the target of CML, despite the above-mentioned reservation.) Further, in order to generate cytotoxic cells aimed at the SD targets, it is helpful, if not necessary in at least some cases, to have an LD difference.[5,6] If the LD difference that activates proliferation in MLC is present during the sensitization phase, then equally good cytotoxicity can be obtained on targets carrying only the SD antigens or both the SD and LD differences of the sensitizing cells. It would thus appear that the LD differences facilitate activation of the system, whereas the SD antigens serve as the target for CML.

One elegant demonstration of the LD–SD interaction, which provides a basis for the PHC test, is illustrated in Table 1. In this case, based on the experiments of Schendel,[6,10] we deal with three cells from unrelated individuals. The three cells have the following relationship to each other with respect to the LD and SD differences of the MHC. If we regard the cells of A as the responding cells in mixed culture, then the cells of B differ from A by only LD differences of the MHC, and the cells of C differ from A by only SD differences of the MHC. On the basis of results previously obtained, if we mix the cells of A with the cells of B (differing from A only by LD) then we might expect in some combinations that there would be an excellent proliferative response in mixed leukocyte culture but that no CML killing will take place. That is, the LD differences themselves do not allow a cytotoxic reaction to take place. If we mix the cells of A with the cells of C in the mixed leukocyte culture, then, since there are no LD differences, little or no MLC activation will take place (little or no additional tritiated thymidine will be incorporated in the allogeneic mixture as compared with the isogeneic control); further no CML will take place, as might be expected in the absence of MLC activation. However, if as demonstrated in the third combination, we mix the cells of A simultaneously with the mitomycin-C-treated or x-irradiated cells of B and C, then the cells of A are confronted with both an LD difference to activate the system and an SD difference against which cytotoxic potential can be developed. In such a combination it can be shown that there will be present killer cells that are directed against target cells carrying the SD differences. Similar results have been obtained by Eijsvoogel et al. in a family in man.

In a recent set of experiments, Mawas and his collaborators[7] obtained evidence in family studies that is consistent with the possibility that in some cases the target for CML cytotoxicity may be determined by genes segregating independently of HL-A. In this particular case, cells of the father were activated against those differences carried by one of the siblings in the family; when the sensitized paternal cells were tested for their ability to kill target cells of two HL-A SD- and LD-identical siblings, cytotoxicity was noted against only one of the sibling's cells. Appropriate controls suggest that this was not a difference in lysability of the two cells. In this particular case the cells that were active against the target cells had been activated with LD differences present on the stimulating cells in the MLC.

To apply this to a general test for detecting CML targets in cases where HL-A SD and LD identity can be established, we would propose the use of a three-cell experiment as depicted in Table 1. Let us take the example of a bone marrow transplant. A is to be the potential donor of bone marrow, with B the potential recipient. B is presumably an individual who is both HL-A SD- and LD-identical with A. The question is whether there are targets on the tissue of B that do not lead to lymphocyte proliferation in MLC but that A might recognize as foreign in the CML test. To investigate this problem in the PHC test, one would activate the system by confronting A responding cells with mitomycin-C-treated cells of a third individual, e.g., C, which differ from A by only LD components of the MHC. (This individual would be unrelated to A and yet carry the same HL-A SD antigens as A. Segall has recently shown[11] that in such combinations, although there is extensive activation in MLC as evidenced by enhanced tritiated thymidine incorporation into the culture, little or no CML occurs—presumably because there is no SD difference between the two cells.) In the same culture we would add mitomycin-C-treated cells of the recipient B. We now have the analogue to the three-cell experiment depicted in Table 1. In the mixture of A stimulated by both B_m and C_m in the same culture, the C_m cells provide the stimulus to proliferating helper cells, thus allowing A to develop cytotoxic lymphocytes directed at any possible foreign antigens on the tissue of B. The resultant sensitized cells could be tested individually against B target cells, the specific test combination, and C target cells to ensure that no cytotoxicity is directed against C.

The probability of finding cells that are HL-A SD-identical with any given donor cell but that will stimulate that donor cell in MLC is very good; the practicality seems assured given the effective freezing of cells to be used in MLC and CML, as well as the lesser needs in terms of cell numbers in microculture systems.

It may be possible to use any allogeneic cell donor in place of individual C in the above model of the PHC test, even an individual differing from A by both LD and SD components of HL-A. At first approximation the problem of cross-reactivity between CML targets of C and B, and thus cross-killing in CML, seems disturbing. On the other hand, since we are interested only in the question whether A, the same bone marrow donor, can recognize CML targets on B cells, and since in the final PHC test combination the A-sensitized cells are tested specifically and individually for their ability to kill ^{51}Cr-labeled B target cells, the use of any third-party cell for C in the three-cell MLC sensitization phase may be acceptable.

REFERENCES

1. Storb R, Buckner CD, Fefer A, et al: Transplant Proc (in press)

2. Solliday S, Bach FH: Science 170:1406, 1970

3. Lightbody JJ, Bernoco D, Miggiano VC, et al: J Bact Virol Immunol 64:243, 1971

4. Trinchieri G, Bernoco D, Curtoni SE, et al: in Dausset J (ed): Histocompatibility Testing, 1972. Copenhagen, Munksgaard, (in press)

5. Eijsvoogel VP, du Bois RS, Melief CJM, et al: Transplant Proc 5:1301, 1972

6. Alter BJ, Schendel DH, Bach ML, et al: J Exp Med 137:1303, 1973

7. Mawas C, Sasportes M, Christen Y, et al: Transplant Proc 5:1683, 1973

8. Bach FH, Widmer MB, Segall M, et al: Science 176:1024, 1972

9. Bach FH, Widmer MB, Bach ML, et al: J Exp Med 136:1430, 1972

10. Schendel DH: unpublished data.

11. Bach FH, Segall M, Zier K, et al: Science 180: 403, 1973

Activation of T Cells by H-2 Factors in the Graft-vs.-Host Reaction

By William L. Elkins, Paula Kavathas, and Fritz H. Bach

LIVNAT et al.[1] and Klein and Park[2] have shown that the MHC antigens responsible for the splenic enlargement of graft-vs.-host disease in neonatal mice map with those responsible for reactivity in MLC. It is thought that some donor-cell proliferation in GvHD is in response to host alloantigens as in MLC and that these antigen-reactive cells somehow trigger the nonspecific proliferation of a variety of host lymphoid, hematopoietic, and reticuloendothelial cells. It is the latter nonspecific response that dominates and is measured in the standard Simonsen spleen assay.[3]

In the present studies we have looked at the proliferative response of the donor T cells, which are thought to initiate the GvH reaction. The proliferative response of thymocytes in the spleens of lethally irradiated allogeneic hosts can be estimated by the incorporation of ^{125}IUdR into DNA, as first described by Bennett.[4] Single-cell suspensions of thymocytes from 4- to 6-wk-old donors were injected intravenously into adult hosts who had received 900 rad from a ^{137}Cs source 2 to 3 hr previously. A 1-μCi pulse of ^{125}IUdR is given i.p. 1 hr before sacrifice. Isotope that is not incorporated into DNA in spleens or lymph nodes is removed by soaking and washing these organs in 70% ethanol with carrier KI (10 g/5 liter) prior to counting in a crystal scintillation spectrometer.

In experiments in which B10.A thymocytes were injected into lethally irradiated (B10.A × B10) F_1, (B10.A × B10.D2) F_1, and (B10.A × B10.BR) F_1 hosts, we studied the cell dose–response relationship by measuring the percentage of radioactivity recovered in the spleen on the fourth day after injection of 0.025–0.4 donor thymus equivalents (TE). The fourth day represents the peak of the response. The incorporation of ^{125}IUdR in (B10.A × B10) F_1 and (B10.A × B10.D2) F_1 hosts in a typical experiment is shown in Fig. 1 and is seen to be about equal in each. The combined data from several experiments are shown in Table 1. There was no significant response in 41 (B10.A × B10.BR) F_1 hosts inoculated with doses from 0.1 to 2.0 TE. The factors that might stimulate donor cells in these reactions include all four regions of the MHC in the B10 hybrids, H-2K–Ir in the B10.D2 hybrids, and Ss–H-2D in the B10.BR hybrids.[2,5] Thus the left side of the H-2 complex (H-2K–Ir) appears to account for most of the activity of the whole complex in these strain combinations, the right side (Ss–H-2D) being virtually inactive.

In order to investigate the possible contribution of H-2K factors we injected 0.5 TE B10.A thymocytes into AQR hosts.[2,5] As shown in Table 2 there was no response on the fourth day relative to syngeneic controls. The same cells responded to the complete H-2 region difference of B10 hosts, but not to the Ir-IgG–Ss–H-2D difference of B10.A(4R). These findings coupled with those discussed above suggest strongly that Ir-IgA (or Ir-1) region differ-

From the Department of Pathology, University of Pennsylvania, School of Medicine, Philadelphia, Pa., and the Departments of Medical Genetics and Surgery, University of Wisconsin, Madison, Wisc.

Supported by NIH Grants AI-07423, AI-08439, AI-06525, and GM-15422; NF-MOD Grant CRBS 246; and ONR Grant N00014-67-A-0128-003.

This is paper No. 1700 from the Laboratory of Genetics, University of Wisconsin, Madison, Wisc.

Abbreviations: T cell, thymus-derived lymphocyte; MHC, major histocompatibility complex; GvHD, graft-vs.-host disease; GvHR, graft-vs.-host reaction; MLC, mixed leukocyte culture; ^{125}IUdR, ^{125}I-iododeoxyuridine; TE, thymus equivalents; Ir, immune response; B, C57BL mice.

© 1973 by Grune & Stratton, Inc.

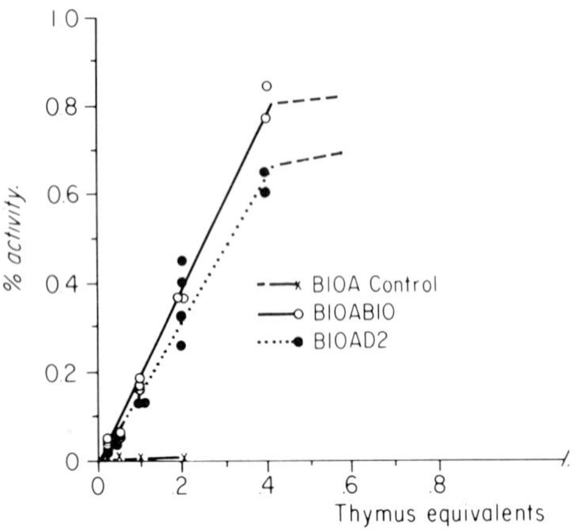

Fig. 1. Cell dose–response relationship for B10.A thymocytes in (B10.A × B10) F_1 and (B10.A × B10.D2) F_1 hosts. Each point represents one spleen. The plateaus indicated are based on data from other experiments and are inserted to indicate the approximate limits of linearity.

ences are of major importance to activate B10.A thymocytes under the conditions of the experiments.

We thus sought for more direct evidence that Ir-region differences alone could stimulate thymocytes. The results of two experiments with 0.5 TE of B10.A(4R) cells are shown in Table 3. A significant response compared to that in syngeneic controls was seen in B10.A(2R) which differs by factors in the Ir-IgG and Ss regions.[2] A similar response occurred in B10.A hosts which differ in the same regions and also in the H-2D region. A somewhat better response was seen in B10 hosts which differ by H-2K and the left-hand portion of the Ir region marked by Ir-IgA and Ir-1;[1] however, the difference was not significant by Mann–Whitney U test. The latter response approximated that seen with a complete MHC difference.

In Table 4 are the results of one experiment with B10.T(6R) thymocytes. A distinct response occurred in (AQR × 6R) F_1 hosts which differ in the Ir–Ss regions only.[2,5] A better response occurred in B10.A hosts, but the difference could be ascribed to a gene-dose effect rather than to a contribution of H-2K factors per se. In this experiment responses were also observed in the lymph nodes of the hosts (cervical, brachial, mesenteric). This suggests that

Table 1. Responses of B10.A Thymocytes in Congenic F_1 Hybrid Hosts Differing for Various Parts of the H-2 Region

Origin of Host Difference*	H-2-Region Differences	Cell Dose	Number of Hosts	Median % Activity in Spleen	Interquartile Range
B10.D2	K–Ir	low†	22	0.34	0.21–0.45
		high‡	16	0.68	0.61–0.79
B10.BR	Ss–D	low	18	0.02	0.02–0.03
		high	23	0.04	0.03–0.07
B10	K–Ir–Ss–D	low	19	0.31	0.19–0.41
		high	11	0.70	0.68–0.77
B10.A	—	low	31	0.01	0.01–0.02
(syngeneic controls)		high	25	0.03	0.02–0.03

*That is, strain crossed to B10.A to produce F_1 hybrid hosts.
†Low dose, 0.10–0.39 TE.
‡High dose, 0.40–2.0 TE.

Table 2. Response of B10.A Thymocytes to Various Regions of H-2 Complex

Host Strain	Number of Hosts	% Activity Recovered in Spleen*	H-2-Region Difference
AQR	6	0.03 (0.01–0.04)	H-2K
B10.A(4R)	4	0.02 (0.02–0.02)	Ir-IgG–Ss–H-2D
B10	6	0.36 (0.17–0.47)	complete
B10.A	5	0.02 (0.01–0.03)	none

*Median (range).

both spleen-seeking and lymph-node-seeking cells can be activated by Ir region differences alone. Similar data were obtained in another experiment.

In summary we find that donor thymocyte proliferation in GvHR can be elicited by factors that seem to correspond to those activating peripheral lymphocytes in MLC[5] and in the Simonsen spleen assay.[3] These factors are found predominantly in the Ir region of the MHC. It should be stressed that the results are preliminary, and that the assay measures proliferation only during the 5-day period after inoculation of the donor cells. Conceivably a response to H-2K and H-2D factors would occur in vivo after this period.

It should be also stressed that the MHC genotype of the donor can be an important factor in determining GvH potential,[7] and that the particular interallelic, i.e., donor–host, relationship also needs to be taken into account.[8] Indeed, we have found combinations in which Ir region differences do not stimulate donor thymocytes in this assay. This matter is currently under investigation.

The possibility that the observed lack of response to H-2D region factors in vivo is due to the hybrid resistance (HR) phenomenon of Cudkowicz is ruled out by his finding that B10.A and B10.BR are alike at the postulated HR locus to the right of H-2D.[6] We have also found that thymocyte proliferation is not blocked by HR under the conditions of our experiments with the C57BL/6 vs. (C57BL/6 × DBA/2) F_1 combination, in which the HR phenomenon was discovered.

Finally, we must caution against the temptation to conclude that the products of the Ir genes themselves are the stimulating factors in GvH and MLC assays. This may only be a matter of extremely close linkage. Moreover, Sprent and Miller showed that the immunogenic, i.e., mitogenic, stimulus is well expressed in T-cell-deprived hosts using an assay similar to that employed here.[9] Their experiment needs, however, to be repeated using combinations differing only in the Ir regions, for it is possible that factors outside the MHC were stimulating in their tests.

Table 3. Responses of B10.A(4R) Thymocytes to Various Regions of H-2 Complex

Host Strain	Number of Hosts	% Activity Recovered in Spleen*	H-2-Region Difference
B10.A(2R)	10	0.17 (0.10–0.27)	Ir-IgG–Ss
B10.A	8	0.15 (0.08–0.37)	Ir-IgG–Ss–H-2D
B10	7	0.35 (0.05–0.59)	H-2K–Ir-IgA
(B10.A × B10) F_1	8	0.54 (0.35–0.64)	complete
B10.A(4R)	11	0.02 (0.01–0.05)	none

*Median (range).

Table 4. Response of B10.T(6R) Thymocytes to Ir–Ss Region Difference

Host Strain	Number of Hosts	% Activity Recovered in Spleen*	% Activity in Lymph Nodes	H-2-Region Difference
(AQR × 6R) F_1	5	0.63 (0.44–0.73)	0.27 (0.18–0.42)	Ir–Ss
B10.A	4	1.21 (1.10–1.44)	0.62 (0.59–0.63)	H-2K–Ir–Ss
B10.T(6R)	2	0.03 (0.02–0.03)	0.03 (0.02–0.03)	none

*Median (range).

REFERENCES

1. Livnat S, Klein J, Bach FH: Nature [New Biol] 243:42, 1973
2. Klein J, Park JM: J Exp Med 136:112, 1973
3. Elkins WL: Prog Allergy 15:70, 1971
4. Bennett M: Transplantation 11:158, 1971
5. Bach FH, et al: J Exp Med 136:1430, 1972
6. Cudkowicz G: International Convocation on Immunology, Buffalo, N.Y., 1968. Basel, Karger, 1969, pp 193–202
7. Longenecker BM, et al: Transplantation 14:424, 1972
8. Lengerova H: Immunogenetics of Tissue Transplantation, Frontiers of Biology Series, vol 16, Amsterdam, North Holland, 1969
9. Sprent J, Miller JFAP: Cell Immunol 3:361, 1972

Relationship of Mixed Lymphocyte Culture Response, HL-A Histocompatibility Antigens, and Renal Transplantation

By J.S. Thompson, R.J. Flink, J.L. Caldwell, C.D. Severson, and W.W. Bonney

A GREAT DEAL of evidence has now been reported and amplified at this workshop that indicates that the factors determining the response in mixed lymphocyte cultures (MLC) are more closely related to lymphocyte-defined (LD) specificities than to serologically defined (SD) HL-A histocompatibility antigens.[1-15] Although there is generally excellent correlation between HL-A compatibility and the absence of MLC stimulation within siblings, several groups have now reported that the lymphocytes of unrelated individuals matched for four HL-A antigens commonly stimulate in MLC tests.[1,3,5,6] Conversely, we and others have noted no stimulation between some siblings mismatched for one HL-A antigen.[4,9]

The opportunity to investigate LD compatibility of apparently SD-identical haplotypes inherited from unrelated individuals arises in families when serologic identity for the HL-A haplotype is demonstrated in both parents, that is, a, b/a′, b′. One of four children will be SD-compatible with a parent (a, b/x, y) by virtue of inheritance of the uncommon haplotype (x, y) from that parent plus the apparently common haplotype from the other (a′, b′). Under these circumstances, parent–child MLC tests may be taken as a measure of LD identity of the common haplotypes.

Another measure of compatibility may be examined when one or more children inherit the same haplotype from both parents and thus are homozygous with respect to these antigens. Mitomycin-treated homozygous cells might not be expected to stimulate cells that possess either the maternal or paternal shared haplotype providing they were compatible for LD as well as SD specificities.

In addition to comparing MLC reactions with serologic typing in a number of families, we have had the opportunity to compare their relative importance to transplantation in some of these same families and in selected unrelated donor–recipient pairs in which genotypic identity of the haplotypes was available.

We believe these selected data provide further evidence for the existence of LD specificities in man, that there may be two or more segregating LD series, and that there is a close relationship between LD compatibility and the prognosis of a renal transplant.

MATERIALS AND METHOD

Lymphocytotoxicity (LCY) and MLC tests are routinely performed as a part of our living-related and cadaveric transplant evaluation. The potential recipient was not on any immunosuppressive drugs, and azotemia was being controlled by hemodialysis at the time of these studies.

Serologic LCY was performed by a slight modification[9] of the two-stage test described by Amos et al.[15] employing 70 or more antisera detecting HL-A antigens 1, 2, 3, 9, 10, 11, 28, W19, W20, W30, AO77, 5, 7, 8, 12, 13, 27, W5, W10, W14, W15, W17, W18, W21, W22, and 4c.

Mixed lymphocyte cultures were performed identically to that previously reported[9] except that the responding cells have been reduced to 1×10^5 and the mitomycin-treated stimulating cells to 3×10^5 in 1.0-ml cultures. All cultures were prepared in 20% pooled human plasma.

To exclude a response by inadequately mitomycin-treated cells, each pair of allogeneic mitomycin-treated cells were cultured together (Rm, Sm). The stimulating index (SI) of each set of triplicate mixed

From the Departments of Medicine, Urology, and Surgery, University of Iowa, and the Veterans Administration Hospital, Iowa City, Iowa.

Work supported by NIH grant AI 10593 and the Veterans Administration.

© *1973 by Grune & Stratton, Inc.*

cultures for each responding cell was expressed as a ratio of sextuplet controls, that is, R, Sm/R, Rm, and statistical analysis was performed by Student's t test to ascertain whether relatively close values were or were not significantly different ($p < 0.01$).

Standard techniques for renal transplantation were employed and immunosuppressive management included azathioprine, prednisone, and local irradiation to the graft bed for a rejection crisis but no antilymphocyte or thymocyte globulin. Months of graft survival, renal function, and death or kidney removal were recorded for SD-compatible transplants performed as a part of this study.

RESULTS

Five families were found in whom a similar HL-A1, 8 haplotype was demonstrated in both parents. Two patterns emerge within these families: one in which parent–child tests were not stimulated and the other in which they were. Family 1-100 exemplifies the first pattern (Table 1). Lymphocyte serologic typing revealed no apparent difference in either the maternal or paternal HL-A1, 8 haplotype. The potential recipient, P, appeared to be homozygous for HL-A1, 8, as confirmed by the fact that all of his children inherited this allele. Mixed lymphocyte cultures were done on all 12 members at the same time. Enclosed in rectangles are those cells that were mutually nonstimulating. Of particular interest is the fact that the father, F, and daughter S_1 were mutually nonstimulating, yet S_1 must have inherited the maternal HL-A1, 8 haplotype. Similarly, the mother, M, and daughters, S_2 and S_3, were mutually nonstimulating where S_2 and S_3 must have

Table 1. Relationship of MLC to HL-A in Family 1-100

Responding Cells (R)		Stimulating Cells (Sm)											
HL-A Haplotypes	Cell Donor*	Pm	Fm	S_1m	Mm	S_2m	S_3m	Bm	SO_1m	D_1m	D_2m	SO_2m	D_3m
1, 8 / 1, 8	P	{124}	76.6	29.5	31.4	95.2	103.5	133.7	76.1	36.8	33.4	63.5	43.5
1, 8 / 2, W28, 12	F	1.9	{397}	0.4	14.2	25.9	9.7	8.1	11.6	12.3	10.6	15.8	14.1
1, 8 / 2, W28, 12	S_1	15.2	1.4	{285}	57.1	114.7	93.2	54.1	54.8	48.3	38.1	78.5	116.8
1, 8 / W19, 4c	M	10.7	203.1	59.8	{103}	2.0	2.1	43.9	88.2	98.5	87.9	134.1	163.1
1, 8 / W19, 4c	S_2	5.6	11.1	3.5	0.9	{485}	0.6	5.1	23.6	23.3	13.9	15.1	12.2
1, 8 / W19, 4c	S_3	7.5	36.4	11.8	0.6	0.7	{372}	6.5	4.7	23.6	12.7	35.3	33.6
W19, 4c / 2, 12	B	23.5	56.7	30.2	51.3	61.4	72.1	{173}	41.9	83.1	66.3	134.2	99.2
1, 8 / W28, 12	SO_1	11.7	160.4	99.7	60.4	316.2	85.0	184.3	{78}	1.1	1.3	23.3	36.6
1, 8 / W28, 12	D_1	4.5	89.0	45.6	54.1	103.6	73.6	108.1	0.9	{132}	0.9	18.4	24.6
1, 8 / W28, 12	D_2	7.1	146.2	46.7	77.3	111.9	87.4	125.1	2.3	2.1	{416}	24.5	17.8
1, 8 / 2, W15	SO_2	3.9	69.1	34.0	41.4	89.5	50.4	67.5	7.9	6.2	6.2	{427}	0.8
1, 8 / 2, W15	D_3	8.1	50.7	20.2	26.1	20.1	33.7	20.4	7.4	7.7	2.2	0.8	{315}

Stimulation index

*M, mother; F, father; B, brother; S_1, S_2, S_3, sisters; P, patient; SO_1, SO_2, sons; D_1, D_2, D_3, daughters; {c.p.m.}, counts per minute; R, Rm.

inherited the paternal HL-A1, 8 haplotype. These observations suggest that the maternal and paternal HL-A1, 8 haplotypes were also similar for LD specificities; however, mitomycin-treated homozygous HL-A1, 8 P cells stimulated every other family member ($p < 0.01$), except the father (SI = 1.9, $p > 0.05$). The degree of stimulation was relatively low grade with the exception of a brother B, who did not inherit either the maternal or paternal HL-A1, 8 haplotype. This observation was confirmed in a second set of cultures with P, F, M, and two sons, SO_1 and SO_2. It is also of interest to note that F and S_1 (1, 8/2, W28, 12) were stimulated by SO_1m, D_1m, and D_2m (1, 8/W28, 12), yet HL-A2 and W28 are thought to be cross-reactive antigens of the first segregant series, and in these cultures there was no apparent positive HL-A antigenic mismatch (Table 1). A similar family in whom HL-A-compatible parent–child mixed lymphocyte cultures were mutually nonstimulated has previously been reported.[9] Transplantation of a paternal-to-son kidney allograft was performed and graft function has remained excellent for 34 mo (Table 2, family 1-50).

In the more common pattern found in three HL-A1, 8 families, mitomycin-treated homozygous HL-A1, 8 cells consistently stimulated haploidentical cells in culture (Table 3, family 1-80) and the degree was generally greater than that observed in 1-100. The other striking difference, with respect to the first pattern, is the observation that maternal or paternal lymphocytes stimulated and were stimulated by their apparently HL-A-compatible children, that is, M, P, and S_4 (1, 8/2, W10) and F and B_2 (1, 8/2, W15). Of special interest is P, because her lymphocytes responded to mitomycin-treated cells from all three HL-A1, 8-haplotype-homozygous siblings but reacted very little with cells from an unrelated genotypically proven HL-A1, 8/1, 8 donor (Table 3). One kidney from this haplotype-homozygous cadaveric donor was transplanted to P (HL-A1, 8/2, W10) and the second into another haploidentical (HL-A1, 8/3, 7) unrelated recipient (Table 2). Low or absent one-way MLC stimulation has correlated with very good function of both allografts for 18 mo.

On the other hand, in family 1-250, haploidentical stimulation by mitomycin-treated HL-A1, 8-haplotype-homozygous paternal donor cells was subsequently associated with severe and irreversible kidney rejection by his haploidentical HL-A1, 8/2, 12 son (Table 2).

Discordance between serologic HL-A typing and mixed lymphocyte culture reactions was even more apparent in the three families that shared HL-A3, 7. Parent–child tests were consistently stimulated, that is, F and P, M and S_1, B_2 in family 1-120 (Table 4) and homozygous HL-A3, 7/3, 7 (B_1m) cells strikingly stimulated haploidentical cells. The patient P received a

Table 2. Relationship Between MLC and Graft Function in HL-A-compatible Renal Transplants

Family	Age of Recipient (yr)	HL-A Genotype		Relationship	MLC* (SI)	Function†	
		Recipient (R)	Donor (Sm)			BEF	Current
1-50	40	1, 8/11, B	1, 8/11, B	father	1.8	75	80 (34)
1-250	12	1, 8/2, 5	1, 8/1, 8	father	10.6	60	R (1½)
1-80	25	1, 8/2, W10	1, 8/1, 8	cadaver	2.7	54	88 (18)
1-81	35	1, 8/3, 7	1, 8/1, 8	cadaver	1.8	58	64 (18)
1-120	18	3, 7/1, 8	3, 7/3, 7	sib	103.1	166	R (1½)

*MLC: one-way mixed lymphocyte culture; SI, stimulation index of R, Sm/R, Rm.

†Function: creatinine clearance in ml/min/1.7 m^2; BEF, best early function; Current, most recent function; R, removed; D, death; numbers in parentheses indicate transplant survival in months.

Table 3. Relationship of MLC to HL-A in Family 1-80

Responding Cells (R)		Stimulating Cells (Sm)										
HL-A Haplotypes	Cell Donor*	B_1m	S_1m	S_2m	S_3m	Pm	Pm	S_4m	Mm	Fm	B_2m	Cm
1, 8 / 1, 8	B_1	{838}	2.7	2.5	12.9	12.5						
1, 8 / 1, 8	S_1	0.2	{495}	0.2	6.5	7.1						
1, 8 / 1, 8	S_2	0.4	0.6	{549}	48.4	29.8						
2, W10 / 2, W15	S_3	54.4	57.2	226.7	{678}	75.1						
1, 8 / 2, W10	P†	19.0	7.4	7.4	40.8	{252}						2.7
1, 8 / 2, W10	P†						{200}	1.1		11.6	28.5	
1, 8 / 2, W10	S_4						2.3	{221}	7.9	33.0	86.5	
1, 8 / 2, W10	M						42.4	72.5	{241}	155.5	344.5	
1, 8 / 2, W15	F						84.1	127.3	132.7	{387}	33.9	
1, 8 / 2, W15	B_2						24.1	28.5	25.8	4.1	{254}	
1, 8 / 1, 8	C‡						45.8					(230)

Stimulation index

*M, mother; F, father; B_1, B_2, brothers; S_1, S_2, S_3, S_4, sisters.
†The cultures in the upper left were performed at a different time than those in the lower right.
‡C, cadaveric donor; genotype based on serologic typing of mother, sister, wife, and four children.
{c.p.m.}, counts per minute, R, Rm.

kidney from B_1m, but progressive irreversible rejection occurred and the transplant was removed after $1\frac{1}{2}$ mo (Table 2).

Three families in whom HL-A2, 7 was the common haplotype were also studied. In one family there was marked parent–child MLC stimulation; in a second there was mutual nonstimulation; in a third, family 1-150, the unidirectional nature of the reactions was particularly informative (Table 5). Whereas mitomycin-treated cells of the patient (Pm) stimulated the cells of W, his two-haplotype-incompatible wife, they failed to stimulate the cells of all other family members with whom he differed by one SD haplotype. P lymphocytes, however, responded to all other cells in culture. The cells of his father F not only failed to respond to Pm, but also did not react with the two daughters (D_1m and D_2m) with whom he shared no common SD haplotype. The cells of his brother B and mother M were mutually nonreactive, implying LD compatibility, yet they differed by one SD haplotype. Genetic recombination would not appear to explain the results in this complex family, and more likely interpretations appear to dictate the existence of similar LD specificities on F, M, and W cells and inheritance by their common relations.

The following theoretical example postulating two independent polymorphic LD segregating series provides one partial explanation for the results in family 1–150. Capital letters depict the specificities of one LD series and small letters a second series: (F) 2*m*, 7*A*/ W19*n*, 27*C*; (M) 2*o*, 7*A*/ 2*n*,

Table 4. Relationship of MLC to HL-A in Family 1-120

Responding Cells (R)		Stimulating Cells (Sm)						
HL-A Haplotypes	Cell Donor*	B_1 m	Fm	Pm	Mm	S_1 m	B_2 m	B_3 m
3, 7 / 3, 7	B_1	{147}	56.7	17.1	61.3	23.1	70.4	81.9
3, 7 / 1, 8	F	404.7	{30}	39.1	228.0	120.5	204.9	167.9
3, 7 / 1, 8	P	103.1	28.9	{111}	54.6	32.2	116.5	71.5
3, 7 / W28, 12	M	30.4	35.0	22.2	{198}	12.4	31.1	44.5
3, 7 / W28, 12	S_1	396.8	179.0	112.2	195.8	{43}	2.2	265.0
3, 7 / W28, 12	B_2	69.3	38.6	19.1	50.7	0.6	{529}	31.6
1, 8 / W28, 12	B_3	51.6	34.6	18.8	19.7	10.9	26.6	{485}
		Stimulation index						

*M, mother; F, father; P, patient kidney recipient; B_1 brother kidney donor; S_1 sister; B_2, B_3, brothers.
{c.p.m.}, counts per minute, R, Rm.

Table 5. Relationship of MLC to HL-A in Family 1-150

Responding Cells (R)		Stimulating Cells (Sm)						
HL-A Haplotypes	Cell Donor*	Fm	Mm	Bm	Pm	D_1 m	D_2 m	Wm
2, 7 / W19, 27	F	{55}	24.2	9.2	0.5	1.3	0.8	8.5
2, 7 / 2, 12	M	41.0	{82}	1.1	0.9	125.5	23.8	58.2
2, 7 / W19, 27	B	30.0	0.6	{75}	0.6	—	—	—
W19, 27 / 2, 12	P	7.9	31.5	30.0	{42}	15.5	18.5	62.5
2, 12 / 9, 12	D_1	9.9	63.0	—	1.6	{207}	0.2	26.0
2, 12 / 9, 12	D_2	4.8	14.6	—	1.8	0.2	{44}	14.0
9, 12 / B1, W17	W	98.0	305.3	—	71.5	364.8	164.3	{93}
		Stimulation index						

*M, mother; F, father; B, brother; P, patient; W, wife; D_1, D_2, daughters.
B1, antigen not demonstrated.
{c.p.m.}, counts per minute, R, Rm.
—, no culture performed.

12*C*; (B) 2*o*, 7*A*/ W19*n*, 27*C*; (P) W19*n*, 7*C*/2*n*, 12*C*; (W) 9*n*, 12*A*/ B1*n*, W17*B*; (D_1 and D_2) 2*n*, 12*C*/ 9*n*, 12*A*. This example predicts that one LD specificity, *A*, is present on F, M, and W cells, but that the three haplotypes carrying this specificity differ by products *m*, *n*, and *o* of a second LD series.

DISCUSSION

According to present information,[16] proliferative reactions in mixed lymphocyte cultures are predominantly under the influence of lymphocyte-defined (LD) and not serologically defined (SD) specificities. Thus, when similar HL-A haplotypes are demonstrable in both parents, HL-A-identical parent–child MLC tests may be taken as a measure of compatibility of LD and perhaps other non-SD determinants on these cells.[16-19] Including some reported herein, Dausset[20] has collated MLC and HL-A studies performed on a number of families with common parental haplotypes that have been investigated by several groups. These combined data demonstrate that mixed cultures were not stimulated approximately 10% of the time when unrelated paternal–maternal HL-A1, 8 or HL-A3, 7 haplotypes were compared in parent–child tests. The more common discordance, moreover, provides further evidence for separation of SD HL-A antigens and LD specificities in man. Incompatibility of LD determinants belonging to a single polymorphic segregating series would explain the observed parent–child and haplotype-homozygous one-way MLC stimulation in families 1–80, 1–120, and 1–250.

Nonreactive parent–child mixed cultures favor compatibility of LD as well as SD determinants in families 1–50 and 1–100, but this conclusion must be tempered in light of the lower but significant stimulation by mitomycin-treated homozygous cells of all but one haploidentical cell spanning three generations of family 1–100. Similar observations have been reported by other investigators.[10,11,14] At least two theoretical explanations cannot be excluded at this time: Cantor and Greaves[21] have advanced the hypothesis that the MLC may be activated by configurational determinants formed by the interaction of closely associated specificities on the cell surface. Adler et al.[22] have demonstrated consistent stimulation of F_1 hybrid lymphocytes by parental strain cells in mouse mixed lymphocyte cultures. Stimulation occurred with parental red blood cell stroma, as well as by x-ray- or mitomycin-treated lymphocytes. The double expression of a truly compatible haplotype, that is, a, b/a, b, may appear conformationally dissimilar to responding haploidentical human cells and provide an analogous situation to the murine observations. Similar to the H-2 complex in the mouse, several investigators at this conference have now proposed that there may be more than one independently segregating LD series associated with the human HL-A complex. The relative strength of these factors on the MLC is uncertain, but their existence may be postulated to interpret the observations in families 1–150 and may partially account for homozygous cell stimulation in 1–100.

An important and related question deals with whether allograft survival, exclusive of hyperacute rejection, is more closely related to SD or LD compatibility.[12,13] Although the sample is too small to be conclusive, the results thus far, with two parent–child and three homozygous to haploidentical transplants matched for HL-A, but not necessarily LD, specificities, support the concept that the latter, as demonstrated by MLC reactions, more critically influence graft function.

SUMMARY

The compatibility of unrelated HL-A-identical haplotypes has been studied in families in whom both parents possessed one serologically defined (SD) haplotype in common, that is, HL-A1, 8; 3, 7; and 2, 7. Commonly, within these families, mixed lymphocyte cultures involving SD-compatible parent–child or haplotype-homozygous cells were stimulated, indicating nonidentity for other lymphocyte-defined (LD) determinants.

Less frequently, parent–child MLC tests were not stimulated, suggesting compatibility for LD as well as SD specificities. In this instance also, however, mitomycin-treated homozygous cells usually stimulated haploidentical cells, suggesting that other factors, including more than one LD segregating series, may influence MLC reactions.

Finally, the results of five SD-compatible parent–child or homozygous to haploidentical transplants support a principal role for LD determinants in allograft survival.

REFERENCES

1. van Rood JJ, Eijsvoogel VP: Lancet 1:698, 1970
2. Sorensen SF, Neilsen LS: Acta Pathol Microbiol Scand 78:719, 1970
3. Bach FH, Day E, Bach ML, et al: Tissue Antigens 1:39, 1971
4. DuPont B, Nielsen LS, Svejaard A: Lancet 2:1336, 1971
5. Johnston JM, Bashir HV: Br Med J 4:581, 1971
6. Koch CT, Frederiks E, Eijsvoogel VP, et al: Lancet 2:1334, 1971
7. Yunis EJ, Plate JM, Ward FE, et al: Transplant Proc 3:118, 1971
8. Siegler HF, Ward FE, Amos DB, et al: J Exp Med 133:411, 1971
9. Thompson JS, Parmely MJ, Flink RJ, et al: J Exp Med 135:596, 1972
10. Sasportes M, Lebrun A, Rapaport FT, et al: Transplant Proc 4:209, 1972
11. Mempel W, Grosse-Wilde H, Albert E, et al: Transplant Proc 5:401, 1973
12. van Rood JJ, Koch CT, van Hooff JP, et al: Transplant Proc 5:409, 1973
13. Cochrum KC, Perkins HA, Payne RO, et al: Transplant Proc 5:391, 1973
14. Lebrun A, Sasportes M, Dausset J: Transplant Proc 5:363, 1973
15. Amos DB, Bashir H, Boyle W, et al: Transplantation 7:220, 1969
16. Bach FH, Widmer MB, Segall M, et al: Science 176:1024, 1972
17. Bach ML, Widmer MB, Bach FH, et al: Transplant Proc 5:369, 1973
18. Klein J, Shreffler DC: J Exp Med 135:924, 1972
19. McDevitt HO, Deak BD, Shreffler DC, et al: J Exp Med 135:1259, 1972
20. Dausset J: Transplant Proc 5:1751, 1973
21. Cantor H, Greaves M: Transplant Proc 4:227, 1972
22. Adler WH, Takiguchi T, Marsh B, et al: J Immunol 105:984, 1970

Correlation of MLC Reactivity After Experimental and Clinical Transplantation. Virus and Cytophilic Antibody: Sources of False Negatives

By Joshua Miller, Richard J. Howard, Brack G. Hattler, and John S. Najarian

WE HAVE previously reported changes in mixed lymphocyte culture (MLC) reactivity occurring in response to kidney transplantation in the dog and human.[1-3] In the absence of other complicating factors, a loss of previously strong MLC reactivity against the donor occurred in a setting of experimental and clinical rejection. This loss of reactivity was attributed to entrapment of MLC reactive cells in the rejecting organ.[2,3] Reactivity returned to preoperative levels in long-term (1-yr) follow-up of these patients and has remained so to date with a good clinical result. It is the purpose of the present report to emphasize the need for close correlation of the clinical status of the patient with the mixed lymphocyte reaction, as there are several factors which may influence it in a clinical or experimental setting that are not associated with changes in immune reactivity against the graft. Two of these variables described in this report that point out the need for frequent testing in a prospective study are (1) the presence of viral infection and (2) the presence of cytophilic antibody directed against the donor attached to the responding cell population.

MIXED LYMPHOCYTE CULTURES

Human and canine peripheral blood lymphocyte separations by density gradients and the macro MLC techniques have been previously described.[1,3] The technique of culturing mouse splenic lymphocytes after density-gradient separation was modified from that of Takiguchi, Adler, and Smith.[4] Reactivity to phytohemagglutinin (PHA) and MLC responsiveness in the mouse were measured by the uptake of tritiated thymidine at 2 and 3 days, respectively, after culture preparations. The detection of cytophilic antibody in dogs in peripheral blood leukocyte populations has also been extensively described elsewhere.[5] The discriminatory mixed lymphocyte assay (DMLC) has been described previously in dogs.[6] The MLC reactivity of patients in this report is part of an ongoing prospective study previously described.[3]

VIRUS INFECTION

Cytomegalic virus carried in vivo and stored at $-40°C$ was injected intraperitoneally at a dose of 10^5 plaque-forming units per mouse in 6-wk-old C57BL/6 and A/J inbred mouse strains. This dose was just below the lethal threshold.

RESULTS

Viral Inhibition of Immune Reactivity in Mice

After injection of a sublethal dose of cytomegalovirus, a partial disruption of lymph node and splenic histological architecture accompanied by a decreased humoral antibody response to sheep red cells occurred, followed by recovery.[7] Responding cells of C57BL/6 mice injected 5 days previously with this dose of virus showed a high degree of spontaneous transformation after 2 and 3 days in culture (Fig. 1) but no significant change in the response to phytohemagglutinin (PHA), compared with vigorous responses of uninfected C57BL/6 mice. In addition, responding cells of infected animals also had no significant pro-

From the University of Minnestoa Medical School, Minneapolis, Minn., and University of Arizona Medical School, Tucson, Ariz.

Supported by VA research grant.

©1973 by Grune & Stratton, Inc.

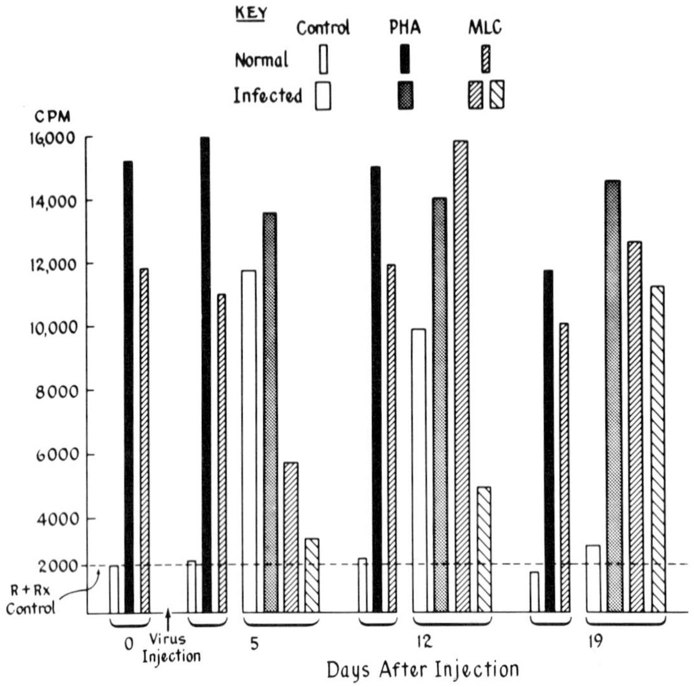

Fig. 1. Inhibition of in vitro reactivity of mouse splenic lymphocytes in response to cytomegalovirus infection. The three narrow bars represent the response of splenic lymphocytes of normal mice cultured before and concomitant with each experimental period. The four wide bars represent activity of infected splenic lymphocytes at intervals after infection. Note that there is a high degree of transformation of cells unstimulated by PHA in infected mice (wide open bars) and that cells that come from infected mice were poor at stimulating (boldly spaced cross-hatched) as well as responding (narrowly spaced cross hatched).

liferative activity against normal A/J x-irradiated stimulating cells in MLC. Moreover, after viral inoculation of A/J mice, stimulating cells of these mice failed to stimulate responding cells from normal C57BL/6 mice, with values of 3000 counts per minute (cpm) compared with 12,500 cpm of normal cultures. By 19 days after viral inoculation, reactivity returned to that of uninfected mice despite the fact that virus could be transferred at this time to infect other mice with subsequent MLC and PHA inhibition.

Viral Inhibition of Immune Reactivity in Humans

Several transplant recipients have been noted to have decreased lymphocyte responses to PHA and mixed culture stimuli in media supplemented with normal (indifferent) plasma at a time when viral illness was overtly present. One example is presented in Fig. 2. The patient received a transplant from a haploidentical sister. Preoperatively there was no MLC reactivity against the sister but strong reactivity against an indifferent individual. There was no change in the reactivity after transplantation due to transplant rejection. However, 2 mo later the patient was exposed to varicella from his children and developed generalized varicella with vesicles containing viral inclusion cells together with fever of 15 days duration. During the phase of active infection there was a loss of responding cell reactivity of R+Ix combinations (R, recipient responding cells; I, indifferent x-irradiated stimulating cells), as well as a loss of stimulating cell activity from the infected recipient (I+Rx). By contrast, response to the haploidentical donor by the indifferent responding cell population remained normally high throughout (not illustrated). Subsequently the patient had fever and cytomegalovirus viremia with repeated transient loss of MLC stimulating and responding cell reactivity. Upon recovery, his reactivity returned to normal. Reactivity to PHA was also decreased by 50% during his overt viral illnesses, but

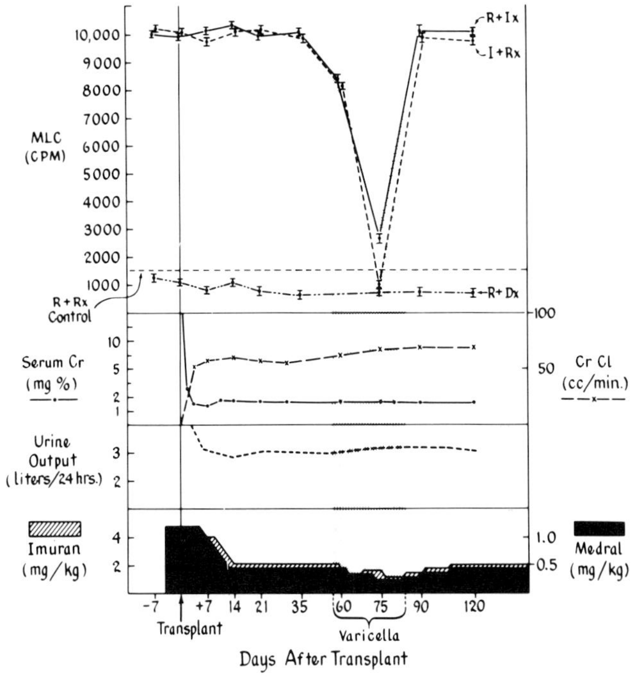

Fig. 2. Clinical course of a patient who received a kidney transplant from a haploidentical sibling. Note that there were no rejection episodes and no changes in MLC reactivity until varicella infection occurred.

there was not a high degree of spontaneous transformation as was observed in the mice in response to cytomegalovirus infection.

Cytophilic Antibody: Blocking vs. Cytotoxic

We have previously reported in dogs[5] that hyperimmunization by allografting of skin and kidneys could lead to a state of nonreactivity of recipient responding cells against donor stimulating cells. This nonreactivity was shown to be a falsely negative reaction, however, due to the presence of alloantibody directed against donor antigens carried by recipient cell cytophilic antibody receptors. This antibody (immunoglobulin G) could be eluted from the responding cell population with return of reactivity. Moreover, IgG obtained from the eluate specifically inhibited this reactivity against donor cells. Moreover, cytotoxic activity could be diluted out from the eluate at concentrations in which MLC inhibitory activity was still present. Using the DMLC cytotoxic activity could be further discriminated from blocking activity of eluates so diluted. In Table 1 donor responding cells cultured in the presence of this cytophilic factor were only temporarily inhibited from responding against indifferent (Ix) cells (first stage). If the factor

Table 1. DMLC of Cytophilic Factor (Cell Combination D+Ix)

Culture Additives		Day of Harvest		
First preparation	Second preparation	3*	5	7
R serum†	I serum	175	255	359
I serum	R serum	132	304	383
R cell eluate	I cell eluate	381	519	16990
I cell eluate	R cell eluate	224	5529	9462
	D + Dx (control)	166	207	237

*Days after second culture preparation.

†High cytotoxic titer.

Table 2. Cytophilic Antibody in an Immunized Human Renal Transplant Recipient

	Cell Combinations*								
	R+Rx	R+Dx	R+Ix	D+Dx	D+Rx	D+Ix	I+Ix	I+Rx	I+Dx
Uneluted cells	324	4826	4178	900	6546	9020	917	3312	7312
Cells eluted and washed +									
1. R cell eluate	271	3641	4380†	657	10058	11603	745	4440	2390†
2. I cell eluate	414	3871	13865	985	11996	19451	568	7968	14952

*All cultures were prepared in media supplemented with indifferent (I) normal plasma.

†MLC inhibition considered to be present if values in counts per minute of cultures containing R cell eluates were 50% or less than control cultures prepared with I cell eluate.

was added 2 days after initial contact with Ix stimulating cells, that is, at a time of repreparation of cultures of D responding cells with fresh Ix stimulating cells (second stage), no inhibition occurred. Conversely, cytotoxic antibody added during the second stage of the DMLC was inhibitory. It is considered feasible therefore that blocking factors can adhere to cells in the absence of increased reactivity against the graft, leading to a false conclusion of nonreactivity due to partial tolerance.

That cytophilic factors can occur in clinical transplantation is illustrated in Table 2. This patient rejected a transplant and developed cytotoxic antibodies which gradually disappeared as antibody titers returned to subthreshold levels over a 1-yr period. His sera obtained before a second transplant inhibited MLC reactivity of an indifferent responding cell population (I+Dx) against which earlier cytotoxicity tests were positive. At the same time, however, this sera did not inhibit reactivity toward a cell population obtained from a second potential donor (D) and there was never cytotoxic reactivity of any recipient (R) sera against this second donor. However, R cells responded very weakly against Ix in I plasma unless R cell cytophilic factor was allowed to detach from these cells. This eluted factor inhibited all cultures in which I cells were present (responding or stimulating). Cytophilic factor was not observed directed against cells of the second prospective donor and no rejection has occurred after transplantation (6 mo).

SUMMARY AND CONCLUSION

It is concluded from these data that the mixed lymphocyte culture can correlate with multifaceted clinical and experimental observations after transplantation. The present report indicates that two additional factors—cytophilic antibody and viral infections—may play a role in altering reactivity. Therefore, before conclusions as to the presence of nonreactivity, i.e., tolerance or rejection, are made, these factors must be ruled out. This can only be done by a thorough knowledge of the clinical status of the patients in an unbiased prospective study.

REFERENCES

1. Miller J, Hattler, BG, Davis M, et al: Transplantation 12:65, 1971
2. Hattler BG, Miller J, Johnson MC: Transplantation 14:47, 1972
3. Miller J, Hattler BG: Surgery 72:220, 1972
4. Takiguchi T, Adler WH, Smith RT: J Exp Med 133:63, 1971
5. Miller J, Rood F, Lifton J, et al: Transplantation 16:142, 1973
6. Miller J, Hattler BG, Johnson MC: Transplantation 14:57, 1972
7. Howard RJ, Kunerth V, Najarian JS: Fed Proc 32:3554, 1973

Further Studies of Genetic Histocompatibility Determinants in Conditioning the Fate of Bone Marrow Allografts in Selectively Bred Dogs

By J. H. Ayvazian, R. Bachvaroff, F. D. Cannon, N. Mollen, D. A. Blumenstock, J. W. Ferrebee, and F. T. Rapaport*

IMPROVEMENTS in the clinical results of transplantation continue to await the development of new techniques capable of inducing permanent host tolerance to allografts without interference with other immunologic defense mechanisms.[1] Definition of the serologically detectable (SD) components of the main histocompatibility complex (DL-A)[2] in selectively bred lines of dogs at the Mary Imogene Bassett Hospital colony in Cooperstown, N.Y., provided a useful marker system for the prospective selection of donor–recipient pairs of animals for bone marrow transplantation on the basis of genotypic identity for the DL-A complex, with evidence of the inheritance of the same DL-A genetic material from the same ancestral source for at least three or four successive generations by each donor and recipient.[3] Although these dogs differed for other genetic markers located on other chromosomes,[4,5] 24 consecutive supralethally irradiated recipients of bone marrow allografts obtained from their prospectively selected donor have had a 100% survival rate for over $2\frac{1}{2}$ yr, including littermate as well as nonlittermate donor–recipient combinations.[6] The bone marrow chimerae have also become permanently tolerant of skin, kidney,[6] and lung[7] allografts obtained from the donor of marrow without any additional treatment. This result stands in marked contrast to the report of Storb, Rudolph, and Thomas,[8] who have shown significant failure rates of bone marrow allografts in dogs matched by serologic testing and by mixed lymphocyte culture (MLC) reactivity, and to the clinical experience of graft failures in recipients of bone marrow obtained from HL-A-identical MLC-negative siblings in man.[9] This difference is most probably a consequence of donor–recipient incompatibilities for as yet unrecognized histocompatibility factors in the latter experimental and clinical situations.[10] The recent development of new in vitro techniques (mixed leucocyte culture tests) for the detection of previously unknown components of the major histocompatibility complex (MHC) in man,[11] mouse,[12] and rat[13] has stimulated the present study of the relative roles of the SD and LD (lymphocyte-detectable)[14] loci of the canine MHC in conditioning the survival of bone marrow allografts in selectivity bred lines of dogs of known DL-A SD genotypes.[3]

MATERIALS AND METHOD

The experimental animals were pairs of male and female littermate and nonlittermate beagles of the Cooperstown colony selected on the basis of genetic and serologic criteria of DL-A SD identity. The DL-A genotypes were routinely confirmed by lymphocytotoxicity tests with a battery of antisera detecting 14 different DL-A specificities.[6] Each donor–recipient pair was genotypically DL-A SD-identical or -compatible, but was not homogenous for a number of other genetic markers, including sex, Swisher erythrocyte group antigens,[4] and the digestive group antigens

---

Irma T. Hirschl Career Scientist Award.

From the Department of Surgery and Institute of Reconstructive Plastic Surgery, New York University Medical Center; the Research Service, Manhattan Veterans Administration Hospital, New York, N.Y.; and the Mary Imogene Bassett Hospital, Cooperstown, N.Y.

Supported by NIH grants AI-10658-01A1 and AM-02215, grants from the John A. Hartford Foundation, the Billy Rose Foundation, and the Irwin Strasburger Memorial Medical Foundation, and USAEC contract AT-(30-1)-2005.

© *1973 by Grune & Stratton, Inc.*

of Zweibaum.[5] Earlier studies by Dausset et al.[3] have identified 23 different DL-A SD haplotypes in the restricted gene pool resulting from the selective breeding of lines of dogs of known DL-A SD genotypes in this colony. These studies have also shown the en bloc transmission of specific DL-A SD haplotypes, i.e., DL-A antigens determined by a single chromosomal unit, from parents to offspring in over 141 consecutive matings. In this regard, the DL-A SD antigens were considered to be effective genetic markers for DL-A-complex genotype identity in these selectively bred lines of dogs.[3] The MLC technique appeared to provide a useful additional in vitro test of this interpretation.

Mixed leucocyte culture (MLC) tests were performed by the method of Hartzman et al.[15] Briefly, lymphocytes were isolated from whole blood by the method of Boyum[16] and were washed three times in balanced salt solution (BSS)[17] containing 50 IU of preservative-free heparin (Thromboliquine) provided by Dr. J. R. A. Simmons of Organon, West Orange, N.J. The cells were resuspended in RPMI-1640 medium containing 6.7 μg/ml of Hepes [4-(2-hydroxyethyl)-1-piperazine-ethane-sulfonic acid] (Aldrich Chemical, Milwaukee, Wisc.), and the pH was adjusted to 7.4 with sodium hydroxide. The medium was supplemented with 20 mM/ml of L-glutamine, 100 IU/ml of penicillin, 50 μg/ml of streptomycin, 50 IU/ml of heparin, and 20% pooled dog serum obtained from 20 normal dogs of the Cooperstown colony. All culture-medium reagents were obtained from the Grand Island Biological Co., Grand Island, N.Y.

The cells were plated on Falcon plastic trays; each well contained 1×10^5 responder and 3×10^5 mitomycin-treated (stimulator) cells in a total volume of 0.2 ml of medium. Mitomycin treatment consisted of incubation of the cell suspensions in BSS with 25 μg/ml of mitomycin-C (Nutritional Biochemicals) for 30 min at 37°C. The mitomycin-treated cells were washed three times in BSS and were then treated in the same manner as the untreated responder cells. The mixture of responding and mitomycin-treated cells was incubated in 5% CO_2-balanced air at 37°C. On the seventh day of incubation, 1 μCi of thymidine methyl (^3H 1.9 Ci/mM) (Schwartz Mann, Orangeburg, N.Y.) was added to each culture well. The cultures were precipitated 16 hr later using an automatic multiple harvester.[18] The radioactivity of each sample was measured in a scintillation spectrometer. The degree of stimulation of responding lymphocytes was measured on the basis of the rate of incorporation of ^3H thymidine expressed in counts per minute. Each MLC test was performed in quadruplicate.

One hundred cell combinations were tested, utilizing four different categories of responding and stimulating cells: (1) donor–recipient pairs that were DL-A SD-identical and -homozygous; (2) pairs that were DL-A SD-identical and -heterozygous; (3) pairs that were DL-A SD-different; (4) pairs that were DL-A SD genotypically compatible but not identical (i.e., the stimulating cells came from a homozygous donor who shared a DL-A SD haplotype with the donor of the responding cells).

Donor–recipient pairs from each category were selected for bone marrow transplantation. Each recipient was exposed to standard supralethal total-body irradiation (1200–1400 R from two opposing ^{60}Co sources)[19] and 12 to 18 hr after irradiation received a bone marrow transplant from his donor. This consisted of the intravenous infusion of 3–3.5 billion nucleated marrow cells obtained by aspiration of the long bones and sternum of the donors, as has been described in detail in previous reports.[20]

RESULTS

As noted in Table 1, MLC tests performed with cells obtained from DL-A SD-identical homozygous (B, F, G, I, J) or heterozygous (A, C, D, E, H) pairs of dogs were uniformly negative. When DL-A SD cells (B, F, G, I, J) were tested with cells from heterozygous donors (A, C, D, E, H), strong MLC reactions occurred, based upon incompatibilities present in the non-shared DL-A haplotype (HL-A SD haplotype *bkcd*) in the stimulating cells. Of greatest interest to the present study is the observation that when heterozygous cells (A, C, D, E, H) were tested with cells obtained from homozygous donors (B, F, G, H, I, J), there was no stimulation in the MLC test. These donors were thus actually DL-A SD-compatible but not -identical with the sources of the responding cells, and in vitro tests showed LD compatibility as well.

The results of bone marrow transplantation performed under the four different genetic conditions of donor–recipient compatibility described earlier are outlined in Table 2. Bone marrow allografts performed in retrospective studies with DL-A SD-identical and MLC-negative dogs are currently surviving uneventfully for an excess of 2 yr in 10 homozygous and in 1 heterozygous donor–recipient pairs. When trans-

Table 1. Mixed Leucocyte Culture Studies in Selectively Bred Lines of Dogs of Known DL-A Genotypes (Cooperstown Colony)

Dog Number	DL-A Genotype	Code	Cells Cultured Alone	One-Way MLC Reactions* Am	Bm	Cm	Dm	Em	Fm	Gm	Hm	Im	Jm
2447	● 1/■ 4	A	605	153	345	144	376	304	209	266	116	80	93
2478	■ 4/■ 4	B	152	9,928	173	5,678	5,679	15,651	178	316	12,381	245	167
2453	● 1/■ 4	C	279	265	517	175	324	209	284	203	296	286	550
2448	● 1/■ 4	D	204	407	348	315	494	379	607	703	186	288	662
2471	● 1/■ 4	E	184	111	146	181	303	379	707	366	271	613	338
2106	■ 2/■ 3	F	200	20,483	224	16,114	20,287	24,498	528	505	30,770	182	192
2479	■ 4/■ 4	G	151	14,463	227	3,130	10,784	45,891	245	430	43,727	606	279
2394	● 1/■ 4	H	135	212	220	563	221	137	585	557	256	314	373
2431	■ 4/■ 2	I	174	40,359	211	18,051	24,307	30,197	443	217	42,738	198	210
2450	■ 4/■ 4	J	196	13,130	320	31,234	28,234	33,865	309	196	46,912	305	299

*MLC reactions expressed as ^{3}H thymidine incorporation (counts/min)
m, mitomycin-treated cells
●, DL-A antigens *bkcd* (haplotype)
■, DL-A antigens *bkhfm* (haplotype)
The numbers opposite each haplotype refer to the different individual origins of these haplotypes.

plants were attempted with marrow from a DL-A SD-homozygous donor (*bkhfm*/*bkhfm*) whose cells reacted strongly in the MLC test against the prospective DL-A SD-heterozygous recipient (*bkcd*/*bkhfm*), there was early engraftment of the bone marrow transplant, followed by graft-vs.-host disease (GvH) within 22 to 30 days later. Three of the four recipients in this group died by the 33rd day of typical severe GvH, and one dog recovered partially by the 40th day but is still in poor condition.*

In three additional experiments, the prospective donor of marrow was DL-A SD-heterozygous (*bkcd*/*bkhfm*) and the recipient was homozygous (*bkhfm*/*bkhfm*). In each instance, the recipient cells did not stimulate the prospective donor lympho-

*This dog died of GvH on the 79th day.

Table 2. Relationship Between DL-A Genotypes, MLC Reactivity, and the Fate of Bone Marrow Allografts in Supralethally Irradiated Recipients Chosen Prospectively from Selectively Bred Lines of Dogs

Donor Code	Recipient Code	Donor DL-A Genotype	Recipient DL-A Genotype	MLC Reactivity* (A + Bm)	Number of Cases	Fate of Bone Marrow Allografts in the Recipients
A	B	■ 4/■ 4	■ 4/■ 4	0	10	Permanent survival (>2 yr)
A	B	● 1/■ 4	● 1/■ 4	0	1	Permanent survival (>2 yr)
A	B	■ 4/■ 4	● 1/■ 4	+	4	GvH in all dogs within 22–30 days (a) 3 dogs died by day 33 (b) 1 dog died on day 79
A	B	● 1/■ 4	■ 4/■ 4	0	3	Failure of graft take with death of all recipients within 10–14 days

*m, mitomycin-treated cells.
●, DL-A antigens *bkcd* (haplotype).
■, DL-A antigens *bkhfm* (haplotype).
The numbers opposite each haplotype refer to the different individual origins of each of those haplotypes.

cytes in the MLC test, but the recipient cells did respond to donor cells in MLC prior to irradiation. Bone marrow allografts showed a total failure to take, with no evidence of cellular regeneration at any time and with death of all three consecutive recipients of typical radiation disease within 10 to 14 days.

DISCUSSION

The results of this study support the existence of a close genetic linkage between the SD and LD components of the canine MHC, in a manner analogous to that observed in man,[11] mouse,[12] and rat.[13] The success of bone marrow transplantation in DL-A SD genotypically identical, MLC-nonreactive (i.e., LD-identical) donor–recipient pairs of dogs are consistent with earlier findings of the usefulness of the DL-A SD marker system in the selectively bred lines of dogs raised at the Cooperstown colony. The appearance of GvH in HL-A-identical, MLC-negative siblings[9] and in DL-A-compatible, MLC-negative littermate dogs obtained from less restricted genetic pools[8] has raised the possibility that the MHC might include, in addition to its currently known components,[14] a number of other closely linked but genetically separable determinants, considering that a modest distance between such determinants and the genes controlling the DL-A antigens could satisfy such a possibility. Such determinants might include not only the SD and LD alleles of the MHC but also the locus (i) detectable by the cell-mediated lympholysis test (CML),[21] an HDR-like system related to cellular immunity, as has been proposed in man by Yunis and Amos,[23] and what, for lack of a better name, the authors have termed a "bone marrow transplantation locus" or BMT,[10] associated with some of the peculiarities of the experimental system.

It is clear that performance of bone marrow allografts across MHC SD and/or LD barriers is associated with an early take, followed by GvH of varying degrees of severity, in the Cooperstown colony as well as in other species.[23] The total failure of take of bone marrow allografts obtained from heterozygous donors of marrow and placed into homozygous recipients, whose cells bore no DL-A SD antigens absent in the donors, may have been due to as yet not well understood factors in the irradiated animals, which retained the capability of reacting against donor DL-A antigens (*c, d*), or other as yet undetermined genetically determined products of the MHC or other chromosomes that were present in the heterozygous donor and absent in the homozygous recipient.[10]

The heterozygous DL-A SD state of the donors in this experiment, taken together with the homozygous state of the recipients for the same criteria, provides certain similarities to the situation that might be encountered in transplantation of marrow from an F_1 hybrid animal into a homozygous parent. Since the prospective donor failed to react in MLC with recipient cells, while the recipient gave a strong MLC reaction against the donor's cells, this particular combination resembles the F_1 hybrid situation for the SD as well as the LD components of the canine MHC. As has been observed in other species,[24–28] marrow allografts performed under such conditions failed to take, and the recipients died of irradiation disease.

In a search for a possible explanation of this result, two additional factors may be deserving of consideration. The first is the possible intervention of as yet unknown histocompatibility determinants present on other chromosomes. In addition, it is not possible to rule out an active immunologic mechanism mustered by the irradiated host. If such a mechanism were to be involved, however, the cells capable of rapidly destroying the transplanted marrow evidently did not need to proliferate; they must have been radiation-resistant and may have been programmed at an earlier time to fulfill this function. Such presensitization may have been due, for example, to previous host contact with bacterial antigens.[29] It is equally possible, however, that no conventional immunologic mechanism was involved and that a variety of as yet undefined genetically determined recognition processes or biochemical differences between donor and recipient[30] may have been involved. In this regard, the results extend to the canine species earlier observations by van Bekkum and associates,[24] McCulloch and Till,[25] Popp et al,[26] and Cudkowicz and Bennett.[27,28]

ACKNOWLEDGMENT

The authors thank Miss E. Kunen for the excellence of her technical assistance.

REFERENCES

1. Lawrence HS: Physiol Rev 39:811, 1959
2. Rapaport FT, Hanaoka T, Shimada T, et al: J Exp Med 131:881, 1970
3. Dausset J, Rapaport FT, Cannon FD, Ferrebee JW: J Exp Med 134:1222, 1971
4. Swisher SN, Young LE: Physiol Rev 41:495, 1961
5. Zweibaum A: private communication
6. Rapaport FT, Watanabe K, Cannon FD, et al: J Exp Med 136:1080, 1972
7. Blumenstock D, Wells E, Sanford C, et al: Transplantation 11:192, 1971
8. Storb R, Rudolph RH, Thomas ED: J Clin Invest 50:1272, 1971
9. Buckley RH: in Amos DB (ed): Progress in Immunology. New York, Academic, 1971, p 1061
10. Rapaport FT, Ozaki A, Cannon FD, et al: Transplant Proc 5:845, 1973
11. Bach FH, Amos DB: Science 156:1506, 1967
12. Dutton RW: J Exp Med 122:759, 1965
13. Silvers WK, Wilson DB, Palm J: Science 155: 703, 1967
14. Bach FH, Bach ML, Sondel PM, et al: Transplant Rev 12:30, 1972
15. Hartzman RJ, Segall M, Bach ML, et al: Transplantation 11:268, 1970
16. Boyum H: Scand J Clin Lab Invest [Suppl 97] 21:1, 1968
17. Mishell RI, Dutton RW: J Exp Med 126:423, 1967
18. Hartzman RJ, Segall ML, Bach FH, et al. Cell Immunol 4:192, 1972
19. Hager EB, Mannick JL, Thomas ED, et al: Radiat Res 14:192, 1961
20. Thomas ED, Plain GL, Graham TC, et al: Blood 23:488, 1964
21. Ceppellini R: in Amos DB (ed): Progress in Immunology. New York, Academic, 1971, p 973
22. Yunis EJ, Amos DB: Proc Natl Acad Sci USA 68:3031, 1971
23. Congdon CC: Science 171:1116, 1971
24. Van Bekkum DW, Vos O: J Cell Comp Physiol 50:139, 1957
25. McCulloch EA, Till JE: J Cell Comp Physiol 61: 301, 1963
26. Popp RA, Cosgrove GE, Popp DM: Ann NY Acad Sci 114:538, 1964
27. Cudkowicz G, Bennett M: J Exp Med 134:83, 1971
28. Cudkowicz G, Bennett M: J Exp Med 134:1513, 1971
29. Rapaport FT: in Kahan BD, Reisfeld RA (eds): Transplantation Antigens. New York, Academic, 1972, p 182
30. Van Bekkum, DW, de Vried MJ: in van Bekkum DW (ed): Radiation Chimeras. London, Academic, 1967, p 22

Phenotypic Expression of the Main Histocompatibility Complex (DL-A) in Randomly Selected Mongrel Dogs: II. Serologically Detectable (SD) Compatibility, MLC Reactivity, and Skin Allograft Survival

By A. Ozaki, R. Bachvaroff, F. D. Cannon, N. Mollen, D. A. Blumenstock, J. H. Ayvazian, J. W. Ferrebee, and F. T. Rapaport*

EVIDENCE has been presented that the canine major histocompatibility complex (MHC) includes DL-A serologically detectable loci, as well as an LD locus or loci amenable to in vitro analysis by the mixed leukocyte culture (MLC) test.[1-3] Earlier studies[2] have provided suggestive evidence of a linkage disequilibrium between the LD locus or loci and the DL-A SD loci in the canine species, similar to that documented in man.[4] In addition, preliminary evidence of a relatively more limited polymorphism of the products of the LD locus or loci has been presented.[2] Although a certain degree of concordance was observed between DL-A SD phenotypes and MLC reactivity in a panel of randomly selected dogs, a significant number of mongrel dogs were not stimulated in the MLC test by cells obtained from donors bearing DL-A SD antigens absent in the responding cells, and the reverse situation was also observed.[2] The recent reports from a number of laboratories of the prolongation of skin allograft survival in related[5] as well as in unrelated subjects[6,7] who were HL-A SD- and LD-identical suggested that it might be of interest to investigate this question further in a panel of unrelated mongrel dogs of known DL-A SD and LD reactivity.

MATERIALS AND METHOD

The reference panel of eight mongrel dogs used in this study, whose DL-A SD phenotypes were determined by standard methods[2] and whose MLC reactivity against each other member of the panel was determined by the technique of Hartzman et al.,[8] has been described in detail in an earlier report.[3] Each animal received full-thickness skin allografts from two different donors. In six recipients, one skin graft was obtained from an LD-negative donor (i.e., a donor whose cells failed to stimulate host cells in the MLC test) and one graft was obtained from an MLC-positive donor. In two other cases, the recipients (878, 881) were tested with skin allografts obtained from two different donors, both of whose cells strongly stimulated the recipients' lymphocytes in the MLC reaction. The techniques of skin grafting and criteria for the detection of skin allograft rejection have been described in detail in a previous publication.[9]

RESULTS

The results of this study are summarized in Table 1. The survival time of all first-set skin allografts performed in this series ranged from 7 to 14 days, with a mean survival time (MST) of 9.06 days. The survival of skin allografts obtained from six MLC-negative donors ranged from 8 to 14 days (MST = 10 days), as compared to a survival of 7–11 days (MST = 8.5 days) for grafts obtained from MLC-positive donors. The presence or absence of DL-A SD incompatibilities between donors and recipients did not appear to have as significant a role in this population of mongrel dogs as compared with the results obtained in selectively bred lines of dogs.[9] The MST of skin allografts obtained from DL-A SD pheno-

---

*Irma T. Hirschl Career Scientist Award.

From the Department of Surgery and Institute of Reconstructive Plastic Surgery, New York University Medical Center; the Research Service, Manhattan Veterans Administration Hospital, New York, N.Y.; and the Mary Imogene Bassett Hospital, Cooperstown, N.Y.

Supported by NIH grants AI-10658-01A1 and AM-02215, grants from the John A. Hartford Foundation, the Billy Rose Foundation, and the Irwin Strasburger Memorial Medical Foundation, and USAEC contract AT-(30-1)-2005.

© *1973 by Grune & Stratton, Inc.*

Table 1. Relationship Between DL-A Compatibility, MLC Reactivity, and the Survival Time of Skin Allografts in Mongrel Dogs

Donor (B) No.	Recipient (A) No.	Donor DL-A Phenotype*	Recipient DL-A Phenotype	DL-A Incompatibility	MLC Reactivity† AAm	MLC Reactivity† ABm	MLC Reactivity† Interpretation	Survival of First-Set Skin Allografts (days)
879	877	kc gne	bkf lgnce	c	1443‡	1,095	0	8
884		kc lgne		c		21,245	+	9
881	878	c lgn	bkc lgne	none	2970	22,144	+	8
882		lge		none		15,553	+	7
883	879	bkc ne	kc gne	b	2124	1,060	0	10
884		kc lgne		l		12,351	+	9
881	880	c lgn	bkc n	l, g	1701	26,298	+	8
883		bkc ne		e		3,885	0	8
880	881	bkc n	c lgn	b, k	350	31,346	+	8
884		kc lgne		k, e		33,441	+	7
879	882	kc gne	lge	k, c, n	362	1,640	0	14
884		kc lgne		k, c, n		42,951	+	8
879	883	kc gne	bkc ne	b, g	490	1,222	0	10
882		lge		l, g		18,151	+	11
879	884	kc gne	kc lgne	l	2309	29,374	+	10
882		lge		none		1,762	0	10

*Phenotypes listed according to population studies in mongrel dogs by Dausset et al., J Exp Med 134:1228, 1971.
†MLC reactivity expressed as rate of incorporation of ^{3}H thymidine (counts/min).
‡Autologous control counts; m, mitomycin-treated cells.

typically compatible donors ranged from 8 to 10 days (MST = 8.66 days), in contrast to a survival time of 9 to 14 days (MST = 9.30 days) in incompatible grafts. The longest skin graft survival time observed in this series occurred in a recipient of a skin allograft obtained from an MLC-nonstimulatory (i.e., LD-compatible) donor (879) who also had major DL-A SD incompatibilities with the recipient. This graft survived for 14 days, while a graft obtained from another donor (884) who was incompatible with the recipient for the same DL-A SD antigens (*k*, *c*, *n*), but whose cells markedly stimulated the host's lymphocytes in the MLC test, was rejected within 8 days.

DISCUSSION

The results of this study confirm and extend to the canine species earlier observations by Koch et al.[6] and van Rood et al.[7] on the importance of products of the LD locus in conditioning the tempo and intensity of skin allograft rejection in unrelated human subjects. It is of interest, however, that the studies by these authors had to be performed in subjects selected first on the basis of HL-A SD phenotypic identity, while the mongrel dogs described in this report were largely incompatible for currently detectable DL-A SD antigens. This difference may be a reflection of the relatively low degree of monospecificity of many of the currently available DL-A SD typing sera.[10] It may also be related to a more limited polymorphism of the products of the LD locus or loci in the canine species. There is, however, a striking difference between the influence of donor–recipient DL-A SD compatibility in mongrel dogs and in dogs from selectively bred lines of known DL-A phenotypes, in which the SD antigens appear to serve as effective marker systems for the entire DL-A complex. This fact has been demonstrated in preselected donor–recipient pairs for transplants of bone marrow, skin, kidney, heart, liver, and lung.[9]

It is of particular interest that under the conditions of this experiment, the survival of skin grafts was slightly but significantly longer (MST = 10 days) in recipients of LD-identical skin grafts as compared with the results of grafts obtained from MLC-stimulatory donors (MST = 8.5 days). This observation did not appear to be conditioned significantly by different donor–recipient states of DL-A SD phenotypic compatibility. The possible greater influence of LD products in conditioning skin allograft survival in mongrel dogs, within the current limitations of methods of serologic testing, was particularly evident in one recipient (882). This recipient was tested with two skin allografts obtained from donors that were both incompatible with the recipient for DL-A SD antigens *k*, *c*, *n*. One graft obtained from the LD-incompatible donor (884) was rejected at 8 days, while the graft obtained from the MLC-nonstimulatory (i.e., LD-compatible) donor (879) survived for 14 days. The possible relevance of this observation to the human situation has recently been shown by the successful bone marrow transplant performed by Dupont et al.[11] using cells obtained from a mother who was HL-A-incompatible with a sibling with immunodeficiency disease but whose cells failed to be stimulated by the sibling's lymphocytes in the MLC test. Taken together with the results presented here, this observation points to the importance of MLC testing as an essential component of the preoperative work-up of prospective clinical bone marrow or kidney transplantations in which living subjects are considered for selection as donors.

REFERENCES

1. Templeton JW, Thomas ED: Transplantation 11:429, 1971

2. Rapaport FT, Bachvaroff R, Cannon FD, et al: Transplant Proc 5:1775, 1973

3. Bachvaroff R, Rapaport FT, Ozaki A, et al: Transplant Proc 5:1561, 1973

4. Dausset J, Sasportes M, Lebrun A: Transplant Proc 5:1511, 1973

5. Sasportes M, Lebrun A, Rapaport FT, et al: Transplant Proc 4:209, 1972

6. Koch CT, Eijsvoogel VP, Fredericks E, et al: Lancet 2:1334, 1971

7. van Rood JJ, Koch CT, van Hooff JP, et al: Transplant Proc 5:409, 1973

8. Hartzman RJ, Segall ML, Bach FH, et al: Cell Immunol 4:192, 1972

9. Rapaport FT, Watanabe K, Cannon FD, et al: J Exp Med 136:1080, 1972

10. Dausset J, Rapaport FT, Cannon FD, et al: J Exp Med 134:1222, 1971

11. Dupont B, Andersen V, Hansen G, et al: Transplantation 14:557, 1972

Segregation Analysis of HL-A Antigens and Haplotypes in 50 Families of Patients With Coeliac Disease

By E. D. Albert,* K. Harms, R. Wank, I. Steinbauer-Rosenthal,* and S. Scholz*

THE study of the correlation of HL-A antigens with certain diseases has become potentially rewarding since the discovery of the close linkage between histocompatibility genes and immune response genes in mice[1] and guinea pigs.[2] In analogy to the situation in the mouse it can be suspected that also in man there are at least some immune response genes located in close proximity of the HL-A loci and that defective immune response genes could be responsible for human diseases which show abnormalities involving the immune system.

The rather disappointing results of numerous correlation studies between HL-A and Hodgkin's disease[3] have suggested to us to investigate diseases only if there is reasonable evidence for the hereditary nature in the form of a significantly higher incidence of the disease among first-degree relatives of a propositus as compared to the incidence in the unrelated population. It has become quite clear that for each observed disease association family studies and segregation analyses should be performed in order to validate the statistical finding in the unrelated patient population.[4]

An unusually high association between the antigens HL-A1 and HL-A8 and coeliac disease (CD) has been reported by Stokes et al.[5] and by Falchuk et al.[6] for adult coeliac disease. It was the objective of the present study to investigate in families a possible joint segregation of HL-A antigens with a gene partly responsible for the occurrence of coeliac disease in children and adults.

MATERIALS AND METHOD

Diagnosis of CD was based on the finding of the typical lesion of a flat small bowel mucosa as assessed by small bowel biopsy.[7] Most patients were biopsied repeatedly at various intervals.

Tissue typing for the presence of 25 established HL-A antigens was performed as previously reported.[8]

RESULTS

Fifty-three patients, 100 parents, and 58 healthy siblings and other relatives were tested for a total of 25 HL-A specificities and compared with a normal control panel of 462 unrelated healthy volunteers.[8]

Phenotype and Gene Frequencies

The antigens HL-A1 and HL-A8 were found in significantly increased frequency among the patients as well as among the parents. All other antigens failed to show any significant differences in the three groups. Phenotype and gene frequencies of HL-A1 and HL-A8 in patients, parents and controls are given in Table 1. From the χ^2 values at the bottom of Table 1 one can see that the most significant deviation is observed for HL-A8.

Haplotype Frequencies

The haplotypes of 100 parents, 50 patients, and 58 siblings and other relatives were deduced by family analysis. Haplotype frequencies were determined for the patients and the parents using the haplotype counting maximum-likelihood method[9]: The haplotype HL-A1–8 was found in a significantly increased frequency of 0.316 among patients as compared to 0.078 in the control group ($\chi^2 = 51.87$, $p < 0.0005$). Also among the parents of the pa-

---

*Members of Sonderforschungsbereich 37, München.

From Kinderpoliklinik der Universität München and Kinderklinik der Universität München.

Supported in part by Deutsche Forschungsgemeinschaft, grant Al 92/7.

© 1973 by Grune & Stratton, Inc.

Table 1. Phenotype and Gene Frequencies of HL-A1 and HL-A8 in Families of Patients with Coeliac Disease

	HL-A1		HL-A8	
	Phenot. Freq.	Gene Freq.	Phenot. Freq.	Gene Freq.
Patients $N = 53$	0.64 (34/53)	*0.377**	0.66 (35/53)	*0.386†*
Parents $N = 100$	0.46 (46/100)	*0.253‡§*	0.46 (46/100)	*0.236¶***
Controls $N = 462$	0.27 (125/462)	0.144	0.19 (88/462)	0.100

*χ^2 patients/controls = 32.01, $p < 0.0005$.
†χ^2 patients/controls = 66.65, $p < 0.0005$.
‡χ^2 parents/controls = 13.05, $p < 0.0025$.
§χ^2 parents/patients = 4.83, $p < 0.05$.
¶χ^2 parents/controls = 27.02, $p < 0.0005$.
**χ^2 parents/patients = 7.09, $p < 0.01$.

Table 2. Segregation Analysis of HL-A Antigens in 50 Families of Children With Coeliac Disease (Segregation in Informative Back-cross Situations)

	Number of Patients at Risk			Number of Healthy Siblings at Risk		
	Positive	Negative	χ^2	Positive	Negative	χ^2
HL-A1	30	9	11.30*	20	19	0.02
HL-A2	14	22	1.78	14	15	0.04
HL-A3	13	14	0.04	14	11	0.36
HL-A9	4	9	1.92	6	5	0.90
HL-A10	2	8	3.60	5	3	0.50
HL-A11	3	2	0.20	0	0	0.00
HL-A28	0	3	2.00	2	1	0.33
W 29	3	1	0.50	1	1	0.00
W 31	1	0	1.00	0	0	0.00
W 32	3	1	1.00	3	3	0.00
HL-A5	6	5	0.09	7	3	1.60
HL-A7	5	11	2.25	7	6	0.77
HL-A8	33	5	20.60†	17	20	0.24
HL-A12	8	7	0.07	6	7	0.77
HL-A13	5	3	0.50	2	3	0.20
HL-A14	3	1	0.50	1	1	0.00
W 15	7	7	0.00	6	6	0.00
W 16	2	7	2.78	7	1	1.50
HL-A17	2	5	1.29	4	3	0.14
W 18	4	9	1.92	8	8	0.00
W 21	1	2	0.33	0	2	2.00
W 22	0	0	0.00	0	0	0.00
W 27	3	2	0.20	4	5	0.11
W 5	5	9	1.14	7	3	1.60
W 10	3	7	1.60	5	7	0.33

*$p < 0.001$. †$p < 0.0005$.

tients the haplotype frequency of HL-A1–8 was 0.186 which is significantly increased over the controls ($\chi^2 = 20.8$, $p < 0.0005$). None of the other haplotypes revealed any significant deviation.

Segregation Analysis

Table 2 presents the results of the segregation analysis of the HL-A antigens in informative backcross situations. The segregation is listed separately for the patients and for the healthy siblings. The only significant deviations could be observed for the antigens HL-A1 and HL-A8 in the patient group, where both antigens were clearly overrepresented. Again, the deviation is stronger for HL-A8 than for HL-A1.

Due to the high degree of polymorphism at the haplotype level there were only few haplotypes frequent enough to be included in a segregation analysis. Table 3 shows that among the seven most frequent haplotypes HL-A1–8 exhibits a strong deviation among the patients, while it is evenly distributed among the healthy siblings.

Numbers of Homozygotes

The incidence of homozygosity was assessed and compared with the expectation based on the gene frequencies of the parents. Homozygosity was found among the patients for the following antigens: HL-A8 (4×), HL-A1 (3×), HL-A2 (2×), HL-A3 (once), and HL-A12 (once). The total number of 11 observed homozygotes did not differ significantly from the combined expectation of 12.79 for all antigens.

Association of HL-A1 and HL-A8 in the Patient Group

It was attempted to decide whether the increased frequency of one of the two antigens HL-A1 and HL-A8 could simply be due to the high linkage disequilibrium that is known for this particular haplotype. In such a case one would expect that the association between both antigens should be higher among the patients than among the controls and this is in fact what one observes: In the patient group 84% of the HL-A1 genes are coupled with HL-A8 as compared to 54% in the controls ($p < 0.005 < 0.001$), indicating that the increased frequency of HL-A1 is caused by the high frequency of HL-A8 by virtue of a strong linkage disequilibrium. In contrast to this, the proportion of HL-A8 genes present in the form of the HL-A1–8 haplotype is almost identical among patients and controls (78% vs. 82%).

Conversely, if one analyzes the frequency of the HL-A1 and HL-A8 genes which are not present as the HL-A1–8 haplotype one finds that the HL-A1 genes are not more common among patients ($g_{1r} = 0.061$) than among controls ($g_{1r} = 0.066$), whereas there is a definitely increased frequency of the (non-HL-A1–8-)-HL-A8 genes among patients ($g_{8r} = 0.07$) as compared to the controls ($g_{8r} = 0.022$; $p = 0.02$).

Table 3. Segregation Analysis of HL-A Haplotypes in 50 Families of Patients With Coeliac Disease

	Patients (N = 50)			Healthy Siblings		
Haplotype	positive	negative	χ^2	Positive	Negative	χ^2
HL-A1-8	31	4	*20.08**	16	16	0.00
HL-A2-12	1	3	0.50	2	3	0.20
HL-A2-W15	4	5	0.11	1	2	0.33
HL-A3-7	4	4	0.00	3	2	0.20
HL-A2-7	1	5	2.67	2	1	0.33
HL-A3-W18	1	3	0.50	1	3	0.50
HL-A3-W5	2	3	0.20	5	2	1.29

*$p < 0.0005$

DISCUSSION

The present study fully comfirms previous reports by Stokes et al.[5] and by Falchuk et al.,[6] although the association observed in our material is not quite as strong as that reported by these authors. This difference can easily be explained by the different populations from which the patients originate.

The family analysis has clearly established the validity of the association between HL-A1 and HL-A8 and CD which was observed in the unrelated patient population. Although this association is so strong and barely needs further confirmation, the family studies are essential to establish a joint segregation between HL-A chromosomes and the disease. It has been suggested by McDonald et al.[10] that CD is inherited through a dominant gene of low penetrance, and in the light of the segregation data presented here it can be assumed that this gene responsible for CD is closely linked with the second HL-A locus. The restricted analysis of the association between HL-A1 and HL-A8 has clearly provided evidence for the orientation of this CD gene in close proximity of the second HL-A locus. It cannot be decided at present whether this gene is located between the HL-A loci or outside, although it seems more likely to be outside. Since it is known that CD involves some degree of immunological disorder such as circulating immune complexes,[11] changes in serum IgA levels,[12] and a higher than normal incidence of malignant tumors,[13] it is quite appealing to speculate that the CD gene could be a defective immune response gene that is—in analogy to the situation in the mouse and the guinea pig—closely linked with histocompatibility genes. The observation of White et al.[14] of a strong association of HL-A8 with dermatitis herpetiformis fits very well with the known relation of this disorder with CD.[11] There are other diseases with immunological implications reported to show an association with antigens of the HL-A system such as childhood asthma,[15] disseminated lupus erythematosus,[16] ankylosing spondylitis,[17-19] and ragweed allergosis.[20]

Although the assumption of defective immune response genes for at least some of these diseases seems to be most appealing, it should be stressed that the possibility of a strong cross-reactivity of the respective HL-A antigens with a pathogenic substance is by no means ruled out. Absorption experiments with gluten preparations have never shown any indication for cross-reactivity with HL-A8.

It should be pointed out that the finding of this unusually high association of HL-A8 with CD cannot be used as a diagnostic criterion since approximately 35% of the patients in our material quite clearly suffer from CD but do not possess the HL-A8 antigen, a finding which must be expected if one assumes linkage of the CD gene with HL-A. On the other hand, if one assumes the over-all frequency of CD as 1 in 2000 = 0.0005 one can calculate that only 0.17% of the HL-A8 positive individuals have CD, which is roughly three times the normal frequency. With these frequencies it is possible to estimate the degree of linkage disequilibrium between HL-A8 and the assumed CD gene as 0.000305. This value seems quite low as compared to values observed in the HL-A and MLC systems,[21] but it must be pointed out that the linkage disequilibrium parameter (Delta) is frequency-dependent so that the degree of gametic association involving a rare gene could be more clearly expressed as the proportion of observed haplotype frequency to expected haplotype frequency, which is in the case of the HL-A8–CD association (0.00033/0.000025 = 13.2). In comparison, the HL-A1–8 association would give the proportion of 0.078/0.014 = 5.5.

Although the CD–HL-A8 association cannot be used as a diagnostic criterion, it may be helpful to point out siblings and relatives of a propositus who are at risk to possess the CD gene. This is particularly important in the light of the reported higher incidence of malignant tumors in CD patients.[13] It has been observed by McDonald et al.[10] that among the relatives of patients there are a number of individuals who upon closer diagnostic scrutiny can be shown to suffer from CD. Quite obviously, if the HL-A8 associated CD gene is the principal genetic condition for the disease, there must be a number of different environmental and/or genetic factors that influence the penetrance of the CD gene. Among these factors there is certainly a strong sex influence[10] as reflected in the 2:1 proportion of female to male patients.

Efforts are currently underway to prove the hypothesis of an HL-A8-associated CD gene by searching for families in which the disease appears in two consecutive generations (one such family, which shows a joint segregation of HL-A8 with the disease, is included in the presented material). Most critical is the investigation of families in which the disease segregates with HL-A genes other than HL-A8. We do not dare to expect the finding of a CD family with an informative crossing-over, which of course could give information as to the exact position of the CD gene within the major histocompatibility complex. While waiting for this lucky event we are taking an alternative approach: After the recent definition of determinants of the MLC locus, which must be located in very close proximity to the second HL-A locus[22] and thus also to the CD gene, we are currently typing CD patients and families for MLC determinants.

ACKNOWLEDGMENTS

The authors wish to express their thanks for the excellent technical assistance of Miss H. Brandenburg, Mrs. M. Hiliopoulos, and Mrs. B. Schiessl.

REFERENCES

1. McDevitt HO, Benacerraf B: Advan Immunol 11:31, 1969

2. Ellman L, Green I, Martin WF, et al: Proc Natl Acad Sci USA 66:322, 1970

3. Joint report of the Fifth International Histocompatibility Workshop, Evian, 1972, Histocompatibility Testing 1972. Copenhagen, Munksgaard, 1973, pp 619–720

4. Bertrams J, Schildberg P, Höpping W, et al: Tissue Antigens 3:78, 1973

5. Stokes PL, Asquith P, Holmes GKT: Lancet 2:162, 1972

6. Falchuk ZM, Rogentine GN, Strober W: J Clin Invest 51:1602, 1972

7. Schmerling DH: Helv Pediatr Acta, Suppl XXII

8. Albert ED, Scholz S, Rosenthal I, et al: Histocompatibility Testing 1972. Copenhagen, Munksgaard, 1973, pp 147–152

9. Albert ED, Mickey MR, Ting A, et al: Transplant Proc 5:215, 1973

10. McDonald WC, Dobbins WO, Rubin CE: N Engl J Med 448, 1965

11. Mowbray JF, Holborow EJ, Hoffbrand AV, et al: Lancet 400, 1973

12. Crabbé PA, Douglas AP, Hobbs JR: in Booth CC, Dowling RH (eds): Coeliac disease. Edinburgh, Churchill Livingstone, 1970, p 134

13. Cooke WT: in Booth CC, Dowling RH (eds): Coeliac Disease. Edinburgh, Churchill Livingstone, 1970, p 198

14. White AG, Barnetson RSC, Da Costa JAG, et al: Lancet 108, 1973

15. Thorsby E, Engeset A, Lie SO: Tissue Antigens 1:147, 1971

16. Grumet FC, Coukell A, Bodmer JG, et al: N Engl J Med 285:193, 1971

17. Schlosstein L, Terasaki PI, Bluestone R, et al: N Engl J Med 288: 704, 1973

18. Brewerton DA, Hart FD, Nicholls A, et al: Lancet, 904, 1973

19. Albert et al., unpublished data

20. Levine BB, Stember RH, Fotino M: Science 178: 1201, 1972

21. Albert et al: Transplant Proc 5:1551, 1973

22. Mempel W, Grosse-Wilde H, Albert ED, et al: Transplant Proc 5: 401, 1973

Histocompatibility-Linked Immune-Response Determinants in Multiple Sclerosis

By Casper Jersild, Bo Dupont, Torben Fog, Grete S. Hansen, Lillian S. Nielsen, Mogens Thomsen, and Arne Svejgaard

OUR GROUP as well as two others have found that the HL-A antigens 3, 7 and W18 are significantly more frequent in patients with multiple sclerosis (MS) than in normal unrelated individuals.[1-3] Furthermore, it has been shown that the antibody titer against measles virus in the serum is increased more frequently in MS patients carrying these HL-A antigens than in those lacking them.[4] There is now considerable evidence in the mouse, the guinea pig, and the monkey[5-7] that at least some immune-response genes (Ir) are located within the major histocompatibility complex (MHC). These findings suggested to us that certain specific immune-response determinants were related to MHC in MS patients and were common between these patients. If this could be shown, it would indicate the existence of a possible genetically determined pathogenic factor in the development of MS. This factor should then be frequent in MS patients, and linkage disequilibrium between Ir and the serologically defined (SD) antigens of the HL-A system could explain the change of some HL-A antigen frequencies in MS.

In this report we describe our preliminary studies on mixed leukocyte culture (MLC) reactions of patients with MS when tested against a selected panel of lymphocytes carrying well-defined HL-A antigens and well-defined MLC-LD determinants.

These results indicate that most MS patients independently of their HL-A haplotypes have at least one specific MLC determinant in common, and that this determinant(s) is identical to those associated with the HL-A7 antigen and possibly also the HL-AW18 antigen in normal unrelated individuals.

MATERIALS AND METHOD

The mixed lymphocyte cultures were performed as previously described.[8] Thirteen MS patients were selected among 150 HL-A typed MS patients. Cells from these 13 patients were repeatedly investigated in the MLC test using stimulator and responder cells from patients as well as from a panel of normal individuals. The HL-A types of patients and controls are shown in Table 1.

The MS patients and the controls were divided into six groups according to their HL-A7-zygosity: HL-A7-homozygote MS patients (group I) and controls (group IV); HL-A7-heterozygote patients (group II) and controls (group V): and HL-A7-negative patients (group III) and controls (group VI).

The lymphocyte test panel consisted of cells from eight normal individuals who were selected according to their HL-A haplotypes and MLC determinants. Because of the increased frequency of HL-A7 and HL-AW18 in MS patients we have selected test cells homozygous for HL-A3, 7 [donors A, B, and C (table 1)]. These cells have previously been shown to be homozygous for the MLC (LD) determinant LD-7a.[9] One test-cell donor (MF) with the HL-A haplotypes 3, 7 and 10, W18 was included in the study. These cells carry the LD determinant LD-7a on the 3, 7 haplotype and the LD determinant LD-W18a on the 10, W18 haplotype. The test cells HL-A3, 7/2, W16 have the LD determinants LD-7a linked to 3, 7 and LD-W18a, W16a on the 2, W16 haplotype. Four other test cells without these LD determinants were also included. Further characterization of the test-cell panel is described in another report in this issue.[9]

MLC tests were performed between all 13 patients and the eight controls on two to four separate occasions, each with new bleedings of all individuals. The tests were performed with equal numbers of responding and stimulating cells as well as with three

From the Tissue Typing Laboratory and Blood Grouping Department, State University Hospital (Rigshospitalet), and the Neuromedical Department, Copenhagen Municipal Hospital, Copenhagen, Denmark.

Study supported by grants from the Research Foundation for Copenhagen, Greenland, and the Faero Islands, the Foundation for Research in Multiple Sclerosis, and the Danish State Research Council, and by AB Gambro.

© 1973 by Grune & Stratton, Inc.

Table 1. HL-A Antigens in Groups I–VI

	Multiple Sclerosis Patients		Four-Locus	Normal Test-Cell Panel		
Group No.	Initials	HL-A Antigens	Antigens	HL-A Antigens	Initials	Group No.
I	EB	3,7/1,7	−7/−7	3,7/3,7	A	IV
	SC	3,7		3,7/3,7	B	
				3,7	C	
II A	VS	3,7,W19,W18	−7/−§	3,7/2,W16	JJ	V A
	PC	3,7,W10				
	AS	3,7,TY				
	OO	3,7/W19,W15				
	EO	3,7/2,W16				
	VD	3,7/2,W16				
II B	KCH	3,7,10,W18	−7/−W18	3,7/10,W18	MF	V B
III	RO	2,W15/2,W16	−§/−§	1,W19,12, TY	JP	VI
	MLR	1,8,11,W5		2,5,10,MK	BD	
	EP	2,W19,W5,W21		2,12,W5	MW	
	IM	1,8,5		11,13,W19,W15	LM	

times increased stimulating cell number. The results obtained with these two methods gave essentially identical results. All values are given as stimulation ratios (SR = cpm in the mixture of A + B_m divided by cpm in the mixture A + A_m).

If four or more combinations were tested in a group (e.g., response of group IV to stimulation with group VI) the results are given as mean values and 95% confidence limits. These calculations were made after logarithmic transformation of the SR values. Logarithms were used in all calculations, but the results are given after retransformation to simple SRs.[10]

The values obtained in the different groups shown in Tables 2 to 5 have been compared to our normal material of two, one, and zero haplotype differences. The mean values and 95% confidence limits in these three groups are: 4.1-*15.2*-58.6; 2.09-*7.95*-30.2; and 0.54-*1.05*-2.07, respectively.[10] In addition to these three groups, we have recently described a fourth group with SRs intermediate between zero and one haplotype (SR: 1.5–3.5). This group will be referred to as the intermediate 0–1 h group.[10] The t test was used to assess the significance of the differences between the average stimulation ratios of test groups and controls.

Table. 2. The LD Determinant (LD-7a) in MS Patients Homozygous for HL-A7

Responding Cells	Stimulating Cells		
	MS Patient EB 3,7/1,7_m	Normal Test Cells: Group IV 3,7/3,7_m	Normal Test Cells: Group VI —/—$_{m*}$
Patient EB 3,7/1,7		0.5	7.8
		0.6	16.7
			32.9
N = 2			N = 6
Group IV 3,7/3,7	0.7	0.9	4.2 – *15.6* – 58.3
	1.2	1.0	
N = 4	7.8	N = 4	N = 6
Group VI ~/~	14.2	4.8 – *8.0* – 13.4	5.5 – *17.9* – 55.7
	32.9		

*m denotes Mitomycin-C treated stimulatory cells. If four or more individuals are included in a combination, the results are given as mean value (italic) and 95% confidence limits. In other cases the individual ratios are given. N = number of combinations.

Table 3. The HL-A7 Linked Common MLC Determinant LD-7a in Patients with Multiple Sclerosis Heterozygote for HL-A7

Responding Cells	Stimulating Cells					
	IIa_m	I_m		IV_m	Va_m	VI_m
		MS	MS			
	$-7/\sim MS_m$	$3-7/17_m$	$3-7/3-7_m$	$3-7/3-7_m$	$3-7/2-W16_m$	$\sim/\sim_m$
II 7/– ~ MS	N = 1 3.0 – 7.4 – 18.6 1h $p \sim 0.65$ 2h $p < 0.001$	1.6 2.4 2.7	3.6 4.2 6.2	N = 11 0.8 – 2.4 – 6.9 < 1 haplotype 0h $p < 0.005$ 1h $p < 0.001$ 2h $p < 0.001$	N = 5 2.6 – 7.9 – 24.2 1h $p \sim 0.99$ 2h $p < 0.05$	N = 16 4.3 – 10.5 – 26.1 1h $p < 0.01$ 2h $p \sim 0.5$
I 7/–7 MS	N = 6 3.2 – 6.6 – 13.5 1h $p \sim 0.3$ 2h $p < 0.005$					
V 3,7/2,W16	N = 5 4.7 – 8.9 – 16.6 1h $p \sim 0.55$ 2h $p < 0.02$					

1h; The MLC responses within this group are compatible with a one HL-A haplotype response.
2h, The MLC responses within this group are compatible with a two HL-A haplotype response.
Legend for the table as in Table 2.
p values give the significance that the stimulation ratios are different from the usual 0, 1, and 2 haplotype differences indicated.

Table 4. The HL-A7 Linked MLC Determinant LD-7A in MS Patients Without HL-A7

Responding Cells	Stimulating Cells			
		$-7/-7\ MS_m$		IV_m
	$III \sim/\sim MS_m$	(3, 7/1, 7)m	(3, 7/3, 7)m	(–7/–7)m
III ~/~ MS	1.5 4.9 18.7 19.3	2.9 4.6	5.1 6.9	N = 6 1.2 – 2.7 – 6.4 ≤ 1 haplotype 0 h $p < 0.01$ 1 h $p < 0.005$ 2 h $p < 0.001$
I 7/7 MS	N = 4 3.1 – 5.5 – 9.8 0 h $p < 0.001$ 1 h $p < 0.1$ 2 h $p < 0.005$			
II 7/~ MS	N = 10 2.3 – 5.4 – 12.3 ≤ 1 haplotype 0 h $p < 0.001$ 1 h $p < 0.01$ 2 h $p < 0.001$			
V a 7/~	N = 4 2.6 – 6.7 – 17.1 0 h $p < 0.005$ 1 h $p \sim 0.6$ 2 h $p < 0.05$			

Legend to table as in Tables 2 and 3.
Groups I–V are defined in Table 1.

Table 5. The HL-AW18 Linked MLC Determinant (LD-W18′) in Patients with Multiple Sclerosis

	MS PATIENTS		NORMALS	
	$3,7/10,W18_m$	$3,7/-§_m$	$3,7/10,W18_m$	$3,7/-§_m$
Group I (MS) −7/−7	0.8 1.7	1h	2.2 1.6	1h
Group II (MS) −7/−§	2.2 2.6 3.7	1h	1.9 2.1 6.0	1h
Group III (MS) −§/−§	2.2 3.7	2h	3.0 4.7	2h

Values given are stimulation ratios. 1h and 2h: See legend to Table 3.

RESULTS

Table 2 shows that the MS patient with the HL-A genotype 3,7/1,7 must carry the same MLC determinant on both haplotypes and that this determinant is identical to the LD-7a determinant present on the two HL-A3,7 homozygous normal controls (A and B). This finding has been further confirmed by family studies performed in our laboratory.

Table 3 gives some of the results obtained in MLC tests between all members in groups I–VI. This table focuses on the MLC reactions of patients heterozygous for HL-A7 (group II). These individuals' lymphocytes respond very poorly to LD-7a homozygous controls ($II\text{-}IV_m$) and respond mutually as a one haplotype difference; this response pattern is also apparent when these MS patients react to HL-A7-heterozygous controls ($II\text{-}V_m$, $V\text{-}II_m$). When group II stimulates the HL-A7-homozygous MS MS patients (group I), a one-haplotype response is obtained again. This suggests that MS patients with HL-A7 have a specific MLC determinant which is identical or very similar to the LD-7a determinant present in most Danes carrying HL-A7.[9] Although genotype data on all these patients are not yet available, it seems reasonable to suggest that the LD-7a determinant is present on the same haplotype as HL-A7.

Table 4 shows that MS patients lacking HL-A7 (group III) also carry the same MLC determinant (LD-7a): When these patients' cells stimulate MS patients with HL-A7 (group I and II) a one-haplotype response is obtained. When MS patients without HL-A7 (group III) respond to normal controls or the MS patients homozygous for the LD-7a determinant (group IV and MS 3, 7/1, 7), only a very weak response is obtained.

All these results indicate that patients with MS most likely have a specific MLC determinant in common and this determinant is identical to LD-7a, which is the characteristic LD-determinant for most Danish individuals carrying HL-A7.

We have then performed experiments with stimulating cells carrying the HL-A haplotypes 3,7 and 10,W18. The test cells were from an MS patient and an HL-A identical normal control (Table 5). This table shows that the HL-A haplotype 10,W18 only contributes very little to the stimulation of all three groups of MS patients. This is also evident when the MS patients' responses to the 3,7/10,W18 cells are compared to the same patients' responses to 3,7 haploidentical test cells which do not have the HL-A10,W18. This shows that the MS patients have a specific lack of recognition of the W18-linked LD determinant (LD-W18a). Only one of the MS patients tested had the Four antigen W18 (patient KCH, Table 1). This indicates that the MS patients included in this study carry the LD-determinants LD-7a and LD-W18a which are characteristic for the Four antigens HL-A7 and W18. This is valid whether or not the patients carry these Four antigens.

These results show that the 13 MS patients studied, irrespective of their LA and Four phenotypes, respond poorly or not at all in the MLC-test to the stimulation with the LD-7a and the LD-W18a MLC determinants. In the normal population these LD-determinants are associated with the Four antigens, HL-A7 and W18, respectively. Furthermore, the MLC reactivity pattern of lymphocytes from these MS patients is in agreement with the assumption that these cells themselves carry the LD-7a and the LD-W18a determinants.

DISCUSSION AND CONCLUSION

In this report we describe a method to identify histocompatibility linked immune response capacities. This is performed by selection of appropriate test cells with well-defined LD determinants and by evaluating the MLC responses of patients belonging to a certain disease unit. In other studies it has been shown that well-defined diseases may be related to certain HL-A antigens, e.g., Mb. Bechterew, psoriasis, gluten allergy, and ragweed pollenosis.[11-14]

Our studies illustrate that multiple sclerosis is not only related to certain HL-A antigen determinants. The relationship between this disease unit and the characteristics of the major histocompatibility complex is further extended by the characterization of LD determinants. It would appear from this preliminary study that the association between these determinants and MS is stronger than that between HL-A3, 7 and W18 and MS, and to our knowledge this is the first demonstration of an association between specific LD-MLC determinants and a disease.

These characteristic lymphocyte-defined determinants (LD) express the individual's ability to identify and react to foreign cells. The LD determinants probably function as Ir factors in a manner similar to the ones described in the experimental animals.[5-7] If this is so, the MLC test would be a tool for recognizing Ir determinants. This test is an in vitro model for cell recognition, but it probably also correlates with the patient's capabilities to eliminate non-self-agents such as viruses, bacteria, and cells infected with these agents.

Further study of MS patients and their families is needed to establish the inheritance and/or acquisition of LD or Ir determinants. But in any case, it appears to us that the observed response pattern reflects a deficiency of the self-recognition mechanism, which could lead to the acceptance of the MS causing agent(s). This would then in turn lead to secondary autoimmune manifestations characteristic of MS.

The method we have employed to study MS patients could also be used to study the MLC determinants present in other disease units associated with particular HL-A antigens. The method of characterization of disease-related LD–Ir determinants can only be performed by selection of an appropriate panel of test cells carrying specific well-defined LD determinants. The HL-A antigen frequency pattern of patients with a particular disease to be studied may indicate which test cells to use to define these LD determinants, characteristic for the disease.

REFERENCES

1a. Jersild C, Svejgaard A, Fog T: Lancet i:1240, t1972

1b. Jersild C, Svejgaard A, Fog T, et al: Tissue Antigens, 3:243, 1973

2. Naito S, Namerow N, Mickey MR, et al: Tissue Antigens 2:1, 1972

3. Bertrams J, Kuwert E, Liedtke U: Tissue Antigens 2:405, 1972

4. Jersild C, Ammitzbøll T, Clausen J, et al: Lancet i:151, 1972.

5. McDevitt HO, et al: J Exp Med 135:1259, 1972

6. Green I, et al: Transplant Proc 5:1849, 1973

7. Balner H, et al: Transplant Proc 5:1555, 1973

8. Dupont B, Andersen V, Hansen GS, et al: Transplantation 14:557, 1972

9. Dupont B, Jersild C, Hansen GS, et al: Transplant Proc 5:1543, 1973

10. Dupont B, Good RA, Hansen GS, et al: Proc Natl Acad Sci USA, in press

11. Caffrey MFP, James DCO: Nature 242:121, 1973

12. Russel TJ, Schultes LM, Kuban DJ: Engl J Med 287:738, 1972

13. Falchuk ZM, Rogentine GN, Strober W: J Clin Invest 51:1602, 1972

14. Levine BB, Stember RH, Fotino M: Science 178:1201, 1972

Some Speculations on the Associations Between HL-A and Disease Based on Studies of Psoriasis Patients and Their Families

By A. Svejgaard, E. Svejgaard, L. Staub Nielsen, and B. Jacobsen

IT was first observed by Russel et al.[1] and later confirmed by White et al.[2] that there is a very significantly increased frequency of HL-A13 and HL-A17 in psoriatic patients. Russel et al.[1] presented evidence that psoriasis may be closely linked to HL-A. In order to study this relationship further we undertook a study of psoriatics and their relatives.

We have typed 80 unrelated patients with psoriasis vulgaris and confirmed the very marked increase in the frequency of HL-A13 (15.0% versus 4.2% in 1541 unrelated controls) and HL-A17 (36.3% versus 8.0%). The relative risks (Woolf[3]) for these antigens are 4.0 and 6.6, respectively. To give an idea of the strength of these associations, we have estimated the relative risks for a number of LA antigens under the assumption that some related Four determinants were responsible for a dominant disease or condition. The highest relative risks obtained in this analysis from the HL-A phenotype distribution in controls are shown in Table 1, and it appears that the relative risks for HL-A13 and 17 in psoriasis compete fairly well with those between LA and Four antigens. Hence, it would seem that psoriasis may be due to genes closely linked to the Four locus.

In our study of eight kindreds with several cases of psoriasis, we found indeed evidence that psoriasis may be linked to HL-A. However, it appeared from these family studies that there would have occurred at least four recombinations between HL-A and psoriasis in a maximum of 30 meiotic divisions. This recombination frequency of 0.13 is certainly larger than suggested by the relative risks. Accordingly we have to abandon the assumption of close linkage between HL-A and psoriasis.

To explain the strong association between HL-A13 and 17 and psoriasis, we then have to postulate that there are additional genes involved in the development of psoriasis. The HL-A genes could then have an "additive" effect on these genes. Evidence in support of this assumption is obtained when analysing the age at onset of psoriasis in patients with HL-A13 and/or 17 and in patients without these antigens. Like White et al.,[2] we noted an earlier age at onset in the HL-A13-17 group (22.3 yr) as compared to the remaining patients (28.1 yr). However, when studying the age at onset distribution more closely, it appeared that the HL-A13-17 group had only one peak as 43% of the cases started between the tenth and 20th year, whereas there were two peaks for the non-HL-A13-17 group: one in the interval from 10 to 20 yr and another between 50 and 60 yr.

If HL-A13 and 17 caused an increased penetrance of other psoriatic genes, one would expect a higher heritability in the HL-A13-17 group than in the remaining patients. Although the difference was not significant there were 69% in the HL-A13-17 group versus 50% in the other group with a positive family history. The same tendency was found by White et al.[2]

The increase of HL-A17 in psoriatics was not continued to the HL-A1,17 haplotype.

From the Tissue Typing Laboratory and Department of Dermatology, State University Hospital, Copenhagen, Denmark.

Study aided by grants from the Danish State Research Council and from the P. Carl Petersen, the F. L. Smidt, and the King Christian the Xth foundations and by AB Gambro, Sweden.

© 1973 by Grune & Stratton.

Table 1. Relative Risks

Antigen	Condition	Relative Risk
HL-A1	HL-A8	19.81
HL-A10	W18	7.15
HL-A11	W5	4.58
W19	HL-A13	3.48
HL-A10	W16	3.30
HL-A3	HL-A7	3.27
HL-A13	Psoriasis	4.01
HL-A17	Psoriasis	6.57

Relative risk = AD/BC where A, B, C and D are the entries of the 2 × 2 table

	Character: Present	Absent
Patients	A	B
Controls	C	D

Eight of our unrelated psoriatics had arthritis psoriatica and five (63%) of these were HL-A27, which is highly significantly different from the frequency (8.1%) in unrelated controls. This observation is relevant in relation to the extraordinary high frequency (96%) of HL-A27 in Bechterew's disease.[4] In addition we have studied 16 patients with Reiter's disease and 11 (69%) of these carried HL-A27. All of these arthropathies are seronegative and thus seronegative arthritis may be related to HL-A27. It is also possible that there is some other relationship between these diseases which can explain the increased frequency of HL-A27.

Finally, we have studied in collaboration with Kissmeyer-Nielsen and Zacchariae[5] 31 patients with pustular psoriasis. In this group there was no increase in the frequencies of HL-A13 and 17, and accordingly, pustular and psoriasis vulgaris may be two different diseases. However, the difference between these two groups could also be explained if HL-A13 and 17 "protect" psoriatics from developing pustulosis.

REFERENCES

1. Russel TJ, Schultes LM, Kuban DJ: N Engl J Med 287:738, 1972
2. White SH, Newcomer VD, Mickey MR, et al: N Engl J Med 287:740, 1972
3. Woolf B: Ann Hum Genet 19:251, 1954–5
4. Caffrey MFP, James DCO: Nature 242:121, 1973
5. Svejgaard A, Kissmeyer-Nielsen F, Zacchariae, et al: in preparation.

Fundamental Characteristics of Histocompatibility-linked Specific Immune-Response (Ir) Genes

By Hugh O. McDevitt*

THE histocompatibility-linked specific immune-response genes control the cellular and humoral immune response to a wide variety of antigens in the mouse, the rat, and the guinea pig, notably to synthetic polypeptide antigens, complex protein antigens, and transplantation antigens.[1] Where detailed mapping studies have been carried out (e.g., reference 2), most of the specific immune-response genes in the mouse map in the region between the H-2K locus and the Ss-Slp loci. As has been pointed out repeatedly in this conference, genetic differences in this region also elicit the strongest reactivity in the mixed lymphocyte culture (MLC) reaction and the graft-vs.-host reaction. Our knowledge of the genetic fine structure of this region of the major histocompatibility complex is insufficient for us to have any reliable estimate of the number of genes which are included in this region, or to have any definitive way of determining whether specific immune-response (Ir) genes and genes eliciting the MLC reaction are the same or, on the other hand, reflect the activity of closely linked loci with separate and distinct functions—that is, recognition of antigenic foreignness on the one hand and recognition of alloantigens on the other. If specific immune-response genes and MLC genes are in fact identical, then it is necessary to understand how these specific recognition structures can themselves function as strong antigens in the MLC reaction. While this could be the result of the summation of the large number of antigenic differences produced by a series of genes coding for specific recognition structures, the resolution of this problem will require a more accurate estimate of the number of gene loci in this region and a more precise understanding of the nature of the gene products coded for by at least some of these loci. A more precise estimate of the number of loci coded for by this region can best be obtained by the production and precise characterization of a large number of recombinants resulting from crossovers between the H-2K and Ss-Slp loci. An understanding of the nature of the gene products coded for by loci mapping in this region will require isolation of gene products, a formidable problem that would be made somewhat less formidable if it were possible to produce antisera against these gene products. Recent results from Klein,[3] Shreffler,[4] and our own laboratory[5] indicate that it may well be possible to produce specific antisera of this type. It is too early yet to state the precise characteristics of these antisera, but they raise the very definite possibility that serological typing may be carried out for MLC antigens and, hopefully, for the Ir gene products as well. Such antisera should also be helpful in efforts to determine whether cell surface antigens eliciting the MLC reaction are structurally or functionally related to structures coded for by the Ir genes.

NATURE AND CELLULAR SITE OF ACTION OF THE Ir GENES

Space does not permit a detailed discussion of the currently available evidence indicating that the Ir genes are expressed in T cells and control antigen recognition by

---

*Senior Investigator of the Arthritis Foundation.

From the Division of Immunology, Department of Medicine, Stanford University School of Medicine, Stanford, Calif.

Research supported by USPHS research grant No. AI 07757 and special fellowship GM 55474 while on sabbatical leave at the University of Oxford, England, in 1973.

© 1973 by Grune & Stratton.

thymus-derived lymphocytes. This topic has recently been discussed extensively in several reviews and communications.[1,6,7] Since histocompatibility-linked immune-response genes control delayed hypersensitivity reactions, antigen-induced tritiated-thymidine uptake in vitro, skin graft rejection, and specific helper functions, there is every reason to believe that these genes affect T-cell function.[1] Definitive evidence that the histocompatibility-linked Ir genes are expressed exclusively in T cells is lacking. Shearer and Mozes[8] have presented evidence which suggests that, for some of the branched synthetic polypeptide antigens, H-linked Ir genes are expressed in B cells as well. However, this evidence is open to alternative explanations, particularly that Ir genes also have an effect on selective T–B-cell interaction. Our own experiments with tetraparental mice[7] indicate that the Ir gene is expressed selectively in some immunocompetent cell other than B cells, and that responder and nonresponder B cells are functionally equivalent. This conclusion is further strengthened by the finding of Schlossman and Williamson[9] that anti-DNP poly-L-lysine antibody produced in PLL responder and PLL nonresponder animals had identical characteristics in isoelectric focusing measurements, indicating that the B-cell products from responders and nonresponders were structurally identical. Finally, the experiments of Shevach, Paul, and Green[10] indicate that antihistocompatibility antisera can selectively inhibit Ir gene function linked to different histocompatibility alleles in an F_1 heterozygote. In these experiments, antihistocompatibility antisera selectively inhibited antigen-induced tritiated thymidine uptake elicited by synthetic polypeptide antigens under histocompatibility-linked Ir gene control. These results suggest that the antisera are interacting with a surface component on T cells, and also indicate that the Ir gene product is in close association with histocompatibility antigens on the T-cell surface.

Taken together, the results of a wide variety of experiments, referred to above, indicate that the Ir genes control the structure and/or function of specific antigen receptors on the surface of antigen-reactive, thymus-derived lymphocytes. The nature of the specific antigen receptor on the surface of T cells remains a puzzling problem. There is as yet no definite resolution of the continuing controversy over the presence or absence of immunoglobulins on the surface of T cells. The available genetic evidence shows quite clearly that the Ir genes are not associated in any way with structural genes coding for the heavy chains of immunoglobulins, since the mouse immunoglobulin allotypes, located on the heavy-chain constant regions, are not linked to the murine major histocompatibility complex. In addition, there is no evidence in man that genes for kappa-chain allotypes are linked with HL-A. Thus, there is every reason to believe that the H-2-linked Ir genes code for structures which are completely unrelated to the immunoglobulin structural genes.

There is also considerable evidence that the specificity of T cells for antigen is not identical with the specificity of B-cell antigen receptors. This is shown clearly in recent experiments of Hämmerling,[11] which are presented in Table 1. This table shows the results of inhibition of specific ^{125}I (T,G)-A–L antigen binding by B cells and T cells from normal and immunized CWB responder mice. B-antigen binding cells (B-ABC) are inhibited equally well by a tenfold excess of (T,G)-A–L, (H,G)-A–L, or (Phe,G)-A–L. This parallels the already-demonstrated extensive serological cross-reactivity between these three antigens.[12] On the other hand, T-ABC are inhibited only by (T,G)-A–L, and not at all by (H,G)-A–L or (Phe,G)-A–L. This lack of cross-reactivity at the T-cell level parallels

Table 1. Inhibition by Chemical Analogs of ^{125}I-(T,G)-A–L Binding to B and T Cells From CWB Mice

		B Cells		T Cells	
Experiment	Inhibitor	ABC/10^4	% Inhibition	ABC/10^4	% Inhibition
A	—	12	—	27	—
	(T,G)-A–L	1	92	2	92
	(H,G)-A–L	3	75	24	11
	(Phe,G)-A–L	2	83	25	7
B	—	44	—	53	—
	(T,G)-A–L	2	95	5	90
	(H,G)-A–L	6	86	52	2
	(Phe,G)-A–L	8	82	49	8

the already-demonstrated lack of cross-immunogenicity between these antigens despite their extensive cross-antigenicity.[12]

Taken as a whole, the available evidence indicates that the Ir genes are selectively expressed in T cells, where they affect or control the structure and/or the function of T-cell antigen-specific receptors. The fact that the Ir genes are located in the center of the murine major histocompatibility complex, and are unassociated with any known immunoglobulin structural genes, combined with the evidence for a different specificity of T- and B-cell antigen binding, raises the possibility that the Ir gene products are in fact a series of antigen-specific receptors on the surface of T cells which are structurally unrelated to the known immunoglobulins, and which may bear a close structural and functional homology with major transplantation antigens and the antigens which elicit the mixed lymphocyte culture reaction and the graft-vs.-host reaction. While studies of the types referred to above utilizing cellular chimerism, and using specific antisera to inhibit antigen-specific T-cell functions may shed further light on this hypothesis, its final resolution will require isolation of Ir gene products with demonstrable specificity for antigens under the control of specific Ir genes.

REFERENCES

1. Benacerraf B, McDevitt HO: Science 173:273, 1972
2. McDevitt HO, Deak BD, Shreffler DC, et al: J Exp Med 135:1259, 1972
3. Hauptfeld V, Klein D, Klein J: manuscript submitted for publication
4. David CS, Shreffler DC, Frelinger JA: manuscript submitted for publication
5. Deak BD, Hämmerling GJ, McDevitt HO: unpublished observations
6. Benacerraf B: Ann Inst Pasteur 1973 (in press)
7. McDevitt HO, Bechtol KB, Freed JH, et al: Ann Inst Pasteur 1973 (in press)
8. Shearer GM, Mozes E, Sela M: J Exp Med 135:1009, 1972
9. Schlossman SF, Williamson AR: in McDevitt HO, Landy M (eds): Genetic Control of Immune Responsiveness. New York, Academic, 1972, pp 54ff
10. Shevach EM, Paul WE, Green I: J Exp Med 136: 1207, 1972
11. Hämmerling GJ, McDevitt HO: manuscript submitted for publication
12. McDevitt HO, Sela M: J Exp Med 126:969, 1967

Histocompatibility-Linked Immune-Response Genes. What Do They Do?

By Marc Feldmann

IN THE past year it has become increasingly fashionable to believe that T-cell receptors for antigen are not immunoglobulin (Ig), but are the products of H-(histocompatibility-) linked Ir (immune-response) genes (e.g., discussion in ref. 1, McDevitt et al., this volume). This discussion examines the above proposition and suggests other possible mechanisms of H-linked Ir gene action. It should be obvious that many of the ideas discussed have been proposed previously by other workers, and that the aim of this discussion is to provoke experimental investigation of other concepts of Ir gene function. No attempt is made to select any one preferred alternative hypothesis, as there is clearly too little experimental evidence.

Despite much controversy (reviewed exhaustively in ref. 1, especially by Cohn, ref. 2) there is evidence that T cells have surface Ig, and that this Ig can under certain circumstances function as a receptor for antigen. T-cell surface Ig has been detected in appreciable amounts by radioiodination by Marchalonis and Cone,[3] Boylston,[4] and by Moroz,[5] but not by Vitetta et al.[1,6] Radiolabeled anti-Ig has been successfully used.[7] More recently Loor, Pink, du Pasquier, and Roelants (personal communication) have shown that a chicken anti-mouse Ig antiserum extensively absorbed against cells (mouse neuroblastoma, fibroblast and red cells, and powders from liver and brain) stained all T-TDL, a population >99% T cells,[8] whereas rabbit anti-mouse Ig does not, suggesting that the exposed portions of T-cell Ig may be the conserved invariant regions.

Many, but not all, T-cell functions have been blocked by anti-Ig. For example, anti-Ig inhibits rosette formation by T cells (e.g. refs. 9, 10) and binding to antigen-coated fibers,[11a] labeled antigen binding by T cells,[11] and induces "capping" of antigen-binding T-cell receptors.[11] After capping induced by anti-Ig, no specific antigen binding cells are found for a few hours. Receptors reappear on the same proportion of cells cultured at 37°C as before anti-Ig-induced loss of receptors, and at the same time in both T and B cells.[11] These results indicate that the only specific receptors for the antigens used, TIGAL and MSH, are Ig in nature. Cell cooperation (e.g., ref. 12), tolerance induction,[13] and radioactive antigen suicide,[14] are inhibited by anti-Ig, but not MLR reactions, and only rarely GvH reactions (discussed in ref. 15). Furthermore, it has been demonstrated that activated T cells release specific cooperative factors which are Ig-like (reviewed in ref. 16). While these studies suggest that some T cells have Ig receptors they do not implicate Ig receptors on all

---

Abbreviations: Ir gene, immune-response gene, IgT, immunoglobulin found on T-cell surface or released by T cells. T-TDL, thoracic duct lymphocytes of irradiated mice repopulated with thymocytes. GvH, graft-vs.-host. MLR, mixed lymphocyte reaction. LD, lymphocyte-defined antigen. SD, serologically defined antigen. PVP, polyvinyl pyrrolidone, MSH, Maro squid hemocyanin. The following are synthetic antigens: PLL, poly-L-lysine. GA, copolymer of L-glutamic acid and L-alanine. GT, copolymer of L-glutamic acid and L-tyrosine. GL, copolymer of L-glutamic acid and L-lysine. PLA, poly-L-arginine. GAT, copolymer of glutamic acid, alanine, and tyrosine. (T-G)-A–L, branched multichain synthetic copolymer of L-glutamic, L-tyrosine conjugated to D,L-alanine side chains coupled to a backbone of L-lysine. TIGAL, iodinated TGAL.

From the I.C.R.F. Tumour Immunology Unit, Zoology Department, University College, London, England.

© *1973 by Grune & Stratton, Inc.*

subpopulations of T cells, or exclude the participation of other, non-Ig receptors in T-cell triggering, even of cells which may possess Ig receptors. It is, of course, possible to reconcile the views that H-linked Ir genes code for T-cell receptors and the results that some T cells have Ig receptors by assuming, as Cohn[2] does, that the H-linked Ir gene product is IgT. Opponents of this view cite the fact that the heavy-chain genes expressed in B cells are in a different linkage group from the H2 and Ir genes. However, since κ and λ genes are in different linkage groups, there is a precedent for two groups of unlinked heavy-chain genes. The view that the H-linked Ir gene product is IgT is attractive, as it reconciles much data which is otherwise conflicting. However, there is increasing experimental evidence that argues that H-linked Ir gene products cannot be the antigen-specific receptors on T cells.

If H-linked Ir genes code for specific T-cell receptors, two deductions can be made: (1) nonresponders, lacking the gene, should have no evidence of T-cell antigen recognition of that antigen; (2) since B cells have specific Ig receptors, H-linked Ir genes should not be expressed in B cells. Let us examine proposition (1), which offers an opportunity to disprove the hypothesis. I know of four documented examples of nonresponders recognizing antigens to which they allegedly have no receptors. Gershon et al.[17] found that DBA/1 mouse thymocytes incorporated ^{125}IUDR in response to the synthetic polypeptide GAT_{10} in irradiated mice, thus demonstrating immunological recognition. In this system B cells do not respond and nonimmunogens, e.g., GT, and thymus-independent antigens, e.g., polyvinyl pyrrolidone (PVP), do not stimulate. Furthermore, Maurer and Gershon (personal communication) have found that nonresponders make good responses to GAT_{10} provided appropriate, often very low, doses of antigen were used. McDonald and Phillips-Quagliata found that lymph node cells from both high- and low-responder mice incorporate just as much tritiated thymidine in response to low doses of ovalbumin or ovomucoid (personal communication). Hammerling, Masuda, and McDevitt (ref. 18, and this volume) measured T cells binding the antigen (T-G)-A–L in responders or nonresponders (CWB and C3H). No differences in the number of binding cells were seen. Roelants and Loor (personal communication) have found no difference in the number of T or B cells binding (T-G)-A–L in CWB or C3H congenic mice over a wide range of antigen concentrations. Antigen-binding T cells were stained directly using a fluorescent anti-θ antiserum. If this technique has any relevance, for which there is much evidence (discussed in ref. 19), then these are strong arguments against H-linked Ir genes coding for "the" T-cell antigen-specific receptor.

Another extrapolation from the specific T-receptor concept of H-linked Ir gene function is that there would be absolutely no T-cell-dependent response in nonresponders. While this is alleged to be so for the PLL gene by Benacerraf et al. (e.g., ref. 1), de Weck's experience is different, provided a more prolonged immunization regime is followed.[20] That should not be the case if a structural gene for a receptor were lacking.

Another argument against H-linked Ir genes being specific T-cell receptors was made by Schlossman[21] on the basis of the exquisite discrimination by T cells of αDNP oligolysines. Recognition of all L-polylysines seems to be under the control of the PLL gene in guinea pigs. Nevertheless, it could be argued that all these genes (e.g., PLL genes) are in reality clusters of genes.

Inhibition of T-cell function by antihistocompatibility antisera has been used to argue that T cells have non-Ig receptors. Shevach et al.[22] described genetic studies in guinea pigs using antistrain 2 and antistrain 13 antisera which inhibited the corresponding genetically linked responses to

DNP GL or GT of peritoneal lymphocytes in vitro. While the initial studies[1,22] could have been interpreted as due to the effect of anti-Ir activity in these antisera, subsequent absorption studies have shown that the inhibitory antibodies are directed against strain 2 or 13 histocompatibility antigens (W. E. Paul, presentation at Cancer Congress, Houston, April 1973). It is interesting that anti-H2 antibody blocks antigen binding by T cells and not by B cells (ref. 18; Basten, unpublished data). However, antisera directed against either the D or K ends of the H2 region both suppressed, eliminating the possibility of the suppression being due to anti-Ir activity. It should be noted that anti-θ also blocked antigen binding.[18] The capacity of any anti-T-cell surface antiserum to inhibit antigen binding suggests that surface structures, apart from high affinity receptors, are involved in T-cell antigen recognition and function. Alternatively, they could suggest differences in antigen handling at the surface of T and B lymphocytes. Recently, Katz et al.[23] presented results involving H-linked Ir genes in cell cooperation. These could be interpreted in several ways, one of which is that B cells also express H-linked Ir gene products. Evidence that B cells express these products has been found (Sachs and Terry, personal communication).

Other considerations on the nature of H-linked Ir gene products depends critically on the degree of immunological specificity of H-linked effects. If it is assumed that there is a very high degree of specificity, just as specific as T-cell recognition,[23] what other functions for these genes would be envisaged? It also becomes important to consider whether Ir gene products are clonally distributed (for which there is as yet no evidence), as is T-cell function in both cooperation[14] and the MLR.[24]

First, it is possible that H-linked Ir genes are regulator genes for another, possibly Ig, receptor. For example, it is possible that it could influence the number of specific receptors displayed. With too few receptors, it could be argued that upon encounter with antigen the only possible consequence may be tolerance. This is compatible with the data of Gershon, Maurer, and Merryman.[17] Other lesions based upon this concept would include an incapacity of surface receptors to translate antigen binding into a signal for stimulation. This could occur if a specific protein (enzyme ?) has to recognize a pattern of receptor interactions at the surface as the stimulus for triggering. It is conceivable, but by no means likely, that there may be subclasses of T-cell receptor. Each subclass may require a different signal-translator molecule which could be under genetic control. Variants of this concept would consider other steps in the antigen recognition and signal-translation pathway. Since we do not know how the cell membrane phenomena are translated into metabolic events, possibilities considered here, such as levels of enzymes involved in the generation or breakdown of possible internal messengers such as cyclic AMP or cyclic GMP,[25] are highly speculative. The above concepts of H-linked Ir genes involve a high degree of specificity due to Ir gene modifying the function of a specific factor. This concept could be extended to cover lesions in the pathway of T/B cooperation. Since this involves two classes of T-cell factors, and at least three cell types, the range of possibilities here is considerable. For example, T cells of nonresponders may produce less specific factor,[16] or even too much of it.[26] Alternatively, even if produced normally, it may be qualitatively abnormal, i.e., it may not be able to bind to cooperative macrophages, or it may bind in a nonimmunogenic manner. For example, an Ir gene product could be the site by which specific cooperative products bind to cooperating macrophages. A considerable degree of specificity could exist, for example if the Ir gene product had anti-idiotypic specificity for IgT.

Conceivably, the Ir-linked defects may be

entirely at the level of the production of nonspecific mediators. T cells could recognize antigen and proliferate (*vide supra*), but if mediators are not released they could be functionless. Since it is only the IgG response to (T-G)-A–L that is under genetic control, it is possible that a defect in production of a nonspecific factor (which augments IgG)[27] may lie at the basis of the nonresponder defect. It is difficult, however, to envisage that there would be multiple allelic forms of nonspecific T factors. Another possible defect in cell cooperation lies in the nature of the cell contacts, if any, which are required. Katz et al.[23] have results which suggest that T and B cells which do not share some surface specificities (H2 and/or Ir) do not cooperate as efficiently. It could be that Ir may be a site for cell contact during triggering. In face of the data from many laboratories that T and B cells do not need to physically interact in order to cooperate, it could be proposed that the Ir contact is expressed at the level of T-cell/macrophage or B-cell/macrophage interaction. In fact, Rosenthal and Shevach[26a] have obtained evidence that in the guinea pig efficient T-cell/macrophage interaction requires identity at the major histocompatibility complex (MHC) and that only macrophages of responder strains could induce responses to genetically linked antigens. These responses were blocked by antisera directed against the MHC. Alternatively, H-linked Ir gene products may act directly as a form of nonspecific stimulus and bind to some but not all B cells with the appropriate receptors. This possibility cannot be ruled out on the available data, as I do not know of any quantitations of nonspecific factors in many genetically disparate recipient cultures. If the H-linked Ir product is one of several such nonspecific factors, it would be difficult to detect in in vitro assays of MLR supernatants, but could be more effective than the others in vivo for a variety of reasons. Another Ir function in T/B cell cooperation could be as a consequence of T-T collaboration[28] in the generation of T helper cells. This concept is attractive at the moment for a variety of reasons. First, Eijsvoogel, Bach, and their colleagues[27,27a] have shown that in the generation of cell mediated cytotoxicity cells which respond to MLR or LD determinants augment the CML of the cells which react against SD specificities. This would be a nice parallel with the situation with T helper cells which do seem to react to serologically defined antigens—just as B cells do. Secondly, it remains to be shown that T/T collaboration, unlike T/B collaboration, does not require cell-to-cell contact.[28] Third, it could reconcile all the results that imply that H-linked Ir genes influence responses to antigen (due to lack of one population of T cells, critical to an optimal response), with the results that indicate that there are T cells in nonresponders that recognize these antigens (*vide supra*). H-linked Ir genes could also be surface sites whereby the two populations of T cells physically interact.

Cross reactivity of an antigen with H antigens would also cause specific, genetic, H-linked, unresponsiveness. While there is one article supporting the cross-tolerance concept,[28] other data argues against it as a general principle in all examples of H-linked unresponsiveness (discussed in ref. 30). Nevertheless, we know that self-tolerance is chiefly manifest in T cells[31] and so logic dictates that there must be H-linked unresponsiveness to antigens which cross react with H2 specificities carried by that strain. But it seems unlikely that all H-linked nonresponsiveness is due to this process.

Results obtained by Gershon, Maurer, and Merryman,[17] cited above, support the concept that nonresponsiveness is due to tolerance induction in the relevant T cells, i.e., upon encounter with antigen the only consequence is tolerance. While there are data in favor of this concept with GAT and possibly a little with (T-G)-A–L (ref. 32;

N. L. Warner, personal communication), the reason why tolerance is so readily induced remains unclear. However, it is known that ease of tolerance induction is a strain-dependent phenomenon[33] and that polymers readily induce T-cell tolerance.[16] It is possible that in nonresponders T cells can only be stimulated to become suppressor T cells, never helper cells. A precedent which provides evidence in support of this possibility has been obtained by Baker et al.[34] They found that while there were few helper T cells for pneumococcal polysaccharide SIII in normal mice, there were a lot of suppressor cells. Responses to SIII in most mice resemble those of nonresponders to (T-G)-A–L with no functional helper cells, i.e., an IgM response with no immunological memory. Recent in vitro studies have indicated that T-cell helper molecules act as suppressors if they do not bind to macrophages, but interact directly with B cells.[26] Thus an abnormality of the specific helper molecule IgT, preventing it from binding to macrophages, would swing the system wholly to suppression.

Clearly the possibility that nonresponsiveness is due to suppressor T cells needs experimental investigation. If suppressor cells are involved in the maintenance of self-nonreactivity (discussed in ref. 35), suppressor-cell activity could be intertwined with cross tolerance as discussed above. Antibody-mediated tolerance, as described by Diener and myself (reviewed in refs. 16, 36) could be well suited to suppressing potentially reactive T cells, since recent work has indicated that T cells are exquisitely sensitive to this form of suppression. It could be argued that the primary IgM response to, say, (T-G)-A–L causes enough antibody to form complexes with antigen upon challenge, and so suppress T-cell function.

At present the exact degree of specificity of H-linked Ir gene effects is not known. The number of identified genes or gene clusters is still small.[1,30] The PLL gene of strain-2 guinea pigs controls responses to basic amino acid polymers, poly-L-lysine, poly-L-arginine (PLA), and copolymers of glutamic- and L-lysine (GL). This gene can be separated from the strain-2 gene for response to the polymer of glutamic/arginine (GA). It is a question of great importance whether the PLL gene is a single gene or a gene cluster. Clearly PLL, PLA, and GL do not cross react for either T or B cells, and if it is a single gene, the specificity of its product would not be that of the specific receptors for these antigens on T cells. PLL, PLA, and GL are all basic polymers, so it could be argued that the PLL gene codes for an accessory binding or triggering site with a broader degree of specificity. There are observations which suggest that accessory binding may be of more importance for T cells than B cells. First, T cells bind and are triggered by lower doses of antigen than B cells, despite the fact that measurements of T-cell receptor affinity or avidity, crude as they are, indicate that it is similar or less than unprimed B cells and much less after priming.[37] Second, T-cell antigen binding is more influenced by antibodies to any T cell surface component (*vide supra*). Third, binding of antigen to T cells seems to be very temperature dependent, more so than for B cells.[38] It thus seems reasonable to use H-linked Ir gene effects to try to account for these phenomena. Antigen capture at low concentrations would be greatly aided by a second set of receptors, even if they were of low affinity. If triggering requires antigen binding at both Ir and Ig receptors, then in view of mobility of membrane components, interference would be readily achieved. The two-receptor concept would also explain greater sensitivity to stimulation—consequences of Ir binding and Ig binding could be summated (integrated) by the cell's metabolic machinery. Furthermore, the differences in the specificity of T-cell functions and B-cell functions, where they occur, could be explained by binding to Ir products, as could the effects of charged antigens on antibody charge which is expressed via T cells.[39] It is also conceivable that some of the reciprocal relationships between cell-mediated immunity and antibody production, as discussed by Parish,[40] may be due to the dichotomy of receptors (Ir and Ig); low-affinity binding (? to Ir) may cause the cells to express delayed hypersensitivity (release mediators, etc.), whereas higher affinity binding (Ig or both) would result in the production of T helper cells and eventually antibody production. This concept would accommodate and may well represent the evolution from the primitive recognition systems of antigen in worms, etc. This receptor pathway may be utilized in the MLR and GvH, and since there are few specificities known, may explain the high frequency of reacting cells.[15]

If it is assumed that there are only a few H-linked Ir genes, where could the products be expressed? Clearly it must be on the surface or near it (*vide supra*). It could be on or in the glycocalyx. This is thicker in T than in B cells,[41] and so the glycocalyx could influence antigen binding by T cells more than in B cells. Furthermore, the same gene product, say an enzyme which adds to or modifies a sugar on the carbohydrate, could be expressed in the glycocalyx of both T and B cells. But effects could be restricted to the former, because its thickness is greater in T cells.

These speculations about H-linked Ir genes obviously did not consider the functions of other Ir genes, e.g., Ir3, which are probably expressed on B cells,[42] nor of Biozzi high- and low-responder lines[43] which are expressed, at least partly, in macrophages.[44]

REFERENCES

1. McDevitt HO, Landy M (eds): Genetics of Immune Responsiveness. New York, Academic, 1972
2. Cohn M: in McDevitt HO, Landy M (eds): Genetics of Immune Responsiveness, New York, Academic, 1972, pp 367–424
3. Marchalonis JJ, Cone RE: Transplantation Rev 14:3, 1973
4. Boylston A: Immunology, 1973, in press
5. Moroz C: personal communication, 1973
6. Vitetta E, Bianco C, Nusserzweig V, et al: J Exp Med 136:81, 1972
7. Bankhurst A, Warner NL, Sprent J: J Exp Med 134:1005, 1971
8. Sprent J, Miller JFAP: Cell Immunol 3:385, 1972
9. Hogg NM, Greaves MF: Immunology 22:967, 1972
10. Ashman R, Raff MC: J Exp Med 137:69, 1973
11. Roelants G, Forni L, Pernis B: J Exp Med 137:1060, 1973; Roelants G, Ryden A, Hagg LB, Lobr F: Nature (in press)
11a. Edelman GM: Science 180:130, 1973
12. Cheers C, Breitner JCS, Little M, Miller JFAP: Nature New Biol 232:248, 1971
13. Feldmann M, Rittenberg MB: unpublished data, 1973
14. Basten A, Miller JFAP, Warner NL, Pye J: Nature New Biol 231:104, 1971
15. Crone M, Koch C, Simonsen M: Transplant Rev 10:36, 1972
16. Feldmann M, Nossal GJV: Transplant Rev 13:3, 1972
17. Gershon RK, Maurer PH, Merryman C: Proc Nat Acad Sci USA
18. Hammerling GJ, Masuda T, McDevitt HO: J Exp Med 137:1180, 1973
19. Ada, GL: Transplant Rev 5:105, 1970
20. de Weck AL: Transplant Rev 10:3, 1972
21. Schlossman SF: Transplant Rev 10:97, 1972
22. Shevach EM, Paul WE, Green I: J Exp Med 136:1207, 1972
23. Katz DH, Hamaoka T, Dorf ME, et al: J Exp Med (in press); Katz DH, Hamoaka T, Benacerraf B: J Exp Med 137:1405, 1973
24. Zoshke D, Bach FH: Science 172:1350, 1972
25. Hadden JW, Hadden EM, Haddox MK, Goldberg ND: Proc Nat Acad Sci USA 69:3024, 1972
26. Feldmann M: Nature New Biol 242:82, 1973
26a. Rosenthal AS, Shevach E: J Exp Med (in press); Shevach E, Rosenthal AS: J Exp Med (in press)
27. Eijsvoogel VP, du Bois R, Melief CJM, et al: Transplant Proc 5:1301, 1973
27a. Bach FH, Bach HL, Sondel PM, Sunpardias G: Transplant Rev 12:30, 1972
28. Ebringer A, Davies DAL: Nature New Biol 241:144, 1973
29. Wagner H: Science, 1973 (in press)
30. Benacerraf B, McDevitt HO: Science 175:273, 1972

31. Weigle WO: Advan Immunol 16:61, 1973
32. Grumet FC: J Exp Med 135:110, 1972
33. Weigle WO, Chiller JM, Habich GS: Transplant Rev 8:3, 1972
34. Baker PJ, Reed ND, Stashak PW, et al: J Exp Med 137:1431, 1973
35. Allison AC, Denman AM, Barnes RD: Lancet ii:135, 1971
36. Diener E, Feldmann M: Transplant Rev 8:76, 1972
37. Moller E, Bullock WW, Makela O: Europ J Immunol 3:172, 1973
38. Brondz BD: Transplant Rev 10:112, 1972
39. Karmely Y, Mozes E, Shearer GM, et al: J Exp Med 137:183, 1973
40. Parish CR: Transplant Rev 13:35, 1972
41. Santer V, Cone RE, Marchalonis JJ, 1973 (in press)
42. Shearer GM, Mozes E, Sela M: J Exp Med 135: 1009, 1972
43. Biozzi G, Stiffel C, Mouton D, et al: Prog. Immunol 1:529, 1971
44. Howard JG, Wiener E: personal communication, 1973

Serologic Detection of Antigens Controlled by the Ir Region of the H-2 Complex in the Mouse

By Vera Hauptfeld, Dagmar Klein, and Jan Klein

THE H-2 complex of the mouse can be visualized as consisting of two peripheral and several central regions.[1] The peripheral regions, H-2K and H-2D, are believed to be accommodating loci coding for the classical H-2 antigens, i.e., antigens present in practically all tissues of the body and detectable by serological and transplantation methods.

Located between the H-2K and H-2D regions are the Ss and Ir regions. The Ss region codes for serum proteins, Ss and Slp.[2,3] The Ir region has been recently associated with the following phenomena:

1. *Genetic Control of Immune Response to a Variety of Antigens.* The quantity of antibodies formed upon immunization with synthetic polypeptides and their hapten conjugates, weak native protein antigens (i.e., antigens that differ only slightly from similar molecules of the host) or strong native protein antigens injected in limited doses, is determined by genes located in the central regions of the H-2 complex (Ir genes; for a review, see ref. 4). At least three Ir genes have been postulated in the H-2 complex: Ir-1, controlling the immune response to a branched synthetic polypeptide (T,G)-A–L[5]; Ir-IgG and Ir-IgA, controlling the response to myeloma proteins (immunoglobulins) of class G and A, respectively.[6] Antibody response to over 30 other antigens has also been associated with the H-2 complex.

2. *Genetic Control of Resistance to Oncogenic Viruses.* Strain differences are known to exist in resistance to murine oncogenic viruses such as Gross virus, Friend virus, Bittner virus, and others (for a review, see ref. 7). In most instances the resistance depends on several genes; in every case, at least one of these genes seems to be H-2-associated and is probably located within the H-2 complex.

3. *Genetic Control of Mixed Lymphocyte Culture Reaction (MLR).* Cocultivation of allogeneic lymphocytes in vitro results in MLR characterized by increased DNA synthesis, morphological transformation, and increased mitotic activity of the cultured cells. The reaction can occur after a mixing of lymphocytes differing only in the central H-2 regions and identical in the peripheral regions.[8]

4. *Genetic Control of Graft-vs.-Host Reaction (GvHR).* Inoculation of allogeneic immunocompetent cells into immunoincompetent recipients leads to a reaction of the grafted cells against the antigens of the host. This GvHR is manifested by a variety of syndromes, of which the most common is enlargement of the host's spleen (splenomegaly). As in the case of MLR, GvHR can also occur across central H-2 region differences in strains that are otherwise genetically identical.[9]

5. *Genetic Control of T–B-Cell Interaction.* Although antibodies are produced by the descendants of bone-marrow-derived lymphocytes (B cells), the events leading to antibody production are in most cases triggered by interaction of B cells with thymus-processed lymphocytes (T cells). The T–B-cell interaction is influenced by the H-2 complex. Recent evidence suggests that disparity in the central H-2 regions is as least one of the factors preventing effective cooperation between T and B cells.[10]

We have recently shown that the central

From the Department of Oral Biology, School of Dentistry, and Department of Human Genetics, Medical School, University of Michigan, Ann Arbor, Mich.

Supported by PHS research grants GM15419 and DE02731.

© 1973 by Grune & Stratton, Inc.

H-2 regions code for antigens that differ from the classical H-2 antigens in that their expression seems restricted to a subpopulation of lymphocytes.[11] Mice of strains B10.T(6R) and B10.AQR, genetically identical except for their central H-2 regions, were cross immunized using spleen and lymph node cells and the resulting antisera tested by a dye-exclusion and immunofluorescence tests. The antisera reacted with only 30%–40% of the lymph node or spleen cells and did not react with thymus or bone marrow cells. It seemed that the antigen(s) detected with the antisera were expressed on only a small fraction of lymphocytes. Testing against a panel of strains representing major H-2 types suggested that the antigen(s) was controlled by the middle portion of the H-2 complex, perhaps by the Ir region. We therefore designated the antigen Ir-1.1. However, to avoid confusion with the Ir-1 locus of McDevitt, we now change the designation to IrR-1.1 (Ir-region antigen 1). Details of this work have already been published.[11] Some additional data are presented in Table 1. These data further support the association of the IrR-1.1 antigen with the H-2 complex. Tests involving the same H-2 types on different genetic backgrounds indicate that presence or absence of the antigen depends on the H-2 type and not on the genetic background of a strain. For example, strains B10.A and A have the same $H\text{-}2^a$ type on two different backgrounds, C57BL/10Sn and A/J, respectively; yet both strains are positive with the B10.T(6R) anti-B10.AQR antiserum. Strains A and A.BY, on the other hand, have the same background but different H-2 types, $H\text{-}2^a$ and $H\text{-}2^b$, respectively. In agreement with this, the A strain is positive and the A.BY negative with the anti-IrR-1.1 antiserum. Similarly, strain B10 ($H\text{-}2^b$) is negative and strain B10.A ($H\text{-}2^a$) positive. Tests with other congenic lines listed in Table 1 also support the conclusion that the IrR-1.1 antigen(s) is controlled by the H-2 complex. The control of this antigen by the Ir region is suggested by the test with H-2 recombinants: The anti-IrR-1.1 antiserum reacts with all recombinants carrying the Ir^k region (the Ir region of the donor) and does not react (or reacts considerably less) with strains carrying other Ir regions. The

Table 1. Cytotoxicity of B10.T(6R) Anti-B10.AQR Antiserum With Cells of Indicated Strains

Strain	H-2 Chromosome	Origin of Regions				% Cytotoxicity at Dilution*			
		H-2K	Ir	Ss	H-2D	1:2	1:4	1:8	1:16
B10.AQR	y-Klj	q	k	d	d	30	30	20	10
B10.T(6R)	y-Sg	q	q	q	d	0	0	0	0
B10.A	a	k	k	d	d	35	40	20	20
A	a	k	k	d	d	25	30	15	5
B10	b	b	b	b	b	0	5	5	5
A.BY	b	b	b	b	b	5	10	5	5
B10.D2	d	d	d	d	d	0	0	−5	−5
DBA/2	d	d	d	d	d	5	−5	0	−5
B10.BR	k	k	k	k	k	25	30	20	15
C3H	k	k	k	k	k	30	20	15	5
B10.A(2R)	h-2Sg	k	k	d	b	40	40	35	20
B10.A(4R)	h-3Sg	k	k/b	b	b	30	20	15	5
B10.G	q	q	q	q	q	5	5	0	5
DBA/1	q	q	q	q	q	10	5	10	10
T138	q	q	q	q	q	10	5	10	5
B10.A(5R)	i-2Sg	b	b	d	d	0	0	−5	5
A.SW	s	s	s	s	s	10	10	5	−5
B10.S	s	s	s	s	s	5	−5	−5	−5

*Percentage of dead cells of the indicated strain minus the percentage of dead cells of the recipient strain.

expression of the IrR-1.1 antigen on T and B cells is currently being vigorously tested.

We also obtained other antisera against the antigens of the central H-2 regions: B10.AQR anti-B10.T(6R), (A.TL × B10) F_1 anti-B10.HTT, (A.TL × B10) F_1 anti-B10.S(7R). These are being investigated. In addition, an antiserum was obtained by Götze and his co-workers[12] by immunization of B10.D2 mice against soluble lymphocyte membrane antigens of B10.A mice. The antiserum detects an antigen controlled by the Ir-1^k region. The antigen seems to be present only on T cells and absent on B cells.

The relationship of the IrR-1 antigens to the functions associated with the Ir region is not yet clear. One is, however, tempted to speculate that the antigens might be identical to those postulated by Katz and his co-workers[10] to explain the failure of T–B-cell cooperation across an Ir-region difference.

REFERENCES

1. Klein J, Shreffler DC: Transplant Rev 6:3, 1971
2. Shreffler DC, Owen RD: Genetics 48:9, 1963
3. Passmore HC, Shreffler DC: Biochem Genet 4:351, 1970
4. Benacerraf B, McDevitt HO: Science 175:273, 1972
5. McDevitt HO, Sela M: J Exp Med 122:517, 1965
6. Lieberman R, Paul WE, Humphrey W, Jr, Stimpfling JH: J Exp Med 136:1231, 1972
7. Lilly F, Pincus T: Advan Cancer Res 17:231, 1973
8. Bach FH, Widmer MB, Bach ML, et al: J Exp Med 136: 1430, 1972
9. Klein J, Park J: J Exp Med 137:1213, 1973
10. Katz DH, Hamaoka T, Dorf ME, Benacerraf B: Proc Natl Acad Sci 70:2624, 1973
11. Hauptfeld V, Klein D, Klein J: Science 181:167, 1973
12. Götze D, Reisfeld RA, Klein J: J Exp Med 138: 1003, 1973

Serologic Detection of Lymphocyte Cell-Surface Antigens Controlled by the Ir Region of the H-2 Gene Complex

By C. S. David, J. A. Frelinger, and D. C. Shreffler

ON THE hypothesis that the Ir region of the H-2 gene complex may control cell-surface structures which are genetically variable and should therefore behave as alloantigens, an extensive series of immunizations with lymphoid cells has been undertaken, using various pairs of strains which are identical in H-2K and H-2D, but different in the Ir and/or Ss-Slp regions. Two examples of such pairs are diagrammed in Table 1. The small letters under each H-2 region indicate the standard haplotype, H-2^{b}, H-2^{d}, H-2^{k}, H-2^{s}, from which that region derived. Note that three different haplotype sources are represented in some cases, because these particular recombinant haplotypes are the results of two or more successive crossover steps.

As a first step in the analysis of these antisera, they were tested for cytotoxic activity against lymph node cells, and, rather to our surprise, in three of the four combinations with the strains in Table 1 cytotoxic antibodies were detected. These three antisera [A.TH anti-A.TL; A.TL anti-A.TH; B10.A(4R) anti-B10.A(2R)] have been analyzed with relatively consistent results.[1-3] The antigens are most readily detectable by the cytotoxic test on lymph node cells, and are therefore referred to as the Lna (lymph node antigen) system. The Lna antigens are also readily detectable on splenic lymphocytes. They are expressed on peripheral blood lymphocytes and thymocytes, but less strongly. The gene(s) controlling these antigens have been localized to the Ir region by analyses of the same H-2 recombinants used to map the immune responses.[1-3] The cytotoxic titers of the A.TH anti-A.TL and A.TL anti-A.TH antisera are very high, more than 2000 in the ^{51}Cr-release test and up to 100,000 in the microcytotoxic dye exclusion test.[1,2] Only 35%–70% of lymph node cells are killed by these antisera. The 4R anti-2R serum has a titer of 640 and kills 40%–50% of lymph node cells.[2] At least two, more or less antithetical, sets of antigens have been defined by the A.TH anti-A.TL and A.TL anti-A.TH sera, one determined by the Ir region of the H-2^{k} haplotype, the other by the Ir region of the H-2^{s} haplotype. The controlling genes are denoted Lna^{k} and Lna^{s}.[1,2] Antibodies directed against the Ir-IgG region of the H-2^{d} haplotype have been identified in the B10.A(4R) anti-B10.A(2R) serum.[3] This observation suggests that the H-2^{d}/H-2^{k} crossover which gave rise to the H-2^{a} haplotype may have occurred within the Ir-IgG region, such that a segment of this region is of H-2^{d} origin (Table 1).

At high dilutions, the A.TH anti-A.TL and A.TL anti-A.TH sera appear to react specifically with Thy-1(θ)-positive lymphocytes (i.e., T cells) (Frelinger et al., unpublished). However, at lower antiserum dilutions, reactions with both T and B lymphocytes are observed.

Anti-Lna antibodies have also been detected in many anti-H-2 reagents, produced in strain combinations differing in the Ir region as well as H-2K and/or H-2D.[4] In general, the titers of anti-Lna antibodies in these antisera are lower than those in A.TH anti-A.TL and A.TL anti-A.TH.

Most of the anti-Lna sera cross-react with H-2 haplotypes other than those used for immunization. For example, A.TH anti-A.TL is an anti-Lna^{k} but also reacts with

From the Department of Human Genetics, University of Michigan, Ann Arbor, Mich.

Supported by USPHS program project grant GM15419 and USPHS career development award K3-HL 24980.

© 1973 by Grune & Stratton, Inc.

Table 1. Composition of the H-2 Complex in Four Intra-H-2 Recombinants.

Strain	Haplotype	H-2 Region					
		H-2K	Ir-1	Ir-IgG	Ss-Slp	H-2D	Tla
A.TL	$H\text{-}2^{tl}$	s	k	k	k	d	d
A.TH	$H\text{-}2^{th}$	s	s	s	s	d	a
B10.A(2R)	$H\text{-}2^{h\text{-}2Sg}$	k	k	d	d	b	b
B10.A(4R)	$H\text{-}2^{h\text{-}3Sg}$	k	k	b	b	b	b

cells of types $H\text{-}2^b$, $H\text{-}2^d$, $H\text{-}2^f$, and $H\text{-}2^q$. These cross-reactive types fail to completely absorb reactivity for A.TL cells, however.[1,2] Likewise, B10.A(4R) which has the Ir-1 sub-region of $H\text{-}2^k$ but the Ir-IgG sub-region of $H\text{-}2^b$, only partially absorbs for A.TL cells, carrying the entire Ir region of $H\text{-}2^k$.[3] These results suggest that the anti-Lna sera are complex, containing multiple antibody specificities which can be fractionated and subdivided by various kinds of approaches. Thus far, at least six different Lna specificities can be identified by such approaches.[4]

It is emphasized that the antigens being detected are not classical H-2 antigens. They are distinct in haplotype distributions from any specificities previously described, they are distinct in tissue distribution—being absent from nonlymphoid tissues and weak on certain lymphoid tissues—and they are present on only a fraction of lymphoid cells—no more than 70% of lymph node cells.[1-4] There is little question that they are new specificities. They have not been detected previously with anti-H-2 sera because the anti-H-2 sera always contained anti-H-2K or anti-H-2D antibodies which obscured the anti-Lna activities. Furthermore, most anti-Lna sera kill 50% or less of lymph node cells and such reactions were often dismissed previously as spurious or nonspecific. The relationship of these antigens to Ir and MLR gene products is not yet clear, but is under investigation. Obviously, these antisera have great potential value for the genetic resolution of the Ir/MLR chromosome region, for the assay, isolation, and characterization of the Lna antigens (which may be Ir- or MLR-gene products), and for the probing of Ir and MLR gene functions.

Note added in proof: An Ir-associated antigen similar to the ones described in this paper has recently been reported.[5]

REFERENCES

1. David CS, Shreffler DC, Frelinger JA: Genetics 74:s58, 1973
2. David CS, Shreffler DC, Frelinger JA: Proc Natl Acad Sci 70:2509, 1973
3. David CS, Frelinger JA, Shreffler DC: Transplantation (in press)
4. David CS, Shreffler DC: Transplantation (in press)
5. Hauptfeld et al: Science 181:167, 1973

Atypical Patterns of Inheritance of the Serologically Detectable (SD) Products of the HL-A Complex in Human Developmental Anomalies

By F. T. Rapaport*, R. Bachvaroff, J. M. Converse, A. P. Raisbeck, J. H. Ayvazian, M. Segall, and F. H. Bach

THE implication of cell surface structure as an important factor in morphogenesis[1] has raised the possibility that the normal progression of ontogeny may be conditioned by the particular cell surface membrane characteristics inherited by the human conceptus. The particularly high density of products of the major histocompatibility complex in man (HL-A) at the cell surface[2] suggested that the inheritance of such products might be worthy of study in family units where one or more members was afflicted with a developmental anomaly. The availability at the Institute of Reconstructive Plastic Surgery of a large patient population with a variety of congenital craniofacial anomalies, including cleft-lip and/or cleft-palate deformities, and of their families, provided a valuable opportunity for the institution of systematic genetic studies of the segregation of currently detectable products of the HL-A complex, and a comparison of the results with those obtained in this laboratory and elsewhere on the segregation of serologically detectable (SD) products of HL-A loci in normal families. Preliminary studies[3] have detected certain atypical patterns of inheritance of HL-A SD alleles in family units with developmental anomalies. The present report extends and confirms these data in greater detail and discusses some of the possible biological implications of the observed results.

MATERIALS AND METHOD

Thirty-six families, including 72 parents and 112 offspring, with 37 patients with cleft-lip/cleft-palate syndromes and 75 developmentally normal siblings were the subjects of this study. Each individual underwent serological HL-A testing in duplicate by two different techniques—the microlymphocytotoxicity test of Terasaki and McClelland,[4] as modified by Dausset et al.,[5] and the method of Kissmeyer-Nielsen et al.;[6] HL-A SD antigens were also tested by the platelet complement fixation test of Colombani and his associates.[7] A standard battery of HL-A typing antisera obtained from Professor Jean Dausset of the University of Paris, the U. S. National Institutes of Health Serum Bank, Professors Kissmeyer-Nielsen and J. J. van Rood, and Dr. Gunnar Nymand was used for serological testing. These antisera had the capability to detect the following HL-A SD antigenic products: (a) first (LA) locus: HL-A1, 2, 3, 9′, 9″, 10′, 10″, 11, W19.6, 28, 29, 30, 31, 32, and FE55/10; (b) second (Four) locus: HL-A5, 7, 8, 12, 13, W5, 10, 14, 15, 16, 17, 18, 21, 22, 27, MK (Da 34), and TYT.[8]

RESULTS

Table 1 summarizes the atypical patterns of inheritance of HL-A SD alleles observed in seven of 36 families with developmental anomalies. These families included 19 offspring, of whom seven were patients and 12 were normal siblings. There were eight instances of atypical HL-A SD allele inheritance in these families, including one family

---

*Irma T. Hirschl Career Scientist Award.

From the Department of Surgery and the Center for Craniofacial Anomalies, Institute of Reconstructive Plastic Surgery, New York University Medical Center, New York, N.Y.; the Research Service, Manhattan Veterans Administration Hospital, New York, N.Y.; and the Departments of Medical Genetics and Surgery, University of Wisconsin Center for the Health Sciences, Madison, Wisc.

This is paper No. 1695 from the Laboratory of Genetics, University of Wisconsin, Madison, Wisc.

Supported by grants from the John A. Hartford Foundation, the Billy Rose Foundation, the Irwin Strasburger Memorial Medical Foundation; National Foundation–March of Dimes grant CRBS 246; NIH grants AI-08439 and GM-15422; and ONR grant M000-67-A-128-0003.

M.S. is an NIH Trainee (grant GM-00398).

© 1973 by Grune & Stratton, Inc.

Table 1. Atypical Patterns of Inheritance of the HL-A SD Antigens in Families With Developmental Anomalies Observed in 7 of 36 Families Studied

	HL-A Haplotypes of:			Normal Siblings of Patient—HL-A Haplotypes		
Family	Father	Mother	Patient	1	2	3
CRU	(a) 1,W10 (b) 9,5	(c) 9,X (d) W19″,W17	(a) 1,W10 (d) W19′,W17	(a) 1,W10 (d) W19″,W17	(b) 9,5 (d) W19″,?†	
DOB	(a) 1,X (b) 2,X	(c) 1,8 (d) 2,7	(b) 2,X (d) 2,7	(a) 1,X (d) 2,7	(a) 1,X (d) 2,?*	
PEN	(a) 3,7 (b) X,W15	(c) 2,X (d) X,12	(a) 3,?* (c) 2,X	(a) 3,?* (c) 2,X		
WAL	(a) 3,7 (b) 10,X	(c) 2,W21 (d) 11,X	(b) 10,X (c) 2,W21	(b) 10,X (c) 2,?†		
GEN	(a) X,W14 (b) X,X	(c) 1,5 (d) 3,7	(b) X,X (d) 3,7	(a) X,W14 (c) 1,5	(a) X,W14 (c) 1,5, + 3*	
RIC	(a) 2,5 (b) 9,W21	(c) 2,W21 (d) 9,5	(a) 2,5 (c) 2,W21	(b) 9,W21 (c) 2,W21 + 5*		
SUL	(a) W29,12 (b) W28,8	(c) X,W5 (d) W28,W14	(a) W29,12 (c) X,W5 + *W14**	(b) W28,8 (d) W28,W14	(b) W28,8 (d) W28,W14	(b) W28,8 (c) X,W5

(a), first paternal haplotype; (b), second paternal haplotype; (c), first maternal haplotype; (d), second maternal haplotype.

HL-A antigens listed by number in accordance with WHO nomenclature and with a prefix W for other specificities accepted at the 1972 Evian Histocompatibility Workshop.

*Instances of gain or loss of a parental antigen.

†Instances that could be alternatively interpreted as recombinational events.

in which two siblings were involved. In three cases, the siblings gave evidence of gain of an HL-A SD antigen; in five other instances, there was a loss of a parental antigen that should normally have been transmitted to that particular sibling. Of the eight cases, only two involved a child with a developmental abnormality; in every other instance, a sibling who appeared to be developmentally normal gave evidence of an HL-A SD antigen gain or loss. In every case of antigen gain, the extra antigen was one determined by one of the transmitted parental haplotypes. The possible mechanisms involved in these instances of HL-A SD antigen gain or loss are illustrated in Figs. 1 and 2, which are reproduced from our initial report.[3] In Fig. 1, three siblings (B, C, and D) showed a normal pattern of inheritance of the HL-A SD antigens, i.e., each sibling inherited one haplotype from each parent (siblings B and C are HL-A SD identical). One sibling, however (sibling A), who was the patient with the cleft-lip/cleft-palate defect, inherited normal haplotype (*a*) from his father, but inherited both antigens associated with the maternal (*c*) haplotype, as well as antigen W14, associated with the mother's second haplotype (*d*).

An example of antigen loss is shown in Fig. 2. A normal en bloc transmission of the HL-A SD alleles (*a, d*) occurred in siblings A and B. Sibling C, however, inherited either haplotype (*a*) from the father and (*d*) from the mother, with a loss of antigen HL-A7, or haplotype (*b*) from the father and (*c*) from the mother, with a loss of antigen HL-A8. Various patterns of inheritance, including recombinational events, might be invoked in attempts to explain these results. In each case, however, loss of a maternal second (Four) HL-A SD locus antigen is involved. It must be noted, however, that not all the HL-A SD antigens

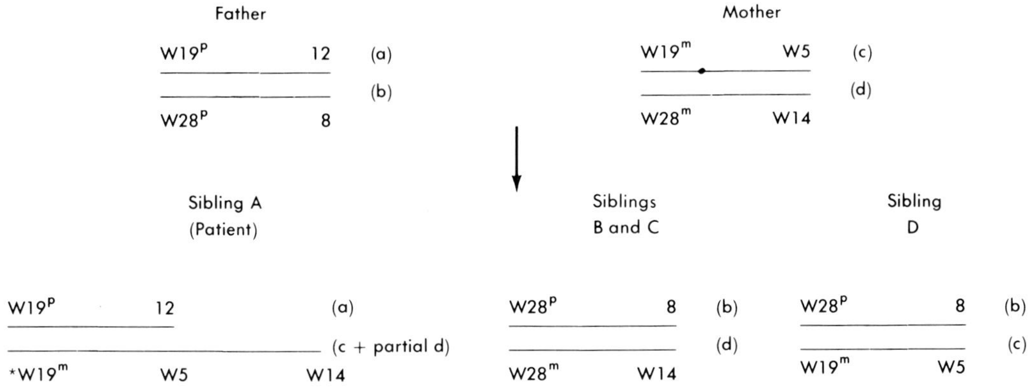

Fig. 1. The two horizontal bars for each individual represent the two HL-A haplotypes. The LA locus antigens are designated to the left of those which are products of the Four locus. Numbers refer to officially named HL-A antigens; numbers preceded by "W" are official Workshop designations.[14] X designates that no antigen was recognized with the battery of sera available (88 antisera capable of detecting 29 different HL-A and "W" antigens). a, first paternal HL-A SD haplotype; b, second paternal HL-A SD haplotype; c, first maternal HL-A SD haplotype; d, second maternal HL-A SD haplotype; p, HL-A SD antigen of paternal origin; m, HL-A SD antigen of maternal origin; * means see text.

could be defined in two other cases of apparent antigen loss (Table 1). In these cases, antigen losses might also be attributable to classical genetic recombinational events.

DISCUSSION

It is generally agreed that the biological role of the major histocompatibility complex (MHC) in man (HL-A) may exceed by far its influence upon the tempo and intensity of allograft rejection, with particular reference to host susceptibility to cancer and a variety of other disease states.[9] The high density of the genetically determined products of the HL-A complex on the cell surface,[2] taken together with the generally accepted importance of cell-to-cell surface interaction in morphogenesis,[1] has raised the possibility that the immunogenetics of the HL-A complex might be deserving of

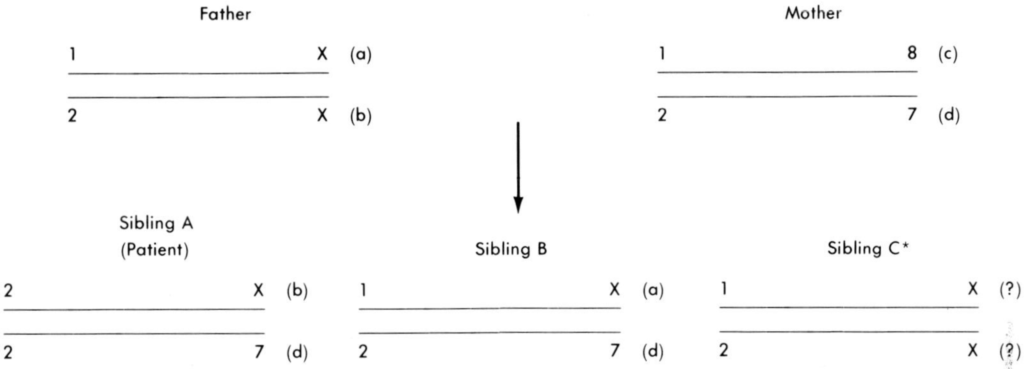

Fig. 2. The two horizontal bars for each individual represent the two HL-A haplotypes. The LA locus antigens are designated to the left of those which are products of the Four locus. Numbers refer to officially named HL-A antigens; numbers preceded by "W" are official Workshop designations.[14] X designates that no antigen was recognized with the battery of sera available (88 antisera capable of detecting 29 different HL-A and "W" antigens). a, first paternal HL-A SD haplotype; b, second paternal HL-A SD haplotype; c, first maternal HL-A SD haplotype; d, second maternal HL-A SD haplotype; p, HL-A SD antigen of paternal origin; m, HL-A SD antigen of maternal origin; * means see text.

further examination in families with developmental malformations. The report by Terasaki et al.[10] of a higher incidence of congenital malformations in offspring of mothers whose sera contained HL-A antibodies appeared to be of possible relevance.

The HL-A complex includes two closely linked loci (the first or LA and the second or Four locus), whose alleles determine antigens (SD) which are amenable to detection by serological techniques. The chromosomal segment bearing these two SD loci is termed a haplotype, and its products have been shown to be inherited en bloc from each parent, so that no human individual bears more than four SD antigens on his or her cell surfaces under normal conditions. Extensive family studies performed in expert laboratories throughout the world[11-15] have shown clear patterns of inheritance of the SD antigens from parents to their offspring, whereby each child normally receives one haplotype from each parent, and both SD antigens associated with an individual parental haplotype are detectable in the child. The only reported exceptions to this normal pattern of inheritance has been detected in cases where a classical genetic cross-over event has taken place between the two SD loci in one of the parents. In such cases, the offspring inherits two antigens from each parent, but the two antigens inherited from one of the parents are determined by one SD allele from one haplotype of that particular parent, and one SD allele from the other haplotype of that same parent. Such cross-overs have an approximate incidence of 1%, and constitute instances of classical genetic recombination. Based upon the incidence of such recombinations in normal families, a distance of 0.8 to 1.0 recombinational units has been calculated to exist between the two SD loci.[16] Although the present study is limited to the inheritance of products of the HL-A SD alleles, it must be noted that other genetic loci have been detected within the human MHC. These include two probable LD loci, which have been implicated in the recognition phase of allograft responses, and are detectable by the mixed leucocyte culture (MLC) test.[17,18]

Progress in the definition of genetic components of the human MHC has provided convincing evidence of great similarities between the HL-A complex and the corresponding H-2 complex located on the ninth linkage group in the mouse.[17,19] The results of the present study, which indicate a significant association between atypical inheritance of HL-A SD alleles in family units in which one or more children has a developmental anomaly, may be of particular interest in this regard. Indeed, these results raise the possibility that the analogy between the chromosomes carrying the major histocompatibility complex (MHC) in man and in the mouse may extend beyond this genetic region. The murine MHC is in relatively close linkage (15 recombinational units) with a gene complex, the T region, which is associated with developmental anomalies, including tail abnormalities and a wide variety of craniofacial malformations.[20] Alleles of this complex region have also been associated with atypical patterns of inheritance of other closely linked portions of the same chromosome.[21] The possibility that the human chromosome bearing the HL-A complex may also contain genetic determinants similar to the murine T complex, and that certain alleles of this region might result in the abnormal inheritance of components of linked complexes, such as HL-A, for example, may therefore be deserving of further investigation.

The atypical inheritance of HL-A SD antigens observed in families with developmental anomalies included instances of both antigen gains and antigen losses. An unequal cross-over event, whereby the resulting chromosomes might carry either one or three antigens (Figs. 1 and 2) may provide a plausible genetic explanation for these observations. What is of particular relevance, however, is the fact that this pattern of HL-A SD antigen inheritance has not been reported thus far in any of the extensive similar studies performed in developmentally normal family units,[11-15] while it has occurred with such unexpected frequency in families with developmental anomalies. An additional observation of potential interest is that most of the atypical patterns of HL-A SD antigen inheritance detected in this study occurred in children who did not have a cleft-lip/cleft-palate syndrome. This result may provide further support to the proposed analogies between the murine ninth linkage group and the corresponding (as yet undetected) chromosome bearing the human HL-A complex. Certain *t* alleles in the mouse have been associated with intrauterine death.[20,22,23] Should the hypothesized analogy with the T gene complex be valid, a portion of the human offspring who carried certain presumed T-locus gene analogs, as well as atypical patterns of inheritance of the closely linked HL-A complex may have died in utero. In this regard, the results of this study may also be of potential interest in studies of intrauterine deaths in the human species.

The preliminary nature of the reported results must be emphasized. Although the HL-A SD determinations reported in each of the families studied have been repeated on several different occasions, the results require confirmation in a sufficiently large group of families with developmental anomalies before they can merit true validity. At this time, however, the observations may be of usefulness as a model for the type of immunogenetic approach which may provide new data on the biological role of cell surface components determined by the HL-A complex and of other systems which may be genetically linked with the human MHC. Studies in progress at this time would appear to militate against the possibility that the cases of "antigen gain" were a consequence of cross reactions between inherited parental antigens, or that the cases of "antigen loss" were due to cellular events inducing a cytotoxic-negative–absorption-positive behavior of the cells tested. Such studies also need to be confirmed and extended in a larger population before any definitive conclusions can be reached. It must be emphasized, however, that the serological studies described in this report suggest that additional insight is also needed with regard to the patterns of inheritance of other components of the HL-A complex in developmental anomalies, with particular regard to the LD loci.[17,18] Karyotype studies of families with developmental anomalies in which significant abnormalities in the inheritance of components of the HL-A complex have been observed are also urgently needed, and may lead to the identification of the human chromosome bearing the HL-A complex, as well as the hypothesized T complex analogy in man.

A final point that may be deserving of mention is that careful studies of the incidence of HL-A SD antigens, haplotypes, and genotypes in the present population, performed in collaboration with Dausset,[24] failed to show any differences between parents and siblings with cleft-lip/cleft-palate syndromes, normal siblings, and comparable groups of similar racial backgrounds with no developmental abnormalities. It was only when the patterns of inheritance of the HL-A SD antigens from parents to offspring in families with developmental anomalies were analyzed[3] that the atypical results described here became evident. This fact may be of relevance to the many extensive studies currently in progress on a worldwide basis on the role of HL-A antigens in a variety of different human diseases, which have recently been reviewed elegantly by Dausset.[9] Most of these investigations have concentrated on a search for associations between a disease and a particular HL-A SD antigen or phenotype. The approach presented here, which is currently being extended to other disease states, raises the intriguing possibility that studies of the intrafamilial pattern of inheritance of HL-A complex alleles in stricken family units might shed further light upon the suggested relationships between the MHC complex and human disease. The results also provide a possible explanation for the conflicting reports that have emanated thus far from different population studies of the same diseases.[9]

REFERENCES

1. Bennett D, Boyse EA, Old LJ: in Silvestri LG (ed): Cellular Interactions. Amsterdam, North-Holland, 1972, p 247

2. Kourilsky FM, Silvestre D, Néauporte-Sauté C, et al: Eur J Immunol 2:249, 1972

3. Rapaport FT, Bach FH: Transplant Proc 5:1139, 1973

4. Terasaki PI, McClelland JD: Nature 206:998, 1964

5. Dausset J, Rapaport FT, Ivanyi P, et al: in Balner H, Cleton FJ, Eernisse JG (eds): Histocompatibility Testing 1965. Copenhagen, Munksgaard, 1965, p. 63

6. Kissmeyer-Nielsen F, Svejgaard A, Hauge M: Nature 219:1116, 1968

7. Colombani J, Colombani M, Benajam A, et al: in Curtoni ES, Mattiuz PL, Tosi RM (eds): Histocompatibility Testing 1967, Copenhagen, Munksgaard, 1967, p 413

8. Dausset J (ed): Histocompatibility Testing 1972. Copenhagen, Munksgaard, 1973.

9. Dausset J: in Schwartz RS (ed): Progress In Clinical Immunology. New York, Grune and Stratton, 1972, p 183

10. Terasaki PI, Mickey MR, Yamazaki JN, et al: Transplantation 9:538, 1970

11. Dausset J, Ivanyi P, Ivanyi D: in Amos DB, van Rood JJ (eds): Histocompatibility Testing 1965. Copenhagen, Munksgaard, 1965, p 51

12. van Rood JJ, van Leeuwen A, Schippers AJM, et al: in Amos DB, van Rood JJ (eds): Histocompatibility Testing 1965. Copenhagen, Munksgaard, 1965, p 37

13. Bach FH, Amos DB: Science 156:1506, 1967

14. Curtoni ES, Mattiuz PL, Tosi R (eds): Histocompatibility Testing 1967. Copenhagen, Munksgaard, 1967

15. Dausset J, Colombani J, Legrand L, et al: Blood 591:35, 1970

16. Svejgaard A, Bratlie A, Hedin PJ, et al: Tissue Antigens, 1:81, 1971

17. Bach FH: Transplant Proc 5:23, 1973

18. Bach FH, Widmer MB, Bach ML, et al: J Exp Med 136:1430, 1972

19. Klein J: Transplant Proc 5:11, 1973

20. Bennett D, Badenhausen S, Dunn LC: J Morphol 105:105, 1959

21. Dunn LC, Bennett D, Beasley AB: Genetics 47:285, 1962

22. Bennett D: Nature, 181:1286, 1958

23. Dunn LC, Bennett D: Science 144:260, 1964

24. Dausset J: personal communication

Genetic Studies of Mixed Leukocyte Culture Reactivity in Human Developmental Anomalies

By F.T. Rapaport,* R. Bachvaroff, J.M. Converse, A.P. Raisbeck, J.H. Ayvazian, M. Segall, and F.H. Bach

THE mixed leukocyte culture test (MLC) of Bain, Vas, and Lowenstein[1] and Bach and Hirschhorn[2] is generally recognized as a useful in vitro expression of the recognition phase of the allograft reaction. It was not until 1968, however, that Amos and Bach[3] and subsequently Bach et al.[4] observed that MLC reactivity may be governed by a locus or loci closely linked to the serologically detectable (SD) loci of the HL-A complex, which is thus a component of the major histocompatibility complex (MHC) in man. The differences in the MHC resulting in lymphocyte activation in the MLC test, which are not yet amenable to definition by serological techniques, are now referred to as lymphocyte-defined (LD) loci. The observations of Amos, Ceppellini, and Bach have been focused and extended by Yunis and Amos,[5] Dupont, Nielsen, and Svejgaard,[6] Gatti, Meuwissen, Terasaki, and Good,[7] Lebrun et al.,[8] and Eijsvoogel et al.[9] Population studies have provided evidence of a linkage disequilibrium between the two HL-A SD loci and the principal LD locus or loci.[10-16] Family studies have also demonstrated the independence of the LD principal locus or loci, probably located outside but in close proximity to the second (Four) locus, from either of the two HL-A SD loci.[5,17,18]

The present report describes further genetic studies of the HL-A complex in families with human developmental anomalies. In view of earlier preliminary data suggestive of an atypical inheritance of HL-A SD alleles in such families,[19,20] it appeared of interest to investigate the same population on the basis of the MLC test. The results suggest that given LD alleles are not necessarily associated with particular SD alleles; individuals who do not share an HL-A SD haplotype may nevertheless share an LD allele as suggested by MLC reactivity between the parents and offspring.[21,27] Comments will also be made with regard to the apparent frequency of shared LD parental alleles in the family units under study.

*Irma T. Hirschl Career Scientist Award.

From the Department of Surgery and the Center for Craniofacial Anomalies, Institute of Reconstructive Plastic Surgery, New York University Medical Center, New York, N.Y.; the Research Service, Manhattan Veterans Administration Hospital, New York, N.Y.; and the Department of Medical Genetics and Surgery, University of Wisconsin, Center for the Health Sciences, Madison, Wisc.

This is paper No. 1693 from the Laboratory of Genetics, University of Wisconsin, Madison, Wisc.

Supported by grants from the John A. Hartford Foundation, the Billy Rose Foundation, the Irwin Strasburger Memorial Medical Foundation; National Foundation–March of Dines grant CRBS 246; NIH grants AI-08439 and GM-15422; and ONR grant M000-67-A-128-0003.

M.S. is an NIH Trainee (grant GM-00398).

© *1973 by Grune & Stratton, Inc.*

MATERIALS AND METHOD

The subjects of this report are patients under treatment for correction of developmental anomalies (cleft-lip/cleft-palate syndromes) at the Center for Craniofacial Anomalies at the Institute of Reconstructive Plastic Surgery at New York University, as well as their parents and normal unaffected siblings. A total of 21 family units (42 parents and 65 offspring, including 21 patients and 44 normal siblings) was studied.

The serologic techniques used for the detection of the HL-A SD antigens in each individual tested have been described in detail in earlier reports.[19,20] Mixed leucocyte culture tests were performed by the method of Hartzman et al.[28] Briefly, lymphocytes were separated from whole blood by the method of Boyum[23] and were washed three times in balanced salt solution (BSS). One aliquot of cells was resuspended in BSS and was treated with 25 μg/ml of mitomycin

C (Nutritional Biochemicals, Cleveland, Ohio) and was then incubated at 37°C for 30 min. The mitomycin-treated cells were washed three times in BSS and were resuspended in Medium 199 supplemented with 20 mM/ml of L-glutamine, 100 IU/ml of penicillin, 5 μg/ml of streptomycin, and 20% pooled human serum obtained from 30 healthy AB human donors. The culture media were obtained from Grand Island Biological Co., Grand Island, N.Y. The cells were plated on Falcon plastic trays, with each well containing 1×10^5 normal untreated (responding) cells and 3×10^5 mitomycin-treated (stimulating) cells, in a volume of 0.2 ml of culture medium.

The prepared Falcon plastic trays were incubated at 37°C for 5 days in 5% CO_2-balanced air. On the fifth day, 1 μCi of thymidine methyl (^3H 1.9 Ci/mM) (Schwartz Mann, Orangeburg, N.Y.) was added to each culture well. All cultures were precipitated 16 hr later using an automated multiple-sample harvester.[24] The radioactivity of each sample was measured in a scintillation spectrometer. The degree of stimulation of responding cells from each individual, when tested against stimulating cells obtained from every other member of his family, was measured in terms of the rate of uptake of ^3H thymidine in counts per minute. Each test was performed in quadruplicate, and each family was studied at least twice at different time intervals. In all important donor–recipient situations, the one-way MLC test was supplemented by simultaneous performance of two-way MLC tests without use of mitomycin C, by the standard technique of Bach and Hirschhorn[2] using thymidine incorporation as an assay.

RESULTS

Fifteen of the 21 families showed the usual type of MLC reactivity seen within families. Recombinational events were not observed for either HL-A SD or LD alleles. Six families were particularly informative, however. Three of these families have been studied repeatedly and are included in this report. Similar preliminary results have been obtained in the three additional families. The three families reported here include six parents (with an HL-A SD- and LD-identical sister of the father in one family, Sull) and 15 offspring, including three children with cleft-lip/cleft-palate syndromes. One of the latter (Donald, in family Sull) also showed evidence of gain of an extra maternal SD antigen.[19,20] The results obtained in these three families are presented in detail in this report.

Family Alm

The specific data obtained in this family, expressed as incorporation of ^3H thymidine in the one-way and two-way MLC tests, are listed in Table I. As noted in Fig. 1, this family includes the father (HL-A SD haplotype *A* = HL-A 3, 7; HL-A SD haplotype *B* = HL-A 2, W5), the mother (HL-A SD haplotype *C* = HL-A1, W21; HL-A SD haplotype *D* = W 19′, HL-A5), two HL-A SD-identical siblings, Rita and Nelly (*B, D*), and four other HL-A SD-identical siblings, Lydia, Louis, Leo, and Nancy (*A, C*). The parents were reciprocally MLC-reactive; Rita and Nelly (*B, D*) were reciprocally MLC-negative, as were Lydia, Louis, Leo, and Nancy (*A, C*). Both Rita and Nelly were reciprocally MLC reactive with all four of the second group of HL-A SD-identical (*A, C*) siblings, Lydia, Louis, Leo, and Nancy.

It is of particular interest, however, that both Rita and Nelly (*B, D*) were reciprocally MLC-reactive with maternal cells (*C, D*) but were reciprocally MLC-nonreactive with paternal cells (*A, B*), while all four siblings bearing parental haplotypes *A, C* (Lydia, Louis, Leo, Nancy) were reciprocally MLC-reactive with the father (*A, B*) but reciprocally MLC-negative with maternal cells (*C, D*). If the parental LD locus or loci, depicted for pictorial purposes as quadrangles (Fig. 1) outside of the second HL-A SD locus, were to determine four different alleles (LD1, 2, 3, 4), the results of the MLC tests described above would be consistent with the hypothesis that HL-A LD alleles 1 and 4 are identical, i.e., that the two unrelated subjects in question (father and mother) share an LD allele, although they are both heterozygous for and do not share any HL-A SD haplotypes. It is of further interest that none of the offspring is HL-A SD-homozygous or compatible with either parent, with regard to either the first or the second HL-A SD loci.

Table 1. Mixed Leukocyte Culture (MLC) Studies in Family Alm

Donor of Reacting Cells	Code Letter	HL-A Genotype†	One-Way MLC Reactions*								Two-Way MLC Reactions*						
			Am	Bm	Cm	Dm	Em	Fm	Gm	Hm	B	C	D	E	F	G	H
Father	A	(a) 3, 7 (b) 2, W5	124	3,858	3,560	3,283	4,976	3,912	176	232	3,890	3,605	3,400	6,224	3,991	298	303
Mother	B	(c) 1, W21 (d) W19′, 5	5,543	310	441	399	328	256	7,012	6,164	—	270	277	324	271	4,436	3,558
Lydia	C	(a) 3, 7 (c) 1, W21	5,558	264	166	148	184	182	7,085	6,873	—	—	422	170	321	4,166	4,525
Louis	D	(a) 3, 7 (c) 1, W21	7,556	389	157	182	104	228	10,922	10,554	—	—	—	212	178	4,033	4,921
Leo	E	(a) 3, 7 (c) 1, W21	8,284	360	167	243	170	172	14,753	16,881	—	—	—	—	231	5,159	3,984
Nancy	F	(a) 3, 7 (c) 1, W21	5,525	350	234	297	251	141	8,422	7,530	—	—	—	—	—	5,371	4,434
Rita	G	(b) 2, W5 (d) W19′, 5	256	5,151	4,460	5,203	5,086	3,567	210	297	—	—	—	—	—	—	268
Nelly	H	(b) 2, W5 (d) W19′, 5	131	6,502	7,194	6,213	4,627	9,097	202	109	—	—	—	—	—	—	—

Subjects C, D, E, F, G, H are children of parents A and B.

*MLC reactions are expressed as equal to the incorporation of ^{3}H thymidine (counts/min). Each value represents the average c.p.m. obtained from quadruple cultures of the same cell–antigen combination.

†a, first paternal HL-A haplotype, b, second paternal HL-A haplotype; c, first maternal HL-A haplotype; d, second maternal HL-A haplotype.

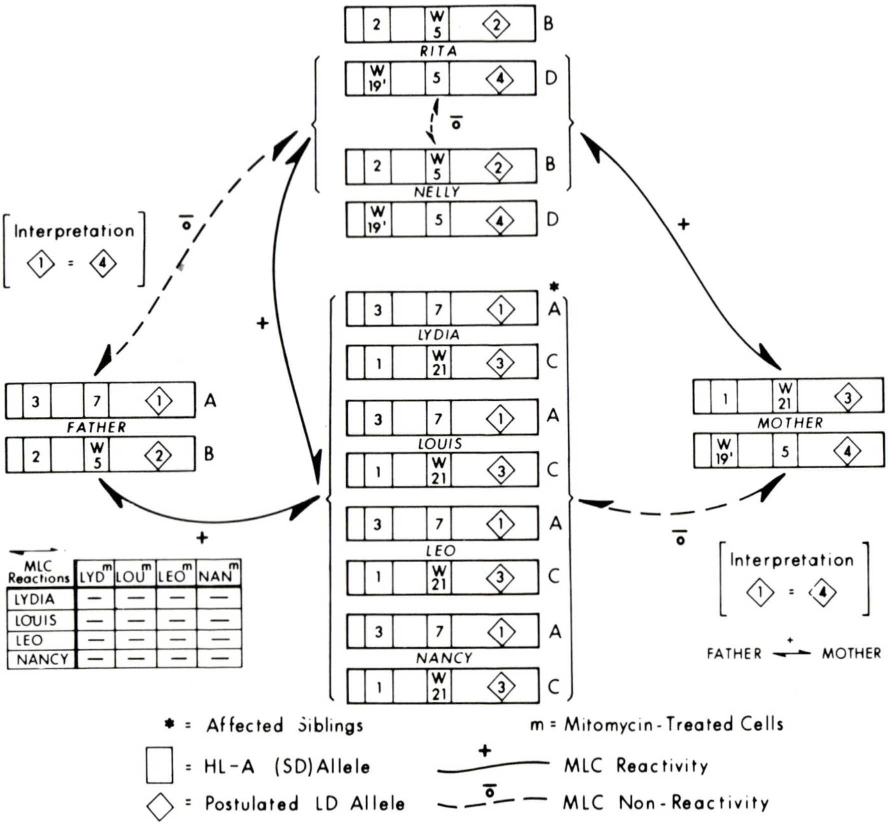

Fig. 1. Family Alm: cleft lip and palate.

Family Sull

The numerical results of one-way and two-way MLC tests in this family are listed in Table 2. As shown in Fig. 2, this family includes the father (HL-A SD haplotype *A* = W 19′, HL-A 12; HL-A SD haplotype *B* = W28, HL-A8), and HL-A identical sister of the father (*A*, *B*), the mother (HL-A SD haplotype *C* = W19″, W5; HL-A SD haplotype *D* = W28, W14), two HL-A SD-identical siblings, James and Charles (*B*, *D*), and two other siblings Donald (*A*, *C* + W14) and Kevin (*B*, *C*).

The parents were reciprocally MLC-reactive; James and Charles (*B*, *D*) were reciprocally nonreactive but both were reciprocally MLC-stimulatory with cells from Donald (*A*, *C* + W14) and Kevin (*B*, *C*). The two latter siblings were also reciprocally MLC-reactive. It is of interest, however, that both James and Charles (*B*, *D*) were reciprocally MLC nonstimulatory with paternal cells (*A*, *B*) or with cells obtained from the father's HL-A-identical sister (the latter was also reciprocally nonreactive with the father's cells). In contrast, Donald (*A*, *C* + W14) was reciprocally nonreactive with maternal cells (*C*, *D*) but was mutually reactive with cells obtained from his father (*A*, *B*) or fro.n the father's sister (*A*, *B*). The fourth sibling, Kevin (*B*, *C*) was reciprocally reactive with cells obtained from father (*A*, *B*), mother (*C*, *D*), and the father's sister (*A*, *B*).

The results obtained in this family provide a further illustration of the points raised with regard to the alleles of the LD locus or loci in family Alm and is consistent with the possibility that the HL-A LD alleles 1 and 4 present on paternal haplo-

Table 2. Mixed Leukocyte Culture (MLC) Studies in Family Sull

Donor of Reacting Cells	Code Letter	HL-A Genotypes†	One-Way MLC Reactions*							Two-Way MLC Reactions*					
			Am	Bm	Cm	Dm	Em	Fm	Gm	B	C	D	E	F	G
Father	A	(a) W19^{1}, 12 (b) W28, 8	1,182	829	15,081	1,120	849	25,052	25,090	389	7,055	640	436	3,359	4,833
Father's sister	B	(a) W19^{1}, 12 (b) W28, 8	628	751	13,432	911	873	23,365	19,653	—	8,128	712	612	4,935	5,167
Mother	C	(c) W19^{11}, W5 (d) W28, W14	9,484	7,321	939	6,132	6,132	1,121	3,380	—	—	5,953	4,930	570	3,197
James	D	(b) W28, 8 (d) W28, W14	900	812	11,155	872	468	25,522	16,108	—	—	—	440	6,812	8,038
Charles	E	(b) W28, 8 (d) W28, W14	816	425	11,378	481	1,062	28,846	16,124	—	—	—	—	6,939	10,391
Donald	F	(a) W19^{1}, 12 (b) W19^{11}, W5	7,985	7,128	657	14,134	14,098	497	8,721	—	—	—	—	—	3,052
Kevin	G	(b) W28, 8 (c) W19^{11}, W5	10,861	9,378	5,460	12,605	11,452	15,421	565	—	—	—	—	—	—

Subjects D, E, F, G are children of parents A and C.

*MLC reactions are expressed as equal to the incorporation of ^{3}H thymidine (counts/min). Each value represents the average c.p.m. obtained from quadruple cultures of the same cell–antigen combination.

†a, first paternal HL-A haplotype; b, second paternal HL-A haplotype; c, first maternal HL-A haplotype; d, second maternal HL-A haplotype.

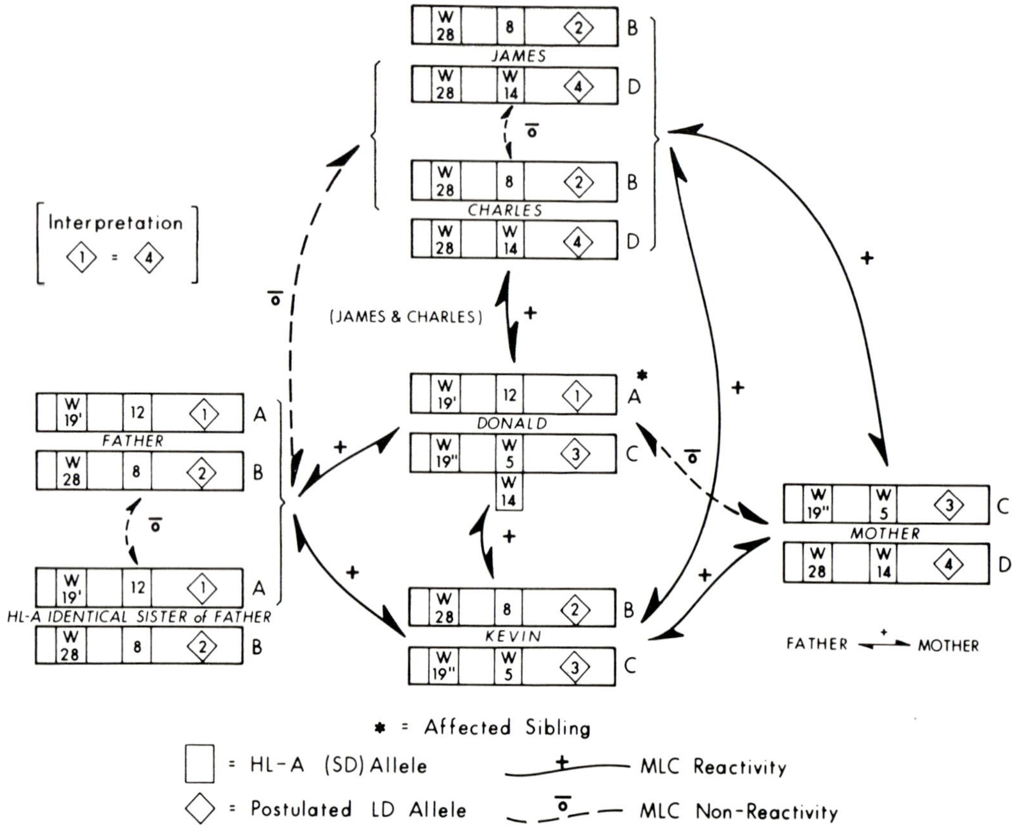

Fig. 2. Family Sull: cleft lip and palate.

type *A* and maternal haplotype *D* may be the same and that this family provides another example of sharing of LD alleles by the unrelated individuals, although they are heterozygous and do not share an HL-A SD haplotype.

Family Yos

The uptake of ^{3}H thymidine in one-way and two-way MLC tests in this family are outlined in Table 3. As illustrated in Fig. 3, this family includes the father (HL-A SD haplotype *A* = HL-A1, 8; HL-A SD haplotype *B* = HL-A2, W27), the mother (HL-A SD haplotype *C* = HL-A1, 8; HL-A SD haplotype *D* = HL-A3, 7), two HL-A SD-identical siblings, Chris and David (*B, C*), and three other offspring, Linda (*A, D*), Paul (*A, C*), and Lisa (*B, D*).

The parents were reciprocally MLC-stimulatory; Chris and David (*B, C*) were mutually nonstimulatory, but both were reciprocally reactive with cells from Linda (*A, D*), Paul (*A, C*), and Lisa (*B, D*). Chris and David were mutually nonreactive with paternal cells (*A, B*) but reciprocally stimulatory with maternal cells (*C, D*). Linda (*A, D*) was mutually reactive with paternal cells but nonreactive with maternal cells. Paul (*A, C*) was reactive to paternal cells as well as to maternal cells, but the father did not react in MLC tests against Paul's cells. Lisa (*B, D*) was mutually reactive against both paternal and maternal cells. Taken together, these data are consistent with the interpretation that father and mother in this family shared HL-A LD alleles 1 and 3, and the results provide further support for the interpretations offered for the data obtained in the first two families.

Table 3. Mixed Leukocyte Culture (MLC) Studies in Family Yos

Donor of Reacting Cells	Code Letter	HL-A Genotype†	One-Way MLC Reactions*							Two-Way MLC Reactions*					
			Am	Bm	Cm	Dm	Em	Fm	Gm	B	C	D	E	F	G
Father	A	(a) 1, 8 (b) 2, W27	178	5,864	644	266	178	4,274	4,424	2,948	168	152	146	1,210	1,371
Mother	B	(c) 1, 8 (d) 3, 7	4,972	374	4,210	6,732	5,604	226	3,864	—	1,636	3,212	2,763	114	2,121
Paul	C	(a) 1, 8 (c) 1, 8	1,970	6,634	156	3,444	3,364	4,222	9,378	—	—	428	534	535	2,173
Chris.	D	(b) 2, W27 (c) 1, 8	116	9,082	1,410	460	124	3,868	5,636	—	—	—	132	3,580	1,889
David	E	(b) 2, W27 (c) 1, 8	200	9,730	1,212	166	130	4,462	8,856	—	—	—	—	2,292	2,023
Linda	F	(a) 1, 8 (d) 3, 7	3,470	306	1,758	6,782	4,586	312	4,286	—	—	—	—	—	2,054
Lisa	G	(b) 2, W27 (d) 3, 7	2,912	3,632	5,950	3,988	3,354	1,756	168	—	—	—	—	—	—

Subjects C, D, E, F, G are children of parents A and B.

*MLC reactions are expressed as equal to the incorporation of ^{3}H thymidine (counts/min). Each value represents the average c.p.m. obtained from quadruple cultures of the same cell–antigen combination.

†a, first paternal HL-A haplotype; b, second paternal HL-A haplotype; c, first maternal HL-A haplotype; d, second maternal HL-A haplotype.

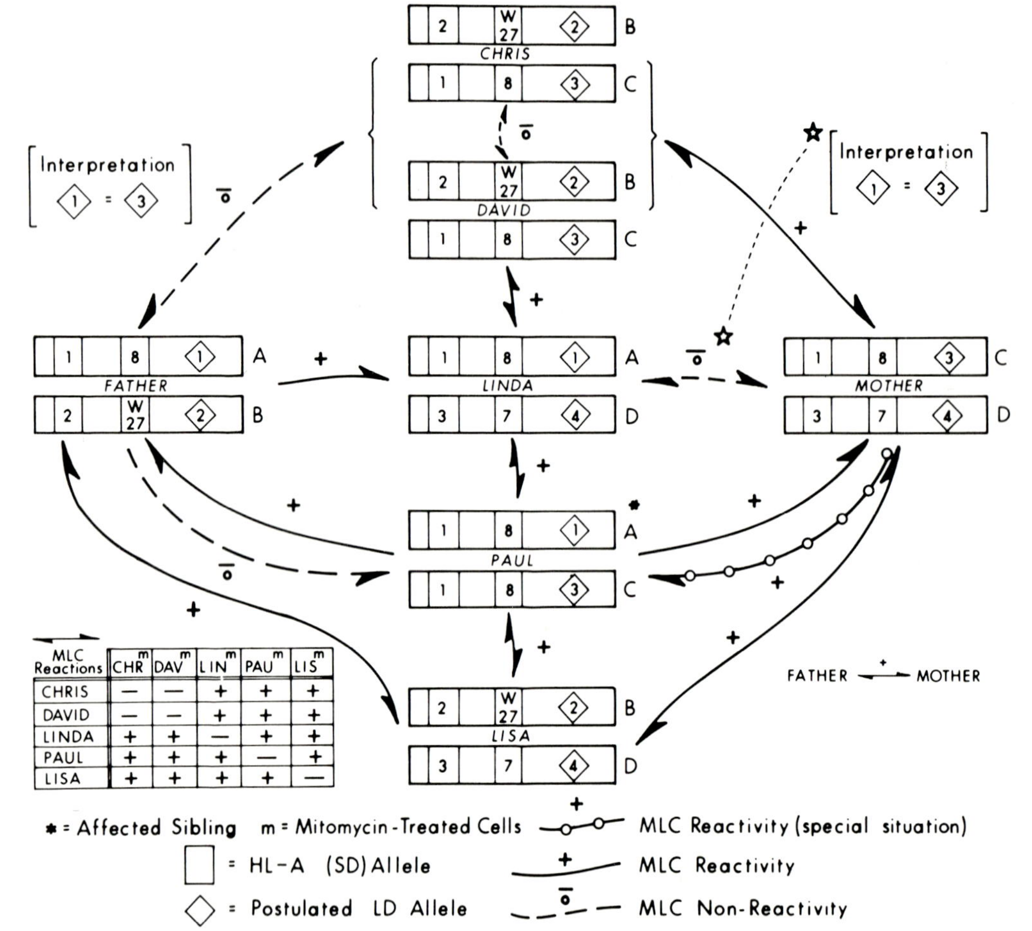

Fig. 3. Family Yos: cleft lip and palate.

In addition, however, it must be noted that Paul is reactive in MLC to both parents; that both the mother and Linda (her HL-A SD- and LD-identical offspring) give positive MLC reactions against Paul, who lacks any detectable HL-A SD or (presumably) LD factors against which Linda or her mother could react; that positive MLC reactions are also seen in a similar genetic situation when cells of Chris or David are stimulated by Paul; and that paternal cells, which also should not have been able to recognize any HL-A SD or LD differences in Paul according to this model, may have been stimulated by Paul's lymphocytes only very weakly. These additional results argue that the genetic control of LD factors may be more complex than involving only a single LD locus in the region depicted or that interactions depending on a variety of factors are taking place.[28] Primarily, these results should warn against simple interpretations of potentially highly complex situations.

DISCUSSION

The MLC family studies described in this report provide further evidence of the existence of an MHC LD locus or loci. The independence of the products of this locus or loci from the products of the SD alleles seen in this study confirms earlier elegant studies of this question from a number of other laboratories.[3-9,15-18] The main relevance of the results presented here to the immunogenetics of the LD components of the human MHC relates to the observation in multiple family units that MLC nonreactivity between parents and siblings can occur in family situations where the parents do not share any HL-A SD haplotypes and the offspring are heterozygous for the HL-A SD loci. In this regard, the results are in agreement with those reported by Dupont et al.,[24] although these authors considered their results as an example of abnormal mixed lymphocyte reactions in the family of a patient with severe immunodeficiency disease. Rather, the data presented in this report support the existence of multiple LD alleles, and of the possible sharing of such alleles by unrelated individuals, regardless of their HL-A SD status.

The studies of Pentycross,[27] van Rood and Eijsvoogel,[13] Koch et al.,[25] and Bach and his associates[15] suggest that the incidence of MLC nonreactivity between pairs of unrelated individuals who differ by HL-A SD antigens is extremely low. These observations, taken together with the findings of Dupont et al.[24] in a family unit afflicted with an immunodeficiency disease in which an X-linked recessive form and an autosomal recessive form occur,[26] raise the possibility that the findings reported here might be related to genetic factors involved in developmental anomalies. The three families described in detail in the present report, taken together with three additional families with preliminary evidence of similar findings, result in a possible incidence of 6 out of 21 pairs of unrelated parents who share a postulated LD allele in family units with developmental anomalies. It is obvious that this observation can only serve at present as a basis for further extensive population and family studies of the LD alleles in man and that data may eventually accumulate to demonstrate an actual limited polymorphism of the products of the LD locus or loci, with a similarly high incidence of shared LD alleles in unrelated parents of developmentally normal families where the parents do not share one or both HL-A SD haplotypes. In the meantime, however, the available evidence suggests that this question may be deserving of further intensive study, particularly in view of the observation of atypical patterns of inheritance of other components of the human major histocompatibility complex, the HL-A SD alleles, in human developmental anomalies.[19,20]

REFERENCES

1. Bain B, Vas MR, Lowenstein R: Blood 23:108, 1964
2. Bach FH, Hirschhorn K: Science 143:813, 1964
3. Amos DB, Bach FH: J Exp Med 128:623, 1968
4. Bach FH, Albertini RJ, Amos DB, et al: Transplant Proc 1:339, 1969
5. Yunis EJ, Amos DB: Proc Natl Acad Sci USA 68:3031, 1971
6. Dupont B, Nielsen LS, Svejgaard A: Lancet 2:1336, 1971
7. Gatti RA, Meuwissen HJ, Terasaki PI, et al: Tissue Antigens 1:239, 1971
8. Lebrun A, Sasportes M, Lebrun D, et al: C R Acad Sci (Paris) 273:2130, 1971
9. Eijsvoogel VP, Koning L, Groot-Kooy L de, et al: Transplant Proc 4:199, 1972
10. Segall M, Omodei-Zorini C, Bach FH, et al: Transplant Proc 5:383, 1973
11. Eijsvoogel VP, Schellekens PThA, Breur-Vriesendorp B, et al: in Terasaki PI (ed): Histocompatibility Testing 1970. Copenhagen, Munksgaard, 1970, p 523
12. Kissmeyer-Nielsen F, Svejgaard A, Sorensen SF, et al: Nature 228:63, 1970
13. van Rood JJ, Eijsvoogel VP: Lancet 1:698, 1970
14. Sorensen FS, Staub-Nielsen L: Acta Pathol Microbiol Scand 78(B):719, 1970
15. Bach FH, Day E, Bach ML, et al: Tissue Antigens 1:39, 1971
16. van Rood JJ, Koch CT, van Hooff JP, et al: Transplant Proc 5:409, 1973
17. Sasportes M, Lebrun A, Rapaport FT, et al: Transplant Proc 4:209, 1972
18. Eijsvoogel VP, van Rood JJ, du Toit ED, et al: Eur J Immunol 2:413, 1972
19. Rapaport FT, Bach FH: Transplant Proc 5:1139, 1973
20. Rapaport FT, Bachvaroff R, Converse JM: Transplant Proc 5:1823, 1973

21. Dausset J, Sasportes M, Lebrun A: C R Acad Sci (Paris) 275(D):2279, 1972

22. Hartzman RJ, Segall M, Bach ML, et al: Transplantation 11:268, 1971

23. Boyum A: Scand J Clin Lab Invest 21 (Suppl. 97):1

24. Dupont B, Anderson V, Hansen GS, et al: Transplantation 14:557, 1972

25. Koch CT, Eijsvoogel VP, Fredericks E, et al: Lancet 2:1334, 1971

26. WHO Committee on Primary Immunodeficiencies: Pediatrics 47:927, 1971

27. Pentycross CR, Klouda PT, Lawler SD: Transplantation 14:657, 1972

28. Segall M, Bach FH: Transplant Proc 5:1595, 1973

Part IV

Cell Membrane Surfaces

Fate of HL-A Antigens and Antibodies at the Lymphocyte Surface

By S. E. Cullen, D. Bernoco, A. O. Carbonara, H. Jacot-Guillarmod, G. Trinchieri, and R. Ceppellini

IT IS generally accepted that many proteic components of the cell membrane, as for instance immunoreceptors of lymphocytes and some classes of transplantation antigens, are floating in the lipid bilayer, where they are oriented according to their physical characteristics[1] and are subjected to active turnover.[2,3]

Potent and specific tools for rearranging cell surface components without necessarily impairing cell viability and disrupting the basic structure of the cell membrane are antibodies directed against some of these products. Aggregation by antibodies of molecules at the outer layer of the cell into caps and spots[4] has become an important technique for exploring the topography of cell surface. For instance, in the case of the HL-A system of man, Bernoco et al.[5,6] have shown by this technique that each one of the three pairs of genes, at the moment known to be expressed as serum-detected antigens (SD), are responsible for the synthesis of single and distinctive physical units, which have, however, multiple antigenic sites. This has also been confirmed by others.[7,8]

In the case of HL-A antigens, their rearrangement at the cell surface is greatly accelerated and magnified by a two-step procedure (strip, in our laboratory jargon), i.e., the cells are first coated with the allogeneic antiserum, then, after washing, they are treated with xenogeneic anti-human Ig. Usually fluorescent reagents are used, and the rearrangement of molecules is observed at the microscope (fluorostrip). However, Bernoco et al.[5] have also observed that rearrangement of HL-A antigen/antibody/anti-human Ig complexes at the lymphocyte surface makes the cell completely and specifically resistant to complement-dependent lysis (CdL), even upon addition of new antibody and excess complement, for all immunodeterminants carried by the molecular population that has been stripped (lysostrip). By contrast, the cell is normally susceptible to CdL for any other antigen. Similar phenomena have been described for other systems under the general term antigenic modulation.[9,10] We prefer, however, not to use this term, because it has been previously employed in immunogenetics for describing the changes in gene expression brought about at the surface of paramecia and other protozoa by antibodies and other factors, which last for some length of time and even after many cell divisions.[11] This is certainly not the case of HL-A and H-2 because the stripped antigens are expressed again in a matter of hours (recovery), even in nondividing lymphocytes,[5] at the same rate as after antigen stripping by enzymes.[12,13]

The pioneer work of Amos et al.,[14] Bernoco et al.,[15] and Miyajima et al.[16] has shown that fixation of antibody on the membrane of living lymphocytes is labile and, besides molecular aggregation, initiates a chain of events that only now begins to be understood. In this article we present additional evidence on the fate of HL-A antigens and antibodies when they interact at the lymphocyte surface.

From the Basel Institute for Immunology, Basel, Switzerland, and Istituto di Genetica Medica dell' Università, Torino, Italy.

The work done in Torino has been supported in part by NIH grant AI 08896 and in part by CNR contract Centro di Studio per l'Immunogenetica e l'Istocompatibilità.

© 1973 by Grune & Stratton, Inc.

MATERIALS AND METHOD

HL-A specificities are indicated according to the joint report of 1972.[17] The terms monospecific, supertypic (public), subtypic (private), cross reacting, and the corresponding symbols are used as described by Richiardi et al.[18] The three loci of the HL-A region, whose products are currently recognized by serology, are here indicated as SD (serum-defined): SD1 = LA, SD2 = Four, SD3 = AJ.

Complement-dependent lysis (CdL) is carried on according to a modification of NIH technique: incubation time 3 hr, strictly at 16°C, in a 0°C to 60°C incubator (Heraeus, Zurich). The strength of HL-A factors is measured by percentage of dead cells in conditions of limiting dilutions of antibody (Ab) and complement (C′).

Lymphocytes are from a panel of donors typed for all HL-A specificities studied at the Fifth International Workshop on Histocompatibility Testing,[17] plus a few new specificities of the third SD locus.[6] Lymphocytes were separated from fresh blood by the method of Boyum.[19] In more recent experiments, Dr. W. Mayr's modification was adopted (personal communication): blood is defibrinated by shaking with glass beads and layered in plastic tubes over a 53% dilution of Urografin 30% (Schering A. G., Berlin, Bergkamen). The tubes are centrifuged 20 min at 1,000 g at 4°C. Mononuclear cells are collected at interface, washed twice with PBS, and resuspended in RPMI-1640 supplemented with glutamin (2 mM) and 10 to 20% autologous heat-inactivated serum (this culture medium is here indicated as RAS). When autologous serum could not be used, a selected pool of human AB serum was used.

For most experiments, cell suspensions in RAS obtained from Urografin centrifugation were layered in 3024 Falcon plastic bottles and incubated 2 to 4 hr at 37°C in humidified 5% CO_2 atmosphere. Nonadherent cells were collected in fresh RAS and stored at 15°C until used. With this precaution, very clean preparations of lymphocytes were obtained, with minimal contamination of other blood cell types and platelets. Viability was 99% within 24 hr and 80 to 90% after 6 days. This is very important because contamination with other blood components (adherent cells and platelets) may greatly influence desensitization and shedding.[20]

In many experiments, all these steps were done under strictly sterile conditions. For metabolic studies no antibiotics were added.

Antisera: All anti-HL-A sera used were absorbed for 4 hr at 0°C with pools of lymphocytes from different donors known to be negative for the desired specificity, with the aim of removing panlymphocytotoxins that could be lytic at 16°C.[21] A 50% cytotoxic unit of Ab (U) is the reciprocal of the titer producing 50% lysis by the CdL technique described above, in complement excess.

Sera to be used for long-range experiments (desensitization, recovery, digestion, etc.) were sterilized through millipore filters and diluted in RAS. More recently, their IgG fraction or eluates from positive platelets prepared as in reference 22 were used. All sera received from outside laboratories were dialyzed for eliminating the possible presence of NaN_3 or other preservatives. Anti-human Ig sera were prepared in rabbits as in reference 5 and contained anti-γ, anti-κ, and anti-λ antibodies. More recently, their $F(ab)_2$ prepared as in reference 18 and repeatedly absorbed with human red blood cells and human thymocytes (obtained from cardiac surgery) were used. They were still able to agglutinate at a 10^{-4} dilution human Rh-positive red cells coated with anti-Rh incomplete antibodies of different origin. The use of $F(ab)_2$ has greatly reduced the percentage of dead cells (10%) in the controls of lysostrip.

Antibody radiolabeling: Serum ToGn is a polyspecific antiserum from a patient with aplastic anemia who received over 100 blood transfusions in the past few years. It induces CdL in over 90% of random donors and has a titer > 10^4 with HL-A12, 5 (4a-homozygous) cells. By absorption/elution studies, the prominent specificities are anti-HL-A2, 5, 12, 4a, but other undefined specificities are also present. It strongly fixes C′ on platelets. From this serum the IgG fraction was prepared and labeled with ^{125}I using lactoperoxidase-catalyzed radioiodination as described by Marchalonis.[23]

Complement was from a pool of rabbit sera, individually selected for showing maximal lytic activity against a standard lymphocytotoxic anti-HL-A system and no lysis against nonsensitized human lymphocytes. A 50% cytotoxic unit of complement (C′) is the reciprocal of the titer producing 50% lysis against standard 4a-homozygous cells coated with 8 Ab U of a standard anti-4a serum (To/1.20).

Desensitization is operationally defined as the loss of susceptibility to lysis upon addition of C′: lymphocytes are coated with excess of anti-HL-A antibody (usually 8 U/10^6 cells/ml) by incubation 2 hr at 0°C; washed twice; resuspended in RAS (10% autologous serum: high protein concentration delays rate of clearance); incubated at 37°C for various lengths of time; washed twice; resuspended in McCoy; C′ is added ranging from 2 U, which gives 80 to 90% killing with fully sensitized cells, to 8 U, which gives 100% killing. When after incubation at 37° cells are treated with additional Ab + C′, they are usually lysed as untreated controls, unless spontaneous resistance has developed.

Spontaneous resistance is operationally defined as the loss of susceptibility to lysis upon addition of Ab + C′ to cells that underwent desensitization. Usually this is observed only with some Ag/Ab combinations and can be better seen by adding suboptimal amounts of lytic reagents.

Shedding[3,15] is the clearance of Ab from the lymphocyte surface visually observed by fading of immunofluorescence (direct or indirect method) or by decrease on cell pellet and increase in the supernatant of radiolabel that has been linked to coating Ab.

Consumption is the disappearance of Ab activity measured as decrease of cytotoxic units from an antiserum incubated in large excess with lymphocytes that are positive for the HL-A specificity of the antiserum.

Strip is removal and aggregation into caps and spots and/or functional incapacity of surface antigens to fix more Ab and C′, obtained through the interaction between alloantibodies coating the cell surface and anti-human Ig.

(*a*) *Lysostrip* is acquisition of specific resistance to CdL:[5] lymphocytes are coated with anti-HL-A serum 2 hr at 0°C; washed three times in serum-free medium at 0°C; incubated 30 min at 0°C with anti-human Ig (as intact rabbit IgG or as its $F(ab)_2$ fragment); washed three times in serum-free medium at 0°C. The cells are then adjusted to 2×10^6/ml in RAS and incubated 30 min at 37°C and quickly cooled to 0°C; 10 mM NaN_3 is added for delaying any further rearrangement of surface components. The cells are then used for typing. With careful handling (i.e., purity of lymphocyte preparations, sterility, use of autologous serum, use of anti-human Ig as $F(ab)_2$ fragment), at the end of treatment, even after addition of C′, controls show less than 10% dead cells. When rabbit anti-human Ig serum was used as such, controls after addition of C′ alone showed 20 to 30% dead cells (possibly B-lymphocyte killing[24,25]).

(*b*) *Fluorostrip* is the corresponding phenomenon observed in immunofluorescence.[5,6]

Recovery is new expression of HL-A antigens after acquisition of spontaneous resistance or strip. It is studied by incubating the cells in RAS at the desired temperature and length of time. Then the cells are washed once with McCoy and tested with C′ alone or with pertinent anti-HL-A sera and C′.

Exhaustion of HL-A antigens by metabolic inhibitors is the disappearance of HL-A determinants from lymphocytes that have not experienced any antibody treatment but are incubated in RAS with drugs. At the end of the incubation period the cells are again typed, and antigen strength is measured against decreasing concentrations of Ab and C′. As metabolic inhibitors, puromycin (10–50 μg/ml), cycloheximide (10–100 μg/ml), and sodium azide (5–15 mM) have been used. For the times of incubation used, these levels of the drugs were not cytotoxic (dead cells in controls, below 20%).

To evaluate the effect of inhibitors on protein synthesis, the incorporation of ^{3}H-leucine by cells cultured in the presence or absence of drugs was measured: medium RPMI-1640, deficient in cold leucine (10% of the normal leucine content = 0.038 mM), implemented with 50 Ci/ml ^{3}H-leucine and 10% human Ab serum (heat-inactivated and dialyzed against leucine-deficient medium).

RESULTS

Typical results, chosen from the many similar experiments carried on by our group in the last 3 yr, are here presented for clarifying the more relevant points.

Desensitization. Loss of susceptibility to lysis upon addition of C′ alone to Ab-coated cells, which takes place at physiologic temperature, has been shown to be mainly, although not uniquely, due to clearance of Ab leaving the cell surface, as was originally suggested by Amos et al.[14] and Bernoco et al.[15] In fact, as shown in Table 1, the ^{125}I label leaves cells (column a) and is found in the supernatant (column b). The separation of radiolabel from cells parallels rather well the loss of sensitivity to C′ (e) and the increasing inability to fix C′ (g). Two modes of clearance can be recognized:

(1) Some loss of ^{125}I, up to 10 to 20% in different experiments, takes place in the first 30 to 60 min of incubation even at 15°C, but at this temperature does not proceed further (compare second and last line). This has also been confirmed by loss of CdL using limiting dilutions of C′ (2U) as shown in Fig. 1 (a). Moreover, a significant part of the radioactivity that has been released can be specifically bound on positive lymphocytes or platelets (column c). Although small as percentage of radioactivity originally bound to the cells, this active radiolabel has been consistently found in many different experiments. This suggests that some Ab molecules, probably of poorer avidity, are released into the medium. Conventionally, this type of release is here referred to as elution.

(2) By contrast, after this initial loss, when the cells are washed once, resuspended in fresh medium (prewarmed at 37°C), and incubated at 37°C (new zero time), the loss starts again and proceeds for the next 24 hr. At that time, in different experiments, only between 15 and 30% of the radiolabel initially fixed on the cell re-

Table 1. Shedding of Inactive Radiolabel From Lymphocytes Coated With Radioactive Allogeneic Antibody

Incubation		% Radioactivity			% Dead Cells			C′ Fx
Time	Temperature	a	b	c	Control d	Only C′ e	Ab + C′ f	% g
0 (1st)	15°C	100	0	0	5	100	100	100
30 min	15°C	90	10	5	5	95	100	100
0 (2nd)	37°C	100	0	0	5	95	100	100
30 min	37°C	90	10	0	5	90	100	80
4 hr	37°C	60	40	0	5	70	100	40
18 hr	37°C	33	67	0	10	23	100	15
24 hr	37°C	30	70	0	10	10	100	0
24 hr	15°C	90	10	7	5	95	100	100

IgG were prepared from serum ToGn (polyspecific anti-HL-A2,5,12,4a) and labeled with ^{125}I.[23] Lymphocytes HL-A2,9,5,12,4a were coated with 8U/ml of ^{125}I IgG from serum ToGn and washed three times; c.p.m./10^6 cells = 5,453 = 100%. Cells were resuspended in nutrient medium implemented with 10% autologous serum (RAS) and, for reasons explained in the text, washed two times, resuspended in fresh RAS (second time zero), incubated at 37°C, and sampled at intervals. An aliquot was left at 15°C. For every sample, radioactivity was measured on the cell pellet (a) and on the supernatant (b). The amount of radioactivity that could be specifically bound to fresh untreated lymphocytes of the same subject was also measured (c). Radioactivity left on cell pellet after the initial loss at 15°C, c.p.m./10^6 cells = 4,963, was again taken as 100% for comparison with following samples. For each sample, control viability (d) and susceptibility to lysis upon addition of C′ alone (e) or C′ + Ab (f) were carried on. Moreover, the ability of coated cells to fix C′ (g) was measured. Initial C′ fixation = 10U/10^6 coated cells = 100%. Lymphocytes were obtained from fresh peripheral blood by defibrination, purification on Urografin, and elimination of adherent cells by incubation at 37°C for 4 hr on a plastic surface. All procedures were under strict sterile conditions. No antibiotic was added.

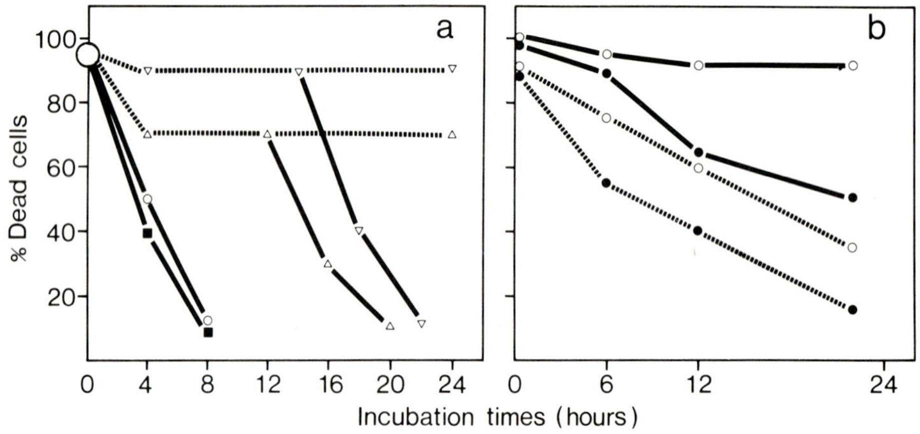

Fig. 1. (a) Effect of temperature and cycloheximide on desensitization of anti-HL-A-coated lymphocytes. HL-A2-positive cells were sensitized with 4U of monospecific anti-A2, washed, resuspended in nutrient medium and incubated at 37°C (continuous lines) or at 15°C (discontinuous lines). At various times aliquots were collected, washed, and mixed with C′. A loss of sensitivity to CdL is observed even at 15°C during the first hours of incubation, barely significant when C′ is added in excess (▽), more marked for suboptimal doses of C′ (△). Circles connected by lines show the typical rate of desensitization at 37°C. It is also unaffected when cells are incubated with 100 μg/ml of cycloheximide (squares and lines). (b) Effect of cycloheximide on clearance of HL-A antigens from the cell surface. HL-A2,5-positive cells are incubated in RAS at 37°C in the presence of cycloheximide. At intervals, aliquots are typed (NIH technique) with anti-HL-A2 (open circles) and anti-HL-A5 (black circles), using either excess of Ab and C′ (8U + 8U) or limiting amounts (2U + 2U). In the first condition (continuous lines), only HL-A5 seems to be partially lost because of the drug. When limiting amounts of reagents are used (discontinuous lines) both antigens show a decreased sensitivity to CdL. In controls (no drug added), sensitivity to CdL at 24 hr is 100% for both antigens.

mains on the cell pellet, probably inside the cell because it cannot be separate from the cell membrane (R. Cone, unpublished results). Moreover, the radiolabeled material released at 37°C is totally inactive because it does not bind specifically to corresponding fresh antigen (c). This second type of release (desensitization, *sensu strictu*) is temperature-dependent. In fact, it begins at 25°C and becomes clearly significant above 30°C.[15] Evidence to be discussed below shows that in particular conditions even the ^{125}I released at 37°C is still linked to an IgG-like protein, albeit inactive as antibody.

Note that *pure* suspensions of platelets allowed elution at 15°C of a small percentage of the same ^{125}I antibody (ToGn) specifically fixed on them, which was still able to bind to antigen on fresh platelets or lymphocytes. Platelets, however, are not able to get rid of the residual antibody even after protracted incubation at 37°C.[20] Similar behavior is well known for red cells.

Resistance of Desensitization to Metabolic Inhibitors. Since optimal desensitization of lymphocytes requires physiologic temperatures, it was thought to depend on some metabolic processes. Several metabolic inhibitors were therefore used in an attempt to block it. As shown in Fig. 1 (a), addition of 100 μg/ml of cycloheximide did not modify desensitization in any way. Puromycin (10 μg/ml) was also ineffective, although at these levels the two drugs blocked protein synthesis (measured as ^{14}C-leucine incorporation) up to 90 to 100%. Also NaN_3 (15 mM) did not significantly affect desensitization. It must be pointed out, however, that these experiments were fortuitously limited to clearance of anti-HL-A1, 2, 9. In view of more recent information, lack of inhibition by these drugs should not be generalized for all HL-A specificities until ad hoc experiments are performed.

Consumption of HL-A Antibodies by Positive Lymphocytes. Clearance of coating antibody seems to be a fundamental property of the living lymphocyte that is not easily impeached in vitro. In fact, not only is it immediately resumed at the same rate when the cell population is shifted from 15°C to 37°C, Fig. 1 (a), but it goes on unabated indefinitely. In the experiment of Table 2, 4b-positive cells were still coated with antibody at day 5 when incubated at either 15°C or 37°C. In fact, after washing and resuspending in fresh medium, both samples were 100% killed upon addition of 4U of C′. However, when they were allowed

Table 2. Antibody Consumption by Positive Lymphocytes in Culture

Cells, 10^7/ml	T, °C	anti-HL-A	Ab Units Found in Supernatants After Days in Culture: 0	1	2	3	4	5	6
none	37°	anti-4a	60	60	60	60	60	60	60
		anti-4b	60	60	60	60	60	60	60
yes	37°	anti-4a	60	60	60	60	60	60	60
		anti-4b	55	35	25	15	5	2	0
yes	15°	anti-4a	60	60	60	60	60	60	60
		anti-4b	55	55	50	50	50	50	50

60U/ml of an anti-4a serum and 60U/ml of an anti-4b serum have been mixed and incubated under sterile conditions with 10^7 lymphocytes/ml of donor HL-A1, W25, W5, 8 (4b/4b). Adherent cells had not been removed in this experiment. The donor of cells is also the producer of the anti-4a serum used in the experiment, Medium RAS (15% autologous antiserum + 25% allogeneic antiserum for obtaining the desired concentration of the two antibodies); incubation in humidified 5% CO_2 atmosphere; shaking three times per day; total volume 0.2/ml per tube. Two tubes for each experimental point. At stated intervals the tubes were centrifuged 30 min at 1000 g; the supernatants were separated and frozen at −70°C. All supernatants were then diluted in 0.33 steps with McCoy and titrated on the same day against two cells (4a- and 4b-homozygous, respectively). The residual U reported are the approximate average of those found in the three tubes for each experimental point.

to incubate at 37°C for 18 hr before addition of C′, they had become completely resistant to lysis. Note that the cells kept at 37°C must have inactivated several times the number of Ab molecules that could be fixed by antigen initially available at the cell surface. Note also that this inactivation is strictly specific and requires interaction between positive lymphocytes and antibody. The innocent bystander anti-4a antibody (produced by the cell donor) was not affected at all. Reciprocal results were obtained, i.e., consumption of anti-4a and preservation of anti-4b, when the mixture of the two sera was incubated with 4a-positive, 4b-negative lymphocytes. It must be mentioned that in this experiment adherent cells had not been removed from the lymphocyte preparation.

Spontaneous Resistance. In our experience desensitization of Ab-coated cells is almost always paralleled by a normal sensitivity to lysis when they are treated with additional antibody. This has brought us to think that in the one-step procedure (i.e., with no strip by anti-human Ig) enough antigenic sites are always available at the cell surface for allowing CdL, either because they have been freed from wornout antibody molecules or because new antigen molecules have substituted the ones that might have shed away with Ab. For instance in Table 1, at any time and for any temperature, 100% lysis was obtained (column f).

Occasionally, however, a few antisera were met, in general multispecific and with a high cytotoxic titer, that gave significantly lower titers upon incubation at room temperature (22°C to 28°C) than at 16°C, even when cold panlymphocytotoxins[21] had previously been adsorbed out. These same sera also showed incomplete lysis when during clearance new Ab + C′ of the same specificity was added. This spontaneous resistance to lysis is more evident when limiting amounts of lytic reagents, e.g., 2U of Ab + 2U of C′ are used (reagents in these amounts give in our standard technique 80 to 90% killing). These observations, even if inconsistent and difficult to repeat, suggested to us that shedding of Ab and/or sequestration by stripping into caps and spots as can be seen in immunofluorescence were probably not the only phenomena causing resistance to lysis. It was then decided to carry on other experiments with a radiolabeled Ab under strict control of temperature, which prima facie seemed to be an important source of variability.

In these new series of observations, the same ^{125}I-labeled antibody (ToGn) already used in the experiment of Table 1 was employed. Note, however, that in the experiment presented in Table 3, lymphocytes were different, namely they were negative with serum ToGn for the products of Sd1 (in fact lysostrip with ToGn did not interfere with HL-A1, W19 specificities). Note the usual elution of labile Ab after 1 h at 15°C. As before, radioactivity left on the cell pellet after this first incubation time has been taken as 100% for comparison with the results obtained after preincubation at other temperatures. After 1 hr preincubation the cells were washed twice at 0°C with chillded McCoy, then lytic reagents (also precooled) were added. Finally, the mixtures were incubated at 16°C for 3 hr.

A significant resistance to lysis upon addition of C′ alone and addition of suboptimal doses of Ab + C′ begins to appear after preincubation at 25°C. After preincubation at 30°C, resistance becomes prominent even when 4U Ab + 4U C′ are added. After 1 hr at 37°C an attenuation of resistance is observed, and at 2 hr, while desensitization and shedding have further progressed (40% dead cells by addition of C′ alone, 74% radioactivity bound to cells), resistance is no longer observed (100% killing by addition of Ab + C′). Note, however, that the amount of radioactive Ab left on the cell pellet (column d) is higher after preincubation at 30°C than after preincuba-

Table 3. Temperature-dependence of Spontaneous Resistance to Lysis of Lymphocytes Coated by Anti-HL-A

Preincubation After HL-A Coating		% Dead Cells (NIH 3 hr at 16°C) Reagents Added			
Time	Temp. °C	2U C′ a	2U Ab + 2U C′ b	4U Ab + 4U C′ c	^{125}I d
0 hr	15°	85%	95%	100%	107%
1 hr	15°	85%	95%	100%	100%
1 hr	20°	80%	85%	100%	100%
1 hr	25°	60%	70%	100%	96%
1 hr	30°	50%	55%	65%	88%
1 hr	37°	50%	70%	90%	82%
anti-Ig strip		10%	10%	10%	93%

HL-A1, W19, 5, 12, T5 lymphocytes have been incubated 2 hr at 4°C with 8U of serum ToGn (anti-HL-A2,5,12,4a) that had been radiolabeled with ^{125}I, washed two times, resuspended in fresh medium, preincubated at various temperatures, and then further incubated (NIH technique, 3 hr at 16°C) with either: (a) suboptimal dose of C′ alone, (b) suboptimal doses of same Ab and C′, or (c) 4U of same Ab and 4U of C′. Aliquots of cells were centrifuged and washed three times, and the pellet was measured for radioactivity still bound to cells. At time zero, c.p.m. = 4,303/10^6 cells. After initial loss at 15°C (see text and Table 1), c.p.m. = 4,022. This amount was taken as 100% for further comparisons (column d). In the last line, lysostrip, i.e., after first coating with anti-HL-A antiserum, cells have been washed three times, incubated 30 min at 0°C with anti-human Ig, washed, incubated 30 min at 37°C, then typed and measured for radioactivity as other samples. Between 25°C and 37°C, a certain amount of resistance to lysis develops even when fresh antibody is added. This is particularly evident when limiting amounts of lytic reagents are used. Strip with anti-Ig, however, is much more effective. Note that above 20°C, resistance to lysis is greater than expected on the basis of loss of radioactive label (d).

tion at 37°C. Thus, paradoxically, a higher amount of Ab at the cell surface parallels increased resistance. Cells subjected to anti-Ig strip (last line), as expected, are completely refractory to lysis. They also show a higher amount of radioactivity linked to cells, in agreement with the observation that anti-Ig strip delays shedding of allogeneic antibody.[20] The interpretation of these findings is discussed below.

Recovery After Anti-Ig Strip. As reported by Bernoco et al.,[5] resistance to lysis is strictly specific for the determinants carried by the physical units involved in the first coating and is rapidly overcome by healthy cells that are able to express again in a matter of hours the specificities sequestered into caps and spots. Actually the rate of recovery of molecules stripped by immunologic treatment is comparable to the rate of reappearance reported after digestion of HL-A antigens at the cell surface by proteolitic enzymes.[13,26]

In the experiment summarized in Fig. 2(a), the rate of recovery, within the accuracy of the technique employed, does not seem to be significantly different for the three antigens tested. Because recovery (as desensitization, *sensu strictu*) is also temperature-dependent[5] and therefore likely controlled by some metabolic process, here again the effects of NaN_3, Fig. 2(b), and cycloheximide, Fig. 2(c), have been tested. As shown in the figure, cycloheximide completely blocks recovery, thus suggesting that this process requires protein synthesis.

The action of NaN_3 is more difficult to interpret because it initially delays, but does not prevent, recovery. After a few hours, however, a loss of expression of some antigens is observed: minimal and nonsignificant for HL-A2, intermediate for HL-A5, and total for FJH.* While our experience is limited for this last antigen (see, however, reference 6), the differential effect of NaN_3 on reexpression of antigens belonging to SD1 and SD2 has been repeatedly observed.

Exhaustion of HL-A Antigens by Cycloheximide. The experiments described above, as well as the block of reexpression

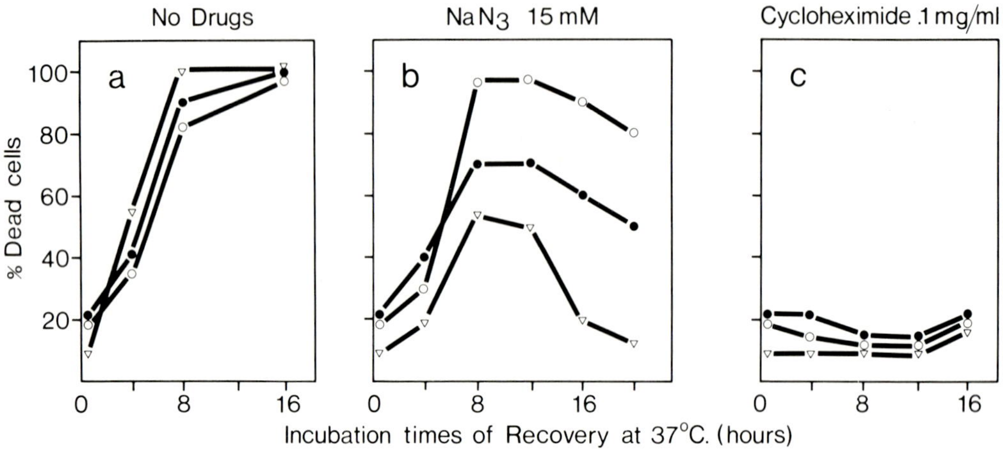

Fig. 2. (a) Recovery after anti-HL-A + anti-Ig lysostrip. Lymphocytes HL-A2,12,FJH*-positive have been divided into aliquots coated with 4U of anti-A2 (open circles), anti-A12 (black circles), or anti-FJH* (▽) for 2 hr at 4°C, washed three times, treated with anti-human Ig 30 min at 37°C, brought to 0°C, and washed again three times. Subsequent addition (time zero) of Ab + C′ (modified NIH technique 3 hr at 16°C) shows that cells have become specifically resistant to lysis. However, when prior to addition of Ab + C′ cells are incubated at 37°C, they quickly recover susceptibility to lysis. Rate of recovery is not significantly different for the three antigens studied. (b) Same as in (a) but incubation at 37°C is carried on in the presence of NaN_3. The drug delays recovery and after prolonged incubation exhausts expression of FJH* and partially that of A12, but not of A2. (c) Same as in (a) but incubation at 37°C is carried on in the presence of cycloheximide. The drug completely inhibits recovery of expression of the three antigens.

after papain removal of HL-A reported by Turner et al.,[13] are firm evidence that protein synthesis is required. They are not, however, informative as to whether a continuous turnover of surface antigens takes place in physiologic conditions, i.e., when the cell membrane is not disturbed by antibody attachment or by enzymatic digestion. To answer this question, lymphocytes that had received no previous Ab treatment were incubated at 37°C for 12 hr with 100 μg/ml of cycloheximide (puromycin in these experimental conditions becomes toxic beyond 12 hr). Initial trials were quite deceiving because expression of HL-A2 after 24 hr was seemingly unmodified when checked by CdL upon addition of excess anti-HL-A2 and excess C′. However, when CdL was repeated with limiting amounts of lytic reagents, a 50% decrease in HL-A2 expression at 24 hr was observed.

Because of the differential results obtained with NaN_3 in the rate of recovery for various antigens, exhaustion by cycloheximide was carried out in parallel, on the same HL-A2,5-positive cells for these two antigens. Fig. 1 (b) shows that expression of HL-A5 seems to be inhibited more promptly and completely.

More recently, these results have been confirmed by using ^{125}I-labeled ToGn serum, appropriately absorbed for separating anti-SD1 and -SD2 specificities and using different cells of appropriate HL-A phenotype. A 50% decrease in radioactivity specifically bound by SD1 antigens and an 85% decrease in radioactivity bound by SD2 antigens after 24 hr incubation with cycloheximide, has been observed. These experiments reported in extenso elsewhere[27] rule out the possibility that the drug should interfere with the lytic action of C′ and not with antigen availability at the cell surface.

DISCUSSION

The study of HL-A is at the moment in a transient phase from simpleminded serology of blood cells toward sophisticated biochemistry of the cell membrane. We are aware of the limitations of the methodology used in the experiments here presented. For instance, serum ToGn was chosen for iodination because of its very high cytotoxic titer even with the standard CdL techniques. Serum ToGn, however, is the least appropriate for studying differential behavior of membrane components owing to the variety of antibody specificities it contains.

For a comprehensive discussion of the phenomena here presented, some additional information, recently obtained by our group, should be given:

(1) Under appropriate conditions, where protein digestion is inhibited (i.e., careful elimination of adherent cells from lymphocyte preparations and addition of protease inhibitors during clearance), the majority of radiolabel initially fixed as Ab at the lymphocyte surface is found in the supernatant, after incubation at 37°C, still linked to a protein that has the general characteristics (molecular weight, antigenicity) of human IgG. However, when the above-mentioned precautions are omitted, radioactivity released is in part bound to molecules of much smaller size.[20]

(2) This seemingly IgG protein, however, does not bind any more to the corresponding antigen on fresh lymphocytes or platelets, as shown for ^{125}I in Table 1. Preliminary experiments with double labeling of coating Ab and of lymphocyte surface (respectively with ^{125}I and ^{131}I) suggest that this inactive Ig is shed off the cell, complexed with some component(s) of the cell surface.[28]

Insusceptibility to Lysis After Sensitization. We have distinguished the terms desensitization, spontaneous resistance, shedding, and lysostrip. Parts of these distinctions have only an operational basis, but parts underline different phenomena and different phases of sequential events.

There is little doubt that shedding, i.e., dispersion without penetrating,[29] of Ab initially fixed at the lymphocyte surface is a well proven fact for both its phases: the initial temperature-independent elution and the second temperature-dependent clearance.[25,30] The data on HL-A,[20,28] as well as the similar data on tumor antigens by Baldwin et al.,[31] show that digestion into small fragments of the coating antibody is not a necessary prerequisite for warm clearance, because both groups of workers were able to recover a rather intact immunoglobulin, although inactive as Ab. These observations are not in contradiction with the possibilities that: (*a*) part of the coating antibody is indeed interiorized and presumably digested by the cell; (*b*) shedding into the surrounding medium may be preceded by a transient phase of inane interiorization (inane because it does not lead to immunoglobulin digestion). Shedding does not require the formation of large caps and spots, because it goes on even with allogeneic antisera that do not show immunofluorescent capping without the help of anti-human immunoglobulin. Microaggregation into particles that cannot be visually recognized is, however, a likely event.

According to the above-mentioned authors,[28,31] inactivity of the shed Ig-like protein, when digestion is prevented, seems to be due to complexation of the antibody combining sites with the antigen molecule or fragments of it. Baldwin et al.[31] have in fact been able to recover active antibody by acid elution of the complex. Thus physical removal of antigen from the cell membrane seems indeed to be one of the consequences of Ag/Ab interaction at the lymphocyte surface and hence a major factor in inducing resistence to lysis upon addition to previously coated cells of both C′ alone (desensitization) or Ab and C′.

The fact that this second type of resistance is usually observed only after strip can easily be explained on the basis of the greater rate and magnitude of antigen aggregation induced by the two-stage treatment (anti-HL-A + anti-human IgG). By contrast, in the one-step process (no intervention of anti-Ig), because of the relative low efficiency of the majority of HL-A/anti-HL-A combinations in inducing microaggregation and spontaneous resistance, enough new molecules of antigen become available (de novo synthesized or derived from a pool waiting at a deeper level of the surface[32]). Therefore the cell can be lysed by additional Ab + C′.

What is not yet clear is why C′ does not lyse the cell in the first phase of the stripping phenomenon, i.e., when Ag/anti-HL-A/anti-Ig aggregation is taking place and the complex has not yet left (inward or outward) the cell surface. Experiments that are to be repeated and extended have shown that at this stage the cells fix twice as much C′ as after anti-HL-A treatment alone. Thus C′ receptors are still available (probably on the rabbit immunoglobulin; experiments with rabbit $F(ab)_2$ remain to be done), and C′ is fixed but is not able to lyse either because of the new geometry acquired by the complex or because of some changes in the nearby areas of the cell membrane where C′ exerts its lytic attack. (Note that these cells are normally susceptible to CdL for antibodies directed against determinants not carried on the same physical units involved in the strip.)

Spontaneous Resistance. Spontaneous resistance has been previously defined as the loss of sensitivity to lysis of previously Ab-coated cells (one-step procedure) even when more antibody of the same specificity is added. As shown in Table 3, it can also be defined as resistance to lysis upon addition of C′ while the first antibody is still present at the cell surface. In fact, on the basis of radioactivity, antibody has not yet shed outward, while it is not yet deeply interiorized because it can be recovered with the cell membrane.[28] The phenomenon is difficult to control and shows best in a restricted range of temperature. More recent data, presented elsewhere in this volume,[6] show that it is more common when antigens of the SD3 series are involved. These antigens are also known to be more easily exhausted by antimetabolites.

These various lines of evidence suggest that a number of events, partly of opposite sign, should coincidentally interact for the manifestation of spontaneous resistance. First, it is likely that the allogeneic antiserum, without the help of anti-Ig, must be able to induce Ag microaggregation at the appropriate rate and of appropriate size such that C′ is unable to lyse. That might depend on the polyvalence of the Ag/Ab system under test and/or on the mobility in the lipid layer of the Ag involved.

Another probable variable is the rate of replacement at the cell surface of the Ag molecules that have been made functionally unavailable. That may depend on the pool of the Ag involved,[32] on the presence of NaN_3 or other preservatives in the serum, or on the suboptimal viability of the cell population. Finally, an increased rate of shedding by accelerating replacement with virgin Ag molecules may contrast the manifestation of spontaneous resistance.

It will be rather difficult to dissect and recognize without the help of refined biochemical techniques the various interacting factors. Most of them, however, seem to be temperature-dependent, albeit at different levels. Thus the results of Table 3 could be interpreted by assuming that microaggregation (hence functional unavailability for lysis) is already efficient between 25°C and 30°C, while replacement of new molecules (recovery) is poor below 30°C, and reaches its optimum at 37°C. These phenomena may be relevant for explaining the marked difference in sensitivity of HL-A typing techniques based on different times and temperatures of incubation.

Action of Antimetabolites. The use of antimetabolites, particularly of cycloheximide, has been informative in many respects. With the reservation already forwarded, namely that all experiments were fortuitously limited to SD1 antigens, the lack of effect of the drugs tested on desensitization suggests that both its components, i.e., (*a*) microagglutination and consequent functional unavailability of

Ag/Ab complexes to the lytic action of C′ and (*b*) physical removal of these complexes from the cell surface, do not depend, at least for the length of time assayed, on protein synthesis. Our feeling is that they depend mainly on the physiochemical properties of the HL-A glycoproteins and the lipidic bilayer.[28] Also of importance might be the activity of membrane-bound enzymes, if shedding requires partial degradation of Ag molecules.

By contrast, the sharp inhibitory effect of cycloheximide and puromycin on recovery after anti-Ig strip shows clearly that the pool of available molecules of antigens is small and that protein synthesis is required for replacing them. This is in agreement with the data of others.[13,33] We have no explanation to offer for the discrepancy between our data and the report of Ferrone et al.,[34] who claim that only puromycin and not cycloheximide prevents synthesis of HL-A antigens. However, these authors were working with different material, i.e., continuously growing lymphoblast lines.

The effect of NaN_3, which initially only delays recovery and later exhausts the expression of HL-A antigens, Fig. 2(b), can be accepted in view of the complex action of this drug on cellular respiration and its difficult entry into living lymphocytes. The use of NaN_3, however, has been very illuminating because it has given us the first hint for suspecting that some biological property of products of the three SD loci (and by extrapolation other loci of the HL-A region) might be different.

This has indeed been confirmed by exhaustive studies on lymphocytes that had not previously been exposed to antibody. As shown in Fig. 1(b), HL-A2 is more resistant to the effect of the drug than HL-A5. Products of SD3 are still easier to exhaust by inhibitors of protein synthesis. This observation, which underlines for the first time a different functional behavior for products of the various SD genes of the HL-A region, has been amply confirmed and is discussed elsewhere.

Finally, our data suggest that a certain degree of turnover of HL-A antigens depending on protein synthesis is taking place also in the so-called small, resting lymphocyte. It remains to be tested with appropriate quantitative methods whether the rate of synthesis in these conditions is of the same order of magnitude or much slower than resynthesis observed after strip by antibody or after enzymatic digestion.[12]

Possible Significance In Vivo. While studying the action of allogeneic antisera upon activation of mixed leucocyte cultures, Bernoco et al.[15] suggested that the products of shedding from the interacting cells could be the most important factor for the observed block of MLC. If this original suggestion is confirmed, this will represent an important in vitro model for studying the effect on immunocytes of Ag/Ab complexes in regard to in vivo situations like allotransplants and cancer immunity. In fact, radiolabeled alloantibody against rat donor, passively given to rat recipients, has been shown to leave the transplanted kidney in a matter of hours.[35] Nonetheless, it is known that one or a few injections of alloantibody may indefinitely protect a kidney graft that otherwise would be rapidly rejected.[36] Evidently passive antibody must have, if any, only a very transient effect at the level of the efferent limb of rejection events. It is more reasonable to suppose that shed antibody may play an important role at the central level for initiating an active process of protection (enhancement and/or tolerance). If this should prove to be true, preparation in vitro of specific products of shedding to be injected into the graft recipient could be envisaged.

Finally, the possibility of controlling by drugs in a differential way the expression at the cell surface of the products of the various genetic units located in the HL-A region might become an important tool for studying their specific biological functions, e.g., the role of SD and LD genes in MLC and CML. Moreover, it might provide a novel approach to the problems of graft rejection[34] and treatment of HL-A associated diseases.[37]

SUMMARY

Fixation in vitro of anti-HL-A antibodies on the surface of living lymphocytes is labile and initiates a complex chain of events: microaggregation of antigen molecules that in particular conditions may lead to resistance to lysis upon addition of further antibody and C′; desensitization of the cell by shedding of the specifically fixed Ig (traced through ^{125}I label) into the medium in an inactive form (probably because complexed with antigen); rapid formation of caps and spots by the two-step process (strip: anti-HL-A + anti-human Ig), which is paralleled by a complete resistance to lysis specifically limited to antigenic determinants involved in the strip; rapid recovery of antigen molecules lost by strip. This last process is completely blocked by cycloheximide and puromycin and delayed by Na-azide. Cycloheximide also exhausts the expression of HL-A antigens at the surface of lymphocytes that have not been treated with either antibody or enzyme. This suggests that protein synthesis is required for maintaining normal HL-A expression at the surface of the cell. Products of SD1, SD2, and SD3 loci are differentially inhibited by antimetabolites.

ACKNOWLEDGMENTS

We are indebted to Dr. E.S. Curtoni, Dr. W. Mayr, and Dr. M. Savi for the generous supply of many sera. The anti-FJH* was a gift from Dr. H. Festenstein. We thank the blood donors of Hoffman–La Roche, Basel, for their invaluable and generous collaboration. We acknowledge the technical help of Mrs. Carla Jacot Guzzi and Mrs. Marietta Bernoco.

REFERENCES

1. Singer SJ, Nicholson GL: Science 175:720, 1972
2. Marchalonis JJ, Cone RE: Transplant Rev 14:3, 1973
3. Vitetta ES, Uhr SW: Transplant Rev 14:50, 1973
4. Taylor RB, Duffus WPH, Raff MC, De Petris S: Nature [New Biol] 233:225, 1971
5. Bernoco D, Cullen S, Scudeller G, et al: in Dausset J, Colombani J (eds): Histocompatibility Testing, 1972. Copenhagen, Munksgaard, p 527
6. Mayr W, Bernoco D, De Marchi M, Ceppellini R: Transplant Proc 5:1581, 1973
7. Neuport-Sautes C, Silvestre D, Kourilsky FM, Dausset J: in Dausset J, Colombani J (eds): Histocompatibility Testing, 1972. Copenhagen, Munksgaard, p 539
8. Svejgaard A, Staub Nielsen L, Ryder LP, et al: in Dausset J, Colombani J (eds): Histocompatibility Testing, 1972. Copenhagen, Munksgaard, p 465
9. Takahashi T: Transplant Proc 3:1217, 1971
10. Old L, Stockert E, Boyse E, Kim J: J Exp Med 127:523, 1968
11. Beale GH: in Boume GH, Danielli JF (eds): International Review of Cytology VI. New York, Academic, 1957
12. Nathenson SG: Ann Rev Genet 4:69, 1970
13. Turner MJ, Strominger JL, Sanderson AR: Proc Natl Acad Sci USA 69:200, 1972
14. Amos DB, Cohen I, Klein WJ: Transplant Proc 2:68, 1970
15. Bernoco D, Mattiuz PL, Miggiano V, Ceppellini R: G Batteriol v irol Immunol 64:272, 1971
16. Miyajima T, Hirata AA, Terasaki PI: Tissue Antigens 2:64, 1972
17. Joint Report of the Fifth International Histocompatibility Workshop, in Dausset J, Colombani J (eds): Histocompatibility Testing, 1972. Copenhagen, Munksgaard, p 619
18. Richiardi P, Carbonara A, Mattiuz PL, Ceppellini R: in Dausset J, Colombani J (eds): Histocompatibility Testing, 1972. Copenhagen, Munksgaard, p 455
19. Boyum A: Scand J Clin Lab Invest [Suppl 21] 1968, p 97
20. Jacot-Guillarmod H, Carbonara A, Ceppellini R: in Peters F (ed): XXI Bruges Colloquia on Protides of Biological Fluids. New York, Harper (in press)
21. Naito S, Mickey MR, Hirata A, Terasaki PI: Tissue Antigens 1:219, 1971
22. Luzzati A, Carbonara A, Tosi RM: J Immunol Methods 1:101, 1971
23. Marchalonis JJ: Biochem J 113:299, 1969
24. Wernet PM, Feizi T, Kunkel HG: J Exp Med 136:650, 1972
25. Knopf PM, Destree A, Hyman R: Eur J Immunol 3:251, 1973
26. Bhandari SC, Singal DP: Tissue Antigens 3: 140, 1973

27. Ceppellini R, Bernoco D, Cone R, Mayr W: to be published
28. Cone R, Bernoco D, Trinchieri G, Ceppellini R: in preparation
29. Webster's Third New International Dictionary. Springfield, Merriam, 1966
30. Wilson JD, Nossal GJV, Lewis H: Eur J Immunol 2:225, 1972
31. Baldwin RW, Bowen JG, Embleton MS, Price MR: Br J Cancer 28:6, 1973
32. Cone RE, Marchalonis JJ, Rolley RT: J Exp Med 134:1373, 1971
33. Cikes M, Klein G: J Natl Cancer Inst 48:509, 1972
34. Ferrone S, Del Villano BG, Pellegrino MA, et al: Tissue Antigens 2:447, 1972
35. French ME, Batchelor JR: Transplant Rev 13: 115, 1972
36. French ME, Batchelor JR: Lancet 2:1103, 1969
37. Ceppellini R: in: Proceedings of the XXIII International Congress of Genetics, Berkeley, 1973 (in preparation)

Inhibition of In Vitro Lymphocyte Proliferation by Alloantisera in Genetically Controlled Immune Systems in Guinea Pigs

By Ira Green, E.M. Shevach, and William E. Paul

AT THIS meeting two spheres of immunological research converge, overlap and hopefully cross-fertilize each other, Fig. 1. The first sphere started at the very beginning of immunology and was and is concerned with the production of antibody and the structure of the antibody molecule, cellular immunity, the nature and chemical basis of immunogenicity, and the mechanisms by which antigens are recognized. The antigens used here were bacteria, bacterial products, soluble protein antigen, hapten protein conjugates, and finally synthetic poly α amino acid antigens. The work of Landsteiner on hapten protein conjugates can be considered an important landmark in this sphere of research.[1]

The second sphere of immunological research also had very early beginnings relating to tissue and tumor grafting. The modern era of this discipline started during World War II and was and is concerned with the nature of the immunity to cellular and tissue grafts. The availability of inbred mice rapidly allowed the discovery that the rejection of cellular grafts was based upon genetically determined antigenic differences between donor and host.[2] Investigation of this area of research received a tremendous stimulus when kidney transplantation in humans became a feasible technical possibility. A very large body of information concerning histocompatibility antigen on cells and their relationship to in vitro graft survival and in vitro lymphocyte responses has rapidly accumulated.

Although these two fields of immunological thinking and research have tended to remain somewhat separate, there are now strong forces which should rapidly bring them together. The first force is the discovery that the ability to form immune responses to both synthetic and complex protein antigens are genetically controlled and that these immune response genes (IR genes) are linked to the major histocompatibility locus of the species.[3-5] The second is the realization that an understanding of the immune process directed against complex cellular and tissue antigens can be obtained by studies of simpler antigens. It should eventually be possible to solubilize, separate, and identify individual cellular antigens and then to determine their role in immune recognition and its consequences.

One of the most pressing problems of modern immunobiology is the mechanism and chemical basis of antigen recognition by T cells and the mechanism of T-cell–B-cell cooperation.[6,7] A closely related question is whether immunoglobulin is present on the surface of T cells and if so, what function these molecules mediate. A number of different approaches have been used to attack these problems. First, can T cells be shown to bind antigen, and if so, by what can this binding be inhibited? Second, do T cells have immunoglobulin on their surface and in what quantity? Third, what type of reagents can inhibit T-cell functions in vivo and in vitro? Our laboratory (Drs. E. Shevach, W. E. Paul, and I. Green) has used the last approach to investigate this problem in an immune system in guinea pigs in which several immune responses to simpler synthetic antigens are determined by the presence of specific immune response

From the Laboratory of Immunology, National Institute of Allergy and Infectious Diseases, National Institutes of Health, Bethesda, Md.
©1973 by Grune & Stratton, Inc.

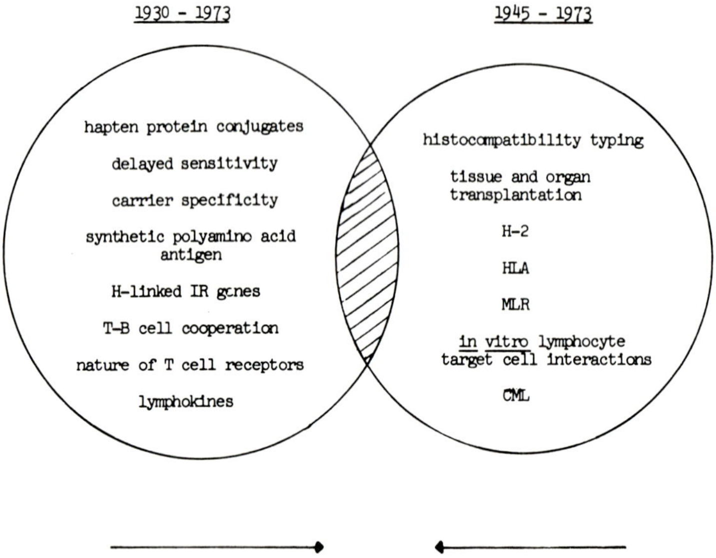

Fig. 1. Spheres of immunological research.

Table 1. Histocompatibility-linked Ir Genes in Guinea Pigs

Antigen	
Poly-L-lysine	Strain 2
Poly-L-arginine	
Protamine	
DNP–poly-L-lysine	
BSA (low dose)	
DNP–BSA (low dose)	
Glutamic acid–alanine copolymer	
Glutamic acid–tyrosine copolymer	Strain 13
DNP–guinea pig albumin (low dose)	

genes.[8-11] These IR genes are linked to genes controlling histocompatibility (H) type of the guinea pig. Since in this species in vitro cellular immune responses of guinea pigs are of considerable magnitude and relatively easy to study, this model is a particularly favorable one in which to explore the meaning of the genetic relationship between H types and IR genes.

The capacity to respond to a 2,4-dinitrophenylated copolymer of L-glutamic acid and L-lysine (DNP-GL) is controlled by an IR gene linked to strain 2 H genes, whereas the response to a copolymer of L-glutamic acid and L-tyrosine (GT) is controlled by an IR gene linked to strain-13 histocompatibility genes. These linkage relationships are shown in Table 1. (2 × 13)F_1 guinea pigs can respond to both DNP-GL and GT. When peritoneal exudate lymphocytes (PEL) from F_1 animals immunized to both DNP-GL and GT are cultured in the presence of either of these antigens, marked stimulation of ^3H thymidine incorporation is observed. The responsiveness of these F_1 cells offers an ideal situation in which to test the effect of various alloantisera on antigen induced in vitro proliferation.[12] As can be seen in Table 2, anti-2 serum can specifically block the transformation induced by DNP-GL in lymphocytes from F_1 animals, whereas an anti-13 serum specifically blocks proliferation induced by GT. Thus alloantisera block only that immune reaction determined by IR gene which is linked to the histocompatibility complex controlling the specificity to which the alloantisera are directed.

There are three general mechanisms which could lead to these results. First, the H-antigens and IR gene products are identical. Second, H antigens are very close to the IR gene product on the cell surface and antibodies to H antigen sterically block the function of the Ir gene product. Third, the alloantisera, in addition to containing

Table 2. Inhibition of Lymphocyte Proliferation, F_1 Animals

		Serum		
Stimulant	Normal	13 Anti-2	2 Anti-13	2 Anti-13 + 13 Anti-2
0	3,499*	1,479	1,484	1,494
DNP–GL	68,361 (1.21)†	1,231 (0.0)	46,385 (1.69)	2,178 (0.02)
GT	17,070 (0.25)	12,147 (0.25)	1,770 (0.01)	3,793 (0.07)
PPD	20,049 (0.31)	12,086 (0.25)	15,159 (0.51)	4,344 (0.09)
PHA	56,887 (1.00)	44,281 (1.00)	28,094 (1.00)	34,940 (1.00)

*Results are expressed as c.p.m./tube; each value is the mean of three determinants.

† Fraction of PHA response.

anti-H antibodies, also contain antibodies to IR gene products.

The following series of experiments was designed to explore these possibilities.[13] The alloantisera were absorbed with a variety of different lymphoid cell populations. Since peritoneal exudate lymphocyte (almost a pure population of T cells)[14] and thymocytes might be expected to have IR gene products displayed on their cell surface, absorbtion with these cells would be expected to be especially efficient in removing anti-IR gene product antibody from our alloantisera. However, the results shown in Table 3 indicate that these cell populations absorb inhibitory activity and cytotoxic activity much less efficiently than L_2C leukemia cells of strain-2 guinea pigs. Since the L_2C cells are derived from B cells, these data suggest that the relevant antigen is more represented on B than T cells,[15] and while this observation does not rule out the possibility that the inhibitory antibody is directed at the IR gene product itself, it makes this possibility somewhat less likely.

Table 3. Effect on Inhibitory Capacity of Alloantisera Following Absorption With Different Lymphoid Cell Populations*

	Δc.p.m.	% Cytotoxicity
Normal	26,567	0
Anti-2	940	33
Ab. with thymus	3,015	27
Ab. with L node	5,283	14
Ab. with PEL	1,250	30
Ab. with L_2C	15,858	0

*The response of F_1 animals immunized with DNP–GL. Δc.p.m. is the difference between the counts in the tubes with antigen minus the counts in the tubes without antigen. The alloantisera used was a 13 anti-2 serum.

Table 4. Associations of H and Ir Genes

Type of Guinea Pig	H	Ir
Inbred	2^+; 13^-	GL^+; GA^+; GT^-
	2^-; 13^+	GL^-; GA^-; GT^+
Outbred	2^+; 13^-	GL^+; GA^+; GT^-
	2^+; 13^+	GL^+; GA^+; GT^+
	2^-; 13^+	GL^-; GA^-; GT^+
	2^-; 13^+	GL^-; GA^+; GT^+

An alternative approach to the analysis of the exact specificity of the alloantisera is to explore the inhibitory capacity of such sera in genetic systems in which Ir and H have been separated by a recombination. Although no recombinant animals have been obtained from known matings, certain populations of random-bred guinea pigs display H-IR relationships consistent with a recombinational event having previously occurred. Table 4 presents linkage relationships between IR genes and H type in some outbred animals. In particular it can be seen that the response to a copolymer of

Table 5. Effect of Anti-2 Serum of GA Response of Hartley Guinea Pigs

	2^+ 13^+ GA^+ PLL^+		2^- 13^+ GA^+ PLL^-	
	Serum		Serum	
Antigen	NL	Anti-2	NL	Anti-2
0	2,989	2,250	845	810
DNP–PLL	37,218	6,284	1,256	1,040
GA	2,428	4,098	40,489	51,740
PPD	29,261	20,118	135,679	144,295

Table 6. Effect of 13 Anti-Hartley Serum on GA Response of Strain-2 Guinea Pigs

Antigen	Normal	13 Anti-2	13 Anti-2^+ GA^+	13 Anti-2^- GA^+
0	3,053	2,621	2,209	3,186
GL	35,044	5,057	1,911	35,862
GA	12,384	4,588	3,744	13,983
PPD	22,179	4,810	11,562	33,405
PHA	98,337	35,335	50,346	96,441

Table 7. Effect of Antiimmunoglobulin Sera on Lymphocyte Proliferation*

	NL Rabbit	Anti-Fab	Polyvalent
0	2,003	3,258	2,695
DNP–GL	53,728	53,623	41,269
GT	7,688	9,252	7,101
PPD	45,331	45,224	35,649
PHA	96,678	97,105	95,123

*Response of F_1 animals immunized to DNP–GL and GT.

L-glutamic acid and L-Alanine (GA) is linked to strain-2 H type in inbred animals but that in outbred Hartley animals, GA responsiveness often occurs in the absence of strain-2 H antigens. Upon testing the in vitro proliferative response to GA of PEL from outbred animals in which GA and 2 H specificity are linked, we observed that GA response is inhibited by an anti-2 alloserum (Table 5). However, if the same alloantiserum is tested with lymphocytes of an outbred animal that is GA responsive but strain-2 negative, the alloantisera fail to inhibit the GA response.

Similarly, if strain-13 guinea pigs are immunized with cells from either 2 positive, GA responsive or 2 negative GA responsive animals, only the anti-2 positive sera inhibit GA responses of strain-2 or (2 × 13)F_1 cells. The 13 anti-2 negative GA positive sera failed to inhibit (Table 6). Taken together these experiments suggest that the inhibitory alloantisera do not contain an antibody to the GA IR gene product, and thus the inhibition observed is probably due to antisera recognizing that H antigen. It would appear therefore, both from the data from the GA system last given and the absorption experiments with various cell populations, that the most likely general explanation for the inhibitory effect of alloantisera is that they have chiefly anti-H specificity and that they inhibit because H antigens and IR gene products are closely placed on the surface of antigen responsive cells.

As a final experiment designed to explore the nature of the recognition factor on guinea pig T cells, we employed various rabbit anti-guinea pig immunoglobulin sera in the in vitro assay. Here 10% rabbit polyspecific anti Ig antisera, anti-Fab antisera, or normal rabbit sera were used in the cultures of PEL with antigen (Table 7). The rabbit anti-immunoglobulin sera failed to inhibit the antigen induced lymphocyte proliferative response. Although the failure to inhibit with guinea pig anti-Ig sera cannot be regarded as definitive evidence that Ig is not the T-cell receptor, this result, together with our demonstration of the potency of alloantisera in such inhibition, strongly suggests that a molecule other than Ig, such as the Ir gene product, may have a crucial role in antigen recognition by T lymphocytes.

REFERENCES

1. Landsteiner K: The Specificity of Serological Reactions. New York, Dover, revised edition, 1962
2. Billingham RE, Brent L, Medawar PE: Phil Trans Roy Soc (Lond) Ser B 239:357, 1956
3. McDevitt HO, Benacerraf B: Advan Immunol 11:31, 1969
4. Ellman L, Green I, Martin WJ, et al: Proc Natl Acad Sci USA 66:322, 1970
5. Benacerraf B, McDevitt HO: Science 175:273, 1972
6. Raff MC, Nature New Biol 242:19, 1973
7. Crone M, Hoch C, Simonsen M: Transplant Rev 10:35, 1972
8. Benacerraf B, Green I, Paul WE: Cold Spring Harbor Symposia on Quantative Biology 32:569, 1967
9. Green I, Ellman L, Martin WJ, et al: in Karper S (ed): in Second International Convocation of Immunology, 1971, p 76
10. Bluestein HG, Green I, Benacerraf B: J Exp Med 134:571, 1971

11. Bluestein HG, Ellman L, Green I, et al: J Exp Med 134:1529, 1971
12. Shevach EM, Paul WE, Green I: J Exp Med 136:1207, 1972
13. Shevach EM, Paul WE, Green I: manuscripts in preparation
14. Rosenstreich DL, Blake JI, Rosenthal AS: J Exp Med 134:1170, 1971
15. Shevach EM, Rosenstreich DL, Green I: Transplantation 16:126, 1973

Modulation of Cell-mediated Lympholysis by Alloantisera

By G. Cordier, H. Betuel, and J.P. Revillard

THE mixed lymphocyte reaction (MLC) and subsequent cell-mediated lympholysis (CML) can be regarded as an in vitro correlate of the allograft reaction including antigenic recognition, sensitization, and destruction of the allogeneic target. Alloantibodies are known to interfere with the cellular response in vivo at different levels from the induction to the effector phase. Alloantibodies can either cooperate with lymphoid cells, in the allograft rejection[1] or inhibit the cellular response; the latter effect is known as immunological enhancement or facilitation.[2] MLC and CML provide appropriate models for the study of the basic mechanisms of interaction between alloantibodies and the cellular response.

MATERIALS AND METHOD

MLC was performed with human peripheral blood lymphocytes according to a technique already described.[3] Stimulating cells (subscript m) were prepared by exposure to Mitomycin C according to Bach and Voynow.[4]

CML was performed according to the original technique of Lightbody et al.[5] with some minor modifications introduced by Bonnard[6] and Miggiano.[7] Chromium-labeled PHA-lymphoblasts were used as targets; the effector cells are the mixture of responding and stimulating lymphocytes (e.g. XYm) after 5 days of coculture and used at ratio of 50 viable cells per target.

Lymphocyte-mediated cytotoxicity (LMC). LMC measures target-cell lysis by peripheral blood lymphocytes from individuals sensitized by blood transfusion or pregnancy. Our technique for LMC is similar to that described by Garovoy et al.[8] although PHA lymphoblasts instead of lymphocytes were used as targets in our experiments.

Lymphocyte-dependent antibodies (LDA) were assessed using again the same target. In this system cytotoxicity is achieved by the addition of alloantibodies directed against the target and unsensitized peripheral blood lymphocytes at a ratio of 50:1.

Alloantisera were obtained from primipara or multipara. All of them had anti HL-A cytotoxic complement-dependent antibodies. Some of them were considered monospecific when tested on a panel of lymphocytes using Terasaki's two steps microlymphocytotoxicity,[9] while others showed broader specificity. They were heat inactivated before use.

RESULTS AND DISCUSSION

Antibody-induced Lymphocyte-mediated Cytotoxicity

Without addition of complement, alloantibodies can induce cytotoxicity in the presence of non phagocytic, nonadherent small lymphocytes bearing a Fc receptor. This reaction is similar to that described in other systems by E. Moller,[10] P. Perlmann,[11] and I.C.M. Mc Lennan.[12] The following observations with LDA are important for the discussion of antibody modulation of CML:

Lysis does not require sensitized lymphocytes; fresh lymphocytes or unsensitized autologous mixture (XXm) can be used as effectors.

Lysis can be achieved with effector cells isogeneic with target in the presence of anti-target antisera.

Antibodies directed against effector cells do not significantly impair cytotoxicity as shown in the following experiment: target HLA (1, 3, W14); effector HL-A (1, 2, W17); specific chromium release was 55.3% ± 5.7% with anti-3, 0.8% ± 2.3% with anti-2, and 57.8% ± 3.8% with anti-3 + anti-2.

These results indicate that antibody-induced cytotoxicity can occur in any system where alloantibodies (LDA) and lymphocytes are present. This effect should therefore be measured using appropriate controls, in order to detect possible block-

From the Laboratoire d'Immunologie, unité INSERM U80, Hôpital de l'Antiquaille, and Centre de Transfusion Sanguine de Lyon, Beynost, France.
©*1973 by Grune & Stratton, Inc.*

Table 1. Modulation of LMC by Alloantisera Target: PHA Lymphoblasts HLA 1, 2, W17

	LDA (Effector 11, W5, 7)	LMC (Effector 1, 3, W14)	% LMC Inhibition
0	0 ± 2.7	32.9 ± 4.8	0
Anti-2 1/40	11.6 ± 5.0	26.3 ± 5.9	−43.3
1/80	16.0 ± 2.5	15.3 ± 3.9	−85.2
Anti-3 1/40	4.2 ± 2.5	9.1 ± 4.3	−62.5
1/80	3.9 ± 5.4	1.7 ± 3.6	−73.4

ing or potentiating effects of alloantisera in the cytotoxic reactions (LMC and CML).

Modulation of LMC by Alloantisera

A typical experiment is represented in Table 1; the same monospecific antisera are tested on the same target in the presence of unsensitized lymphocytes (LDA) or sensitized lymphocytes (LMC) from a multiparous woman. Sensitized lymphocytes induce significant lysis in normal AB serum; anti-2 antiserum has little LDA activity at the dilutions tested, anti-3 has no significant LDA activity on a 3-negative target. Addition of antibodies against the target or against the effector cells in the LMC test significantly reduces the lysis. If one assumes that cytotoxicity induced by LDA and by sensitized lymphocytes are independent phenomena, it is then possible to define an inhibition index which measures the blocking effect of alloantibodies in LMC. If s stands for spontaneous chromium release, t for chromium release with sensitized lymphocytes and normal serum, a for release with sensitized lymphocytes and antiserum and b for release with normal lymphocyte and antiserum (LDA), the inhibition index is

$$\frac{(a - s) - [(t - s) + (b - s)]}{(t - s) + (b - s)} \times 100.$$

A negative index reflects a blocking effect whereas a positive index indicates a potentiating effect of the antiserum.

In most cases antitarget antibodies inhibit LMC as expected from the results obtained from animal systems.[13] In addition, antisera against sensitized effector lymphocytes may block the reaction as shown in Table 1.

Modulation of CML by Alloantisera

When alloantibodies directed either against stimulator or responding lymphocytes are added at the beginning of the MLC the proliferative response is suppressed.[14,3,15,16] The subsequent lysis performed in normal serum is also inhibited, indicating that the proliferative response is important for the differentiation of the effector cells. These results are in agreement with those of Phillips et al. in the mouse[17] and of Trinchieri et al. in man.[18] Inhibition of the sensitizing phase can be achieved with highly diluted antisera (>1 : 1000); it is likely to be attributed to non-HL-A as well as HL-A antibodies.[3,15] When antisera are introduced during the proliferation phase, 3 days after the beginning of the MLC, blocking effect can still be achieved providing higher concentrations of antisera are used.

The possible role of LDA in blocking MLC by reciprocal killing of the lymphocytes cannot be definitely excluded though it seems quite unlikely since the proliferative response to phytomitogens by lymphocytes incubated 6–9 days with blocking antisera remains normal.

When alloantibodies are introduced at the effector stage, after in vitro sensitization by MLC in normal serum, several independent effects can be observed as described after in vivo sensitization in LMC. Inhibition index is defined according to the above-mentioned formula adapted to the in vitro system where XYm represents the

Table 2. Modulation of CML by Alloantisera: +Potentiating Effect; −Blocking Effect

AS	5^{-1}	25^{-1}	100^{-1}
309	+108.0	+ 2.9	
309	+ 23.0	+19.1	
226	+ 51.0	+12.0	− 3.0
297	+ 53.0	+23.0	
226	− 31.0	−57.0	−73.0
297	− 66.2	−77.2	−36.0
291	− 75.1	−73.1	
291	− 60.9	−67.3	

sensitized lymphocytes tested on a target Y and XXm or YYm the unsensitized lymphocytes used to measure the LDA effect. In this system LDA activity was found whenever the antiserum was direct against the target. This confirms similar observations reported by Trinchieri et al. as the lymphocyte antibody lympholytic interaction (LALI) phenomenon.[18] After correction for LDA, alloantisera can either inhibit or potentiate the CML as shown on Table 2. The blocking effect is similar to that observed in LMC but differs in several features from MLC inhibition: Blocking of effector stages requires higher concentrations of antisera, and it has not been so far observed when the antiserum was not directed against the HL-A specificities carried by the target. We do not yet know whether antibodies restricted to effector cells specificities have any blocking effect in this system. Conversely, in several experiments, addition of antisera against effector and target resulted in an increased cytotoxicity. This might be attributed to an improved cell-to-cell contact between effectors and targets due to agglutination. However, other as-yet unknown mechanisms for cooperation between antibodies and sensitized lymphocytes cannot be excluded as suggested by in vivo experiments.[19,20]

If these in vitro models are not artifactual, they might provide relevant data to the possible use of alloantibodies in attempts to modulate the cellular response elicited by allografts in vivo. It would seem indeed that inhibition of the induction of the immune response (afferent blocking) would be more readily achieved that interference of effector cells with the target (efferent blocking).

REFERENCES

1. Voisin GA: in Amos DB (ed): Progress in Immunology. New York, Academic, 1971, p 193
2. Voisin GA, Prog Allergy 15:328, 1971
3. Robert M, Betuel H, Revillard JP, Tissue Antigens 3:39, 1973
4. Bach FH, Voynow NK: Science 153:545, 1966
5. Lightbody J, Bernoco D, Miggiano VC, et al: J Bact Virol Immunol 64:243, 1971
6. Bonnard GD, Lemos L: Transplant Proc IV:177, 1972
7. Miggiano VC, Bernoco D, Lightbody J, et al: Transplant Proc IV:231, 1972
8. Garovoy MR, Franco V, Zschaeck D, et al: Lancet 1:573, 1973
9. Mittal KK, Mickey MR, Singal DP, et al: Transplantation 6:913, 1968
10. Möller E: Science 147:873, 1965
11. Perlmann P, Perlmann H: Cell Immunol 1:300, 1970
12. Mc Lennan ICM, Loewi G, Harding B: Immunology 18:397, 1970
13. Brunner KT, Mauel J, Cerottini JC, et al: Immunology 14:181, 1968
14. Ceppellini R, Bonnard GD, Coppo F, et al: Transplant Proc III:58, 1971
15. Revillard JP, Betuel H, Robert M: Cell Immunol 8:339, 1973
16. Revillard JP, Robert M, Dupond E, et al: Transplant Proc V:331, 1973
17. Phillips SM, Strom TB, Corson JM, et al: Daguillard F (ed): Proceedings of the Seventh Leucocyte Culture Conference. New York, Academic, 1973, p 601
18. Trinchieri G, Bernoco D, Curtoni SE, et al: in Dausset J (ed): Histocompatibility Testing. Copenhagen, Munksgaard, 1972, p 509
19. Batchelor JR, Boyse EA, Gorer PA: Transplant Bull 26:449, 1960
20. Voisin GA, Toullet F: in Immunology and Reproduction, International Planned Parenthood Fed, London, 1969, p 93

Specificity of Antibodies That Inhibit the MLC Response

By E. Thorsby and B. G. Solheim

As FIRST shown by Ceppellini and coworkers,[1] HL-A antisera can inhibit the MLC response. This has later been confirmed in several laboratories. It is largely unknown, however, whether the antibodies having HL-A specificity are responsible for the inhibitory effect, or whether this is a function of other (nonlymphocytotoxic) antibodies in the sera, recognizing the MLC locus product. Our own studies have been particularly directed towards this question, and the following is a short summary and discussion of some of our results. Most of our methods have been described previously in this series.[2]

RESULTS

(1) We recently reported some studies on a monospecific anti-HL-A12 serum, as determined by complement-dependent lymphocytotoxicity (CDL), which was able to completely inhibit both stimulating and responding cells in MLC tests.[2] The blocking activity was not only confined to HL-A12 positive cells; MLC tests involving HL-A12 negative combinations were also often inhibited. The serum was investigated by an antibody-dependent cell-mediated cytotoxicity test,[3] using different lymphocytes preincubated with the serum as target cells.[4] By this more sensitive method, it could be demonstrated that the serum was multispecific and contained more lymphocyte reactive antibodies than shown by CDL. However, we do not yet know whether these other antibodies are weak HL-A antibodies, or directed against the MLC locus product or other cell membrane components.

From the Tissue Typing Laboratory, Rikshospitalet University Hospital, Oslo, Norway.

Financial support from Anders Jahre's Fund for the Promotion of Science.

©1973 by Grune & Stratton, Inc.

To study whether antibodies having HL-A specificity were responsible for at least some of the inhibitory effects of the serum, it was absorbed with an excess of buffy coat cells from different HL-A12 positive and negative individuals.[2] The result of one experiment is given in Fig. 1. It can be seen that absorption with HL-A12 positive cells grossly impaired the inhibitory activity of the serum, while absorption with HL-A12 negative cells had no effect. If the antibodies causing inhibition were directed against MLC locus products, one would have expected that absorption with some HL-A12 negative cells also removed inhibitory antibodies, and that absorption with some HL-A12 positive cells not always removed inhibitory antibodies. Thus, our results indicate that antibodies directed against HL-A antigens of stimulating or responding cells, can inhibit the MLC response.

(2) HL-A typing and MLC data in a family (I.K.) are given in Table 1. It can be seen that the mother and father share the HL-A2, 12 haplotypic combination, but are different at their MLC loci of both haplotypes (x/y and z/v, respectively). If the 2, 12 haplotypes had been identical at their MLC loci, cells from the father should not be able to stimulate lymphocytes from child No. 5 and vice versa. The mother was reimmunized with leucocytes from the father, and strong cytotoxic anti-HL-A11 and anti-W5 antibodies were detected in maternal serum, which was then used as serum source in MLC tests. The table shows that maternal serum was able to inhibit strongly combinations which involved cells carrying the paternal haplotype 11, W5, y. However, only a very slight or no inhibitory effect was observed in combinations of cells which only carried the other haplotype from the father; 2, 12, x. Thus, the blocking

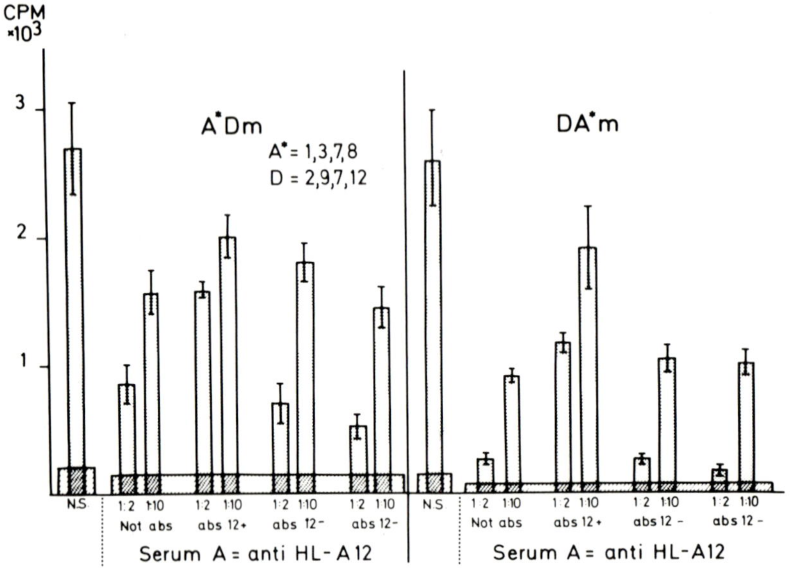

Fig. 1. Result of MLC tests between two unrelated individuals A* and D, expressed as mean cpm of triplicates ± SE. The shaded areas at the bottom of the columns are the mean cpm in the autologous controls (A*A*m and DDm). As serum source is used either normal AB serum (N.S.), or serum A before and after absorption with third-party HL-A12 pos. and neg. cells, diluted 1:2 and 1:10 in AB serum. The serum concentration is kept constant at 20% in the culture medium.

antibodies most probably have HL-A specificity, and/or only react with products of MLC locus allele *y*.

Note that the MLC response between cells from the father and child No. 5, which both possess the 11, W5, y haplotype, is inhibited to a lesser degree by the immune serum. We have also observed in other experiments that MLC inhibition may sometimes be less pronounced when both stimulating and responding cells share the HL-A antigen(s) which are recognized by a given HL-A antiserum.

(3) To study whether all antibodies which react with lymphocyte cell membrane components, irrespective of their specificity, can block the MLC response, we used a hyperimmune blood group anti-A serum. Neither the whole serum nor the IgG fraction from it was able to inhibit MLC tests involving either stimulating or responding cells from individuals of blood group A; see Fig. 2. To remove possible noncytotoxic HL-A antibodies from the serum, it was first absorbed with the lymphocytes from individual E (blood group 0), and then used for preincubation of lymphocytes from the individuals E and F. The cells were washed after incubation, and re-incubated with fluorescein labelled anti-Ig. We then observed immunofluorescence of lymphocytes from blood group A positive individuals with aggregation and some caps, while this was only observed on about 5% of the lymphocytes from individuals of blood group 0.

COMMENTS

We were not able in our experiments, therefore, to demonstrate that all antibodies that react with the lymphocyte cell membrane and cause redistribution of its components are able to inhibit the MLC response. On the other hand, antibodies having HL-A specificity seem to be able to cause MLC inhibition.

It must be emphasized that our results certainly do not exclude the possibility that many antisera owe their inhibitory activity, at least partly, to antibodies directed against the MLC/Ir loci or other products. In studies by Dorf et al.,[5] extensive immunization in HL-A identical MLC positive unrelated combinations did not give rise to antibodies which were able to inhibit the MLC response. However, HL-A differences may also be needed for production of antibodies against the MLC locus

Table 1. MLC Data in Family I.K. in Normal and Immune Maternal Serum

Stimulating Cells		Responding Cells													
		F		M		C_1		C_2		C_3		C_4		C_5	
F	2,12,x/11,W5,y	283	41	9379	1368*	3411	681*	2982	288*	4287	184*	4218	576*	1494	830
M	1,5,z/2,12,v	7060	147*	270	260	3950	3093	3219	2361	4066	2930	3210	2826	2859	199*
C_1	2,12,x/2,12,v	4130	328*	3002	1664	261	249	2853	1938	3034	2343	150	88	2621	514*
C_2	2,12,x/1,5,z	2869	124*	2884	1792	2204	2145	155	82	190	85	3151	1646	5214	549*
C_3	2,12,x/1,5,z	4152	105*	4069	2929	3526	2713	200	183	257	168	3978	3132	4083	255*
C_4	2,12,x/2,12,v	3969	329*	2886	1419	236	225	2630	1102(*)	2565	1809	147	118	2290	619*
C_5	11,W5,y/2,12,z	3816	493*	6243	492*	4489	289*	6284	477*	4493	189*	2982	513*	59	42

x, y, z, and v designate alleles at the hypothetical MLC locus (loci).

The first entry in each column is mean cpm of triplicates in normal serum, the last entry values in maternal immune serum. The values marked with an asterisk represent inhibition of the MLC response by maternal serum to less than 50% of the response in normal serum.

Mitomycin controls: Fm Mm: 218, Mm C_1m: 132.

SE: Usually less than 10% of the mean.

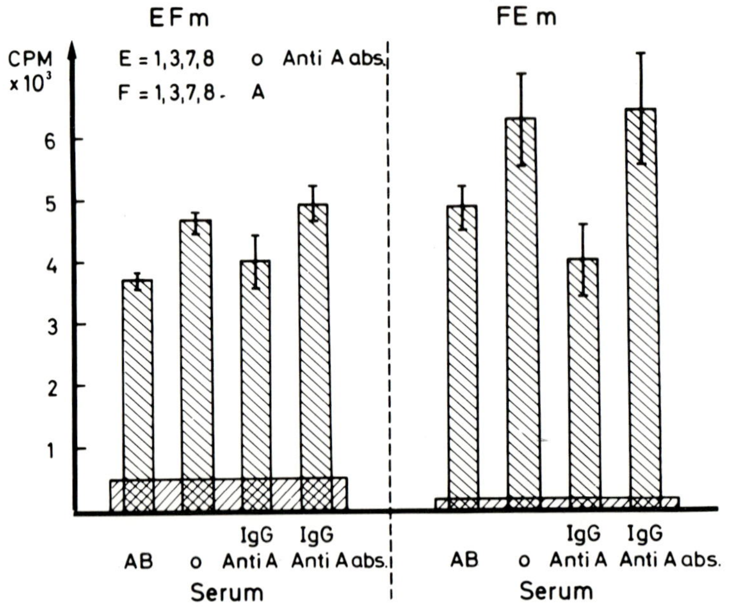

Fig. 2. Result of MLC tests between two HL-A identical unrelated individuals, E being blood group O, and F being blood group A, expressed as in Fig. 1. As serum source is used either normal AB serum (AB) normal O serum (O), or the IgG fraction from the anti-blood-group A serum resuspended in AB serum.

product. On the other hand, our studies of family I.K. demonstrate that HL-A differences do not always give rise to antibodies against incompatible MLC locus products.

If HL-A antibodies are able to inhibit the MLC response, one might have expected that the inhibitory activity of a given serum follows more closely the HL-A specificity of the serum, as detected by CDL. However, a lower concentration of antibodies seems to cause inhibition of the MLC interaction than that needed for complement dependent lymphocytotoxicity. Thus, while CDL tests may not be able to detect all anti HL-A antibodies in a given serum, tests involving MLC inhibition might be able to pick up weaker antibody components also of possible HL-A specificity. This might explain at least some of the observations of strong MLC inhibition also by sera which are negative in CDL tests. On the other hand, it would be an argument against this interpretation if cytotoxic HL-A antisera were found that were not able to inhibit MLC tests involving either stimulating or responding cells possessing the corresponding HL-A antigen(s). However, the possibility still exists that the various Ig classes or subclasses differ in their lymphocytotoxic and MLC blocking efficiency. The lymphocytotoxic HL-A antisera we have tested so far have all inhibited the MLC response involving stimulating or responding cells possessing the corresponding HL-A antigens, with the exception that inhibition may be weak when *both* stimulating and responding cells possess the corresponding HL-A antigen(s). The nature of this latter phenomenon is currently under study.

Further studies are needed to confirm that antibodies having HL-A specificity are able to inhibit the MLC response. If this is shown to be the case, it will strongly suggest that the products of the HL-A and MLC loci are closely linked also in the cell membrane, possibly as different components of a molecular complex.

REFERENCES

1. Ceppellini R: in Amos DB (ed): Progress in Immunology. New York, Academic, 1971, p 973
2. Thorsby E, Bondevik H, Solheim BG: Transplant Proc 5:343, 1973
3. MacLennan ICM: Transplant Rev 13:67, 1973
4. Kaakinen A, Kiss E, Thorsby E: to be published
5. Dorf ME, Eguro SY, Flye MW, et al: Transplantation 15:253, 1973

Phenotypic Expression of the Main Histocompatibility Complex (DL-A) in Randomly Selected Mongrel Dogs: III. Inhibition of the Mixed Leukocyte Culture Reaction During and After Sensitization to Skin Allografts

By R. Bachvaroff, A. Ozaki, F.D. Cannon, N. Mollen, D.A. Blumenstock, J.H. Ayvazian, J.W. Ferrebee, and F.T. Rapaport*

A RAPIDLY growing array of evidence has accumulated to indicate that antibodies directed against major histocompatibility antigens have the capability of inhibiting in vitro reactions between lymphocytes and target cells.[1-3] Such results have been obtained with HL-A-specific antisera produced in response to host immunization by repeated transfusions of whole fresh blood from the same donor,[4] as well as with sera obtained from human renal allograft recipients and multiparous women. The specificity of the induced blocking effect has been highlighted particularly by the observations of Ceppellini and his associates[4] and by the findings of Revillard et al.[6] that sera from human kidney transplant recipients could inhibit the response of recipient lymphocytes against donor cells but not against the cells obtained from some other recipients. This serum blocking factor was identified as a 7S IgG by chromatographic analysis[7] and appears to be mainly directed against kidney donor's lymphocytes, although occasionally also against cells from other sources.[7] Thorsby, Bondevik, and Solheim[8] have provided additional evidence of the inhibitory effect of HL-A-specific typing antisera on the MLC reaction.

A particularly interesting feature of the inhibition of in vitro lymphocyte transformation by HL-A-specific antibodies has been the observation by Ceppellini et al.,[4] Grumet and Leventhal,[9] and Buckley, Schiff, and Amos,[10] that treatment of the responding cells with HL-A SD-specific antisera also interferes with their response to PHA, as well as to a variety of soluble antigens, such as tuberculin, tetanus toxoid, diphtheria toxoid, or candida albicans, if cells are obtained from donors who are sensitive to these antigens. Lueker and Williams[11] have also observed decreased lymphocyte reactivity in MLC tests performed with cells obtained from patients with acute rheumatic fever, even when such cells were mixed with lymphocytes obtained from normal patients. The possibility that the decreased reactivity of lymphocytes observed in such studies was related to the presence in the serum of donors with acute rheumatic fever of streptococcal antibodies cross-reacting with human tissues was supported by the demonstration of strong reactions against myocardium[12] by the sera of three of the six patients reported in that study. The recent demonstration of the ability of soluble extracts of group-A type-12 streptococcal membranes (TGCM) to bind tightly to the lymphocyte membrane surface[13] and to inhibit absorption of HL-A and of species-specific antibodies to cell surfaces treated in this manner[14] may provide an alternative explanation for these findings and is in keeping with earlier find-

*Irma T. Hirschl Career Scientist Award.

From the Department of Surgery and Institute of Reconstructive Plastic Surgery, New York University Medical Center; the Research Service, Manhattan Veterans Administration Hospital, New York, N.Y.; and the Mary Imogene Bassett Hospital, Cooperstown, N.Y.

Supported by NIH grants AI-10658-01A1 and AM-02215, grants from the John A. Hartford Foundation, the Billy Rose Foundation, and the Irwin Strasburger Memorial Medical Foundation, and USAEC contract AT-(30-1)-2005.

© 1973 by Grune & Stratton, Inc.

ings of the ability of HL-A-specific antibodies to interfere with in vitro cellular responses to PHA and to soluble antigens.[4,9,10] The close spatial relationships reported to exist between HL-A-specific, species-specific, and TGCM binding sites on the lymphocyte surface[13-15] may also be of direct relevance to this question.

In spite of the potential importance of these data in transplantation and in the study of variables conditioning host resistance to disease, there has been a relative paucity of studies designed to provide in vivo correlations to the in vitro findings—particularly in experimental transplantation under conditions permitting the performance of serial MLC tests before, during, and after allograft rejection. Among studies of this type performed thus far, there has been relative disagreement on the effects of allograft rejection upon subsequent MLC reactivity of recipient cells against the donor,[16-21] in contrast to the consistent in vitro data described above.[1-10] These findings prompted the present study of the evolution of the MLC test in a panel of unrelated mongrel dogs of known DL-A SD phenotypes and known preoperative MLC reactivity against each other's cells.[22] The results indicate that early sensitization to skin allografts and allograft rejections are regularly associated in dogs with marked inhibitions of MLC reactivity of host cells against lymphocytes obtained from the graft donor(s), as well as against cells from some but not all other dogs tested. The inhibition of MLC reactivity persisted for as long as 19 days after the rejection of first-set grafts, i.e., after complete healing of the graft recipient site. The state of MLC nonreactivity does not interfere with the host's ability to exhibit donor-specific second- and third-set skin allograft rejection responses or with the hyperacute rejection of a renal allograft obtained from the same donor.

MATERIALS AND METHOD

The experimental animals were members of a panel of eight mongrel dogs whose DL-A SD phenotypes were determined by standard lymphocytotoxicity tests utilizing a battery of antisera detecting 12 different DL-A specificities.[22] Baseline MLC reactions were performed in quadruplicate by the method of Hartzman et al.[23] utilizing lymphocytes of each member of the panel as responder cells against stimulating cells obtained from the remaining seven dogs. Full-thickness first-set skin allografts obtained from two donors of known DL-A SD phenotypes and MLC reactivity with the recipients were then performed,[24] and all MLC tests were repeated on the third to the fifth day after transplantation and at 17–19 days after skin graft rejection. The techniques of skin transplantation and criteria for the determination of graft rejection have been described in detail previously.[25] Fourteen second-set grafts from the same donors were performed within 17 to 29 days after first-set skin allograft rejection, and 11 third-set grafts were transplanted to the same recipients within 5 to 9 days after second-set rejection.

Within 6 to 11 days after rejection of the third-set skin grafts, seven of the recipients underwent bilateral nephrectomies and were transplanted with a kidney allograft obtained from one of their specific skin graft donors. All renal allografts were placed into the pelvis of the recipients by a standard technique.[26] The criteria for kidney transplant rejection have also been described in detail in previous publications.[25,26]

RESULTS

Table 1 summarizes the survival of skin and kidney allografts in this series of mongrel dogs. First-set skin grafts had a mean survival time (MST) of 9.06 days (span, 7–14 days). Second-set grafts given within 17 to 29 days after first-set rejection had an MST of 6.79 days (span, 6–8 days). When the interval between second- and third-set grafts was reduced to 5 to 9 days, the MST of third-set grafts from the same donors was 4.09 days (span, 3–5 days); three of the third-set grafts had the characteristics of mixed white graft reactions.[27-33] None of the seven kidneys obtained from one of the specific skin graft donors and transplanted into the recipient within 6 to 11 days after third-set skin graft rejection functioned beyond the third postoperative day. Three of the recipients were sacrificed on the second day, and the remainder were autopsied on the third day. All transplants had the gross and microscopic features of the type of allograft re-

Table 1. Results of Skin and Kidney Allograft Survivals in a Panel of Mongrel Dogs of Known DL-A SD* Phenotypes and MLC† Reactivity

				Survival of Skin Allografts					Survival of Kidney Allografts	
Donor (B) No.	Recipient (A) No.	Serologic Incompatibility for DL-A SD‡ Antigen(s)	MLC Reactivity of Donor Cells to Recipient §	1st Sef (days)	Interval Before 2nd Set (days)	2nd Set (days)	Interval Before 3rd Set (days)	3rd Set (days)	Interval Before Kidney Allografts (days)	Survival Time of Kidney Allografts (days)
879	877	c	ō	8	28	6	8	5	6	3
884		c	+	9	27	5	9	3	—	—
881	878	ō	+	8	28	8	6	4	9	3
882		ō	+	7	29	7	7	3	—	—
883	879	b	ō	10	25	8	—	—	—	—
884		l	+	9	26	8	5	4	10	2
881	880	l,g	+	8	27	6	8	4	11	2
883		e	ō	8	27	6	—	—	—	—
880	881	b,k	+	8	27	6	8	4	11	2
884		k,e	+	7	28	6	—	—	—	—
879	882	k,c,n	ō	14	21	7	7	5	—	—
884		k,c,n	+	8	27	6	8	4	8	3
879	883	b,g	ō	10	—	—	—	—	—	—
882		l,g	+	11	—	—	—	—	—	—
879	884	l	+	10	25	8	5	4	10	3
882		ō	ō	10	17	8	—	5	—	—

*Serologically detectable.

†Mixed leucocyte culture

‡DL-A SD antigenic differences are expressed by the terminology of Dausset et al.[38]

§Criteria of MLC reactivity are expressed in accordance with the criteria of Bachvaroff et al.[22]

sponse commonly associated with hyperacute kidney transplant rejection.[34–36]

As noted in Fig. 1, the levels of MLC stimulation of host responder cells by lymphocytes obtained from the skin graft donors ranged from 15.25 × 10^3 (dog 879) to 49.95 × 10^3 counts per minute (c.p.m.) of ^{3}H thymidine incorporation (mean rate of incorporation, 26.85 × 10^3 c.p.m.) compared with control rates ranging from 350 to 2970 c.p.m. (mean rate of incorporation, 1468 c.p.m.). Within 3 to 5 days after application of the first-set skin allograft, MLC tests performed with the same cells and under the same conditions had a rate of ^{3}H thymidine incorporation that ranged from 125 to 3246 c.p.m. (mean rate of incorporation, 1074 c.p.m.). At 17 to 19 days after first-set graft rejection, the same MLC tests had a rate of ^{3}H thymidine incorporation that ranged from 61 to 8369 c.p.m. (mean rate of incorporation, 1455 c.p.m.). Note that recipient 881 is listed twice, since he was tested with skin allografts obtained from two donors, both of whose lymphocytes stimulated cells obtained from recipient 881 in the MLC.

Studies of the specificity of the inhibition of MLC reactivity observed after first-set skin allograft sensitization indicated that the recipients' lymphocytes were hyporeactive or nonreactive to cells obtained from the specific donors of skin as well as to cells obtained from some but not all other donors, as one would anticipate in view of the evidence of shared histocompatibility antigens in outbred mammalian populations.[37,38] It must also be noted that all MLC tests were done with repeatedly BSS-washed cells that were cultured in pooled serum obtained from normal dogs and that the same pool of normal serum was used in each of the experiments presented in this report. This consideration and the repeated washing of reactive and stimulator cells in BSS prior to each MLC

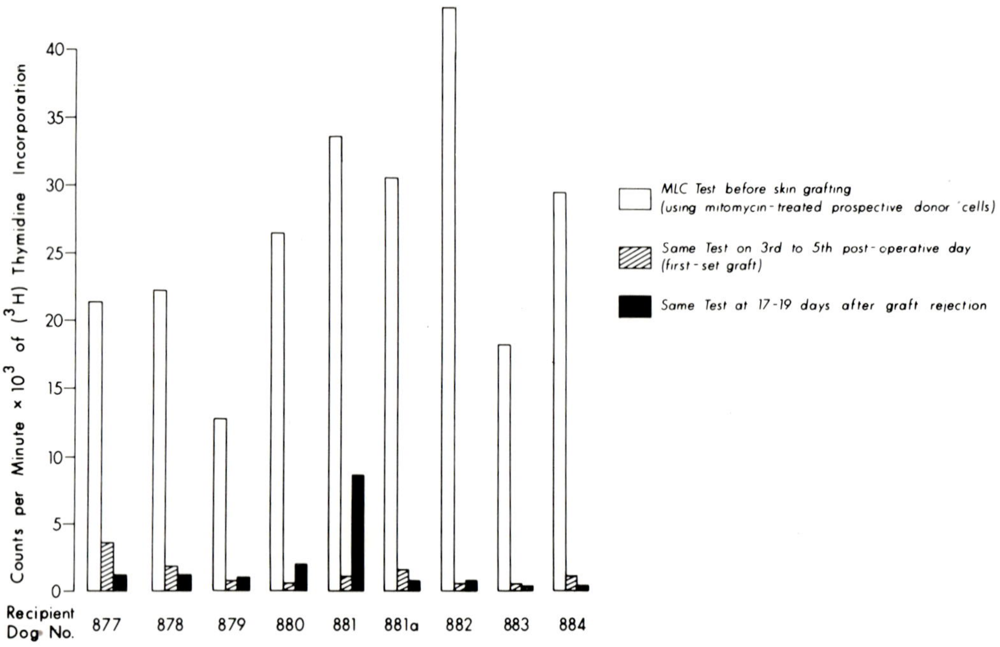

Fig. 1. Alterations in MLC reactivity during and after sensitization to skin allografts in mongrel dogs.

test militate against interpretation of the results as a consequence of the presence in the cultures of significant levels of antibodies directed against the donor's histocompatibility antigens. The test system used does not, however, rule out the potential effectiveness of such serologic factors in the inhibition of the same type of MLC tests under different experimental conditions (i.e., by addition of host serum instead of normal pooled serum.[18,20]

DISCUSSION

The results of this study present convincing evidence that the events of sensitization to and rejection of skin allografts are associated with a marked inhibition in the ability of host cells to develop MLC reactivity against lymphocytes obtained from the graft donor or from some but not other donors.[37,38] The inhibition of MLC reactivity was observed as early as the third to the fifth day after the application of a first-set skin allograft and is in keeping with earlier reports that exposure of the host to skin allografts for as little as 48 hr can induce sensitivity to subsequent skin grafts obtained from the same donor.[39-41]

The observations are in general agreement with earlier reports that some of the serologic consequences (HL-A antibodies) of allosensitization in man result in products capable of inhibiting MLC reactivity in man.[4-8] They are also in harmony with similar findings by Miller et al.[18] after the placement of renal allografts into the neck of canine recipients, although the inhibition of MLC reactivity in the present study was not dependent upon the presence of recipient plasma in the culture media. All of these results are at variance, however, with the reports of Oppenheim, Whang, and Frei[16,17] of increases in host lymphocyte proliferation in the MLC test after first- and second-set skin allografts in human subjects.

The observation that there is still a strong inhibition of host MLC reactivity as late as 17 to 19 days after the rejection of a first-set skin allograft, i.e., at a time when the graft receptor site has become fully healed, would appear to militate against the general interpretation[19] that decreased lymphocyte reactivity in the MLC test may be a consequence of the sequestration of immunoreactive cells at the graft site. It is also of interest that the inhibition in MLC reactivity observed in the present study did not appear to interfere with the ability of the host to muster accelerated rejection responses to second- or third-set skin grafts from the same donor or to reject a kidney allograft from the same donor in hyperacute fashion.

The loss of MLC reactivity at a time when the host is evidently capable of rejecting tissues from the same donor at an accelerated rate is in keeping with the suggestion that the MLC reaction constitutes an expression of the recognition phase of allograft rejection.[42] It is possible that once the cell population involved in the MLC response has served its function and has transmitted the required information to killer lymphocytes, it may undergo membrane surface changes or other alterations (including cell death) that make such cell clones no longer available for further MLC tests with lymphocytes from the same donor. The classical studies of Billingham, Brent, and Medawar,[43] Mitchison,[44] and Gowans[45] demonstrating the ability of lymphocytes obtained from specifically sensitized donors to destroy skin allografts are in keeping with the postulated role of lymphocyte killer population in this regard. The in vitro studies of Miggiano et al.[46] and of Lightbody and Bach[47] have provided evidence pointing to the fact that MLC stimulation is followed in vitro by the production of killer lymphocytes detectable by the cell-mediated lympholysis (CML) test. Ceppellini[48] and Bach[42] have presented cogent arguments to support the thesis that the CML test constitutes an in vitro expression of the effector phase of allograft rejection.

It must be noted, however, that immunoglobulins (HL-A antibodies, placental extracts, etc.) have been shown to have the capacity to inhibit MLC activation.[4-9] The possibility arises, therefore, that inhibition of the MLC test in the course of allograft reactions may occur by two different mechanisms—the first based upon the processes of cell-to-cell surface interaction reviewed earlier.[42,46,47] The second inhibitory phase of the MLC test may, however, be a consequence of the appearance in the increasingly sensitized host of circulating antibodies directed against the donor's histocompatibility antigens. The occurrence of responses such as mixed white graft reactions and hyperacute kidney allograft reactions (i.e., of putatively antibody-mediated responses) in association with negative MLC responses would appear to provide in vivo support for this interpretation. These findings are also in keeping with the inhibition of lymphocyte activation produced in vitro by antibodies directed against major histocompatibility antigens.[1-10]

ACKNOWLEDGMENT

The technical assistance of Miss E. Kunen is greatly appreciated.

REFERENCES

1. Moller E: J Exp Med 122:11, 1965

2. Brunner KT, Mauel J, Schindler R: Nature (Lond) 213:1246, 1967

3. Mauel J, Rudolf H, Chapuis B, et al: Immunology 18:517, 1970

4. Ceppellini R, Bonnard GC, Coppo F, et al: Transplant Proc 3:63, 1971

5. Ceppellini R, Bonnard GD, Coppo F, et al: Transplant Proc 3:58, 1971

6. Revillard JP, Robert M, Betuel H, et al: Transplant Proc 4:173, 1972

7. Revillard JP, Robert M, Dupont E, et al: Transplant Proc 5:331, 1973

8. Thorsby E, Bondevik H, Solheim BG: Transplant Proc 5:343, 1973

9. Grumet FC, Levanthal BG: Transplantation Proc 2:405, 1970

10. Buckley RH, Schiff RI, Amos DB: J Immunol 108:34, 1972

11. Leuker RD, Williams RC: Circulation 46:655, 1972

12. Zabriskie JB, Hsu KC, Seegal BC: Clin Exp Immunol 7:147, 1970

13. Rapaport FT, Bachvaroff R, Markowitz AS: J Immunol 110:1058, 1973

14. Bachvaroff R, Markowitz AS, Rapaport F: Transplantation 15:586, 1973

15. Bachvaroff R, Rapaport FT: J Immunol 109: 1081, 1972

16. Oppenheim JJ, Whang J, Frei E III: Blood 24: 859, 1964

17. Oppenheim JJ, Whang J, Frei E III: J Exp Med 122:651, 1965

18. Miller J, Hattler B, Davis M, et al: Transplantation 12:65, 1971

19. Hattler BG, Miller J, Johnson MC: Transplantation 14:47, 1972

20. Miller J, Hattler BG, Johnson MC: Transplantation 14:57, 1972

21. Shons AR, Etheredge EE, Schmidtke JR, et al: Transplant Proc 4:337, 1972

22. Bachvaroff R, Ozaki A, Cannon FD: Transplant Proc 5:1561, 1973

23. Hartzman RJ, Segall M, Bach ML, et al: Transplantation 11:268, 1970

24. Ozaki A, Bachvaroff R, Cannon FD, et al: Transplant Proc 5:1781, 1973

25. Rapaport FT, Watanabe K, Cannon FD, et al: J Exp Med 136:1080, 1972

26. Rapaport FT, Hanaoka T, Shimada T, et al: J Exp Med 131:881, 1970

27. Rapaport FT, Converse JM: Ann Surg 147: 273, 1968

28. Rapaport FT, Chase RM Jr: Science 145:407, 1964

29. Rapaport FT, Dausset J, Converse JM, et al: Transplantation 3:490, 1965

30. Rapaport FT, Chase RM Jr, Solowey AC: Ann NY Acad Sci 129:102, 1966

31. Rapaport FT, Converse JM: Rapaport FT, Dausset J (eds): Human Transplantation. New York, Grune and Stratton, 1968, p 304

32. Rapaport FT, Dausset J, Legrand L, et al: J Clin Inves 47:2206, 1968

33. Rapaport FT, Markowitz AS: J Exp Med 129: 623, 1969

34. Williams GM, Hume DM, Hudson RP, et al: N Engl J Med 279:611, 1968

35. Milgrom F, Kano K, Klassen J: Transplant Proc 1:1013, 1969

36. Rapaport FT, Chase RM Jr, Markowitz AS, et al: Transplant Proc 3:89, 1971

37. Rapaport FT, Lawrence HS, Thomas L et al: J Clin Invest 41:2166, 1962

38. Dausset J, Rapaport FT, Cannon FD, et al: J Exp Med 134:1222, 1971

39. Converse JM, Ballantyne DL Jr, Woisky J; Ann NY Acad Sci 73:693, 1958

40. McKhann CF, Berrian JH: Transplant Bull 6:428, 1959

41. Henry L, Dammin GJ: Immunology 89:393, 1962

42. Bach FH, Bach ML, Sondel PM, et al: Transplant Rev 12:30, 1972

43. Billingham RE, Brent L, Medawar PB: Proc Roy Soc B 143:58, 1954

44. Mitchison NA: J Exp Med 102:157, 1955

45. Gowans JL, Br Med Bull 21:106, 1965

46. Miggiano VC, Bernoco D, Lightbody J, et al: Transplant Proc 4:231, 1972

47. Lightbody J, Bach FH: Transplant Proc 4:307, 1972

48. Ceppellini R: Amos DB, (ed): Progress in Immunology. New York, Academic, 1971, p 973

Ligand-induced Movement of Lymphocyte Surface Molecular Binding Sites for Soluble Extracts of Streptococcal Membranes (TGCM)

By R. Bachvaroff, A. S. Markowitz, and F. T. Rapaport*

THE ligand-induced displacement of lymphocyte surface molecules and the resulting segregation of complexes into pearllike collar formations at the cell surface, followed by cap formation, has been described for a variety of membrane components, including surface immunoglobulins,[1] histocompatibility antigens,[2] membrane surface antigens reacting with heterologous antilymphocyte antibodies,[3] theta alloantigens,[1] and the concanavallin A receptor.[3] The displacement of lymphocyte surface molecular components requires active cellular metabolic processes, minimum bivalence, and sufficient concentrations of the ligand, as well as a close distance between the membrane surface molecules involved, to permit effective linkage with the combining sites of the ligand.[1,2]

Recent studies have indicated that a water-soluble dialyzable extract of Group A Type 12 nephritogenic streptococcal membrane (a glycoprotein of molecular weight < 10,000), which has previously been shown to have transplantation antigenlike activity in mice[4] and has induced nephritis in rhesus monkeys[5] and in dogs,[6,7] can protect human lymphocytes from the complement-dependent cytotoxic effects of isospecific HL-A typing antisera.[8] This protective effect has been shown to be a consequence of the firm binding of streptococcal extracts (TGCM) to the lymphocyte surface in a manner that resists repeated attempts at dissociation by vigorous washing. Further studies have indicated that TGCM binding sites are distributed in diffuse fashion on the normal human blood lymphocyte surface and occur in approximately 80 to 90% of such lymphocytes.[8] Additional data have also pointed to the existence of a close spatial relationship between HL-A, species-specific, and TGCM binding sites on the human lymphocyte surface.[8] It is the purpose of the present communication to demonstrate that the TGCM binding molecules present on the normal human lymphocyte surface can undergo active displacement and form polar caps, following linkage with specific anti-TGCM antibodies.

MATERIALS AND METHOD

The method of isolation of TGCM from a nephritogenic strain of Group A Type 12 streptococci has been described in detail in a previous report.[5] Rabbit anti-TGCM serum was prepared in standard fashion,[9] and the indicator system used was sheep anti-rabbit IgG serum coupled with fluorescein isothiocyanide[10] in 1:2 dilutions.

Human peripheral lymphocytes isolated from the blood of healthy donors of known HL-A phenotypes by the method of Boyum[11] were washed in balanced salt solution (BSS)[12] and were incubated for 30 min at 37°C in a BSS solution containing 10 mg/ml of TGCM. The cells were centrifuged and washed three times in excess BSS, each washing being done for 10 min at 37°C employing vigorous shaking. The washed cells were incubated with rabbit anti-TGCM antiserum (1:2 dilution) for 30 min at 37°C; they were washed three more consecutive times in the same manner as described above.

The TGCM–anti-TGCM serum-treated lymphocytes were incubated with sheep anti-rabbit IgG preparations (1:2 dilutions) coupled with fluorescein isothiocyanide. After incubation for 30 min at room temperature, the cells were washed three times with

---

**Irma T. Hirschl Career Scientist Award.*

From the Transplantation and Immunology Division and the Institute of Reconstructive Plastic Surgery, Department of Surgery, New York University Medical Center, New York, N.Y., and the Hektoen Institute for Medical Research of the Cook County Hospital, Chicago, Ill.

Supported by a grant from the John A. Hartford Foundation and supported in part by the Billy Rose Foundation, the Irwin Strasburger Memorial Medical Foundation, and USPHS grant AM-04459.

© 1973 by Grune & Stratton, Inc.

BSS at 37°C and were then transferred to microscope slides. Four different controls with lymphocytes obtained from the same donors were used, including: (1) cells treated in the same manner, except that after the first incubation with TGCM, normal rabbit serum was used instead of rabbit anti-TGCM serum; (2) cells were incubated with the same concentration of bovine glycoprotein, instead of TGCM, before exposure to rabbit anti-TGCM serum and conjugated sheep anti-rabbit IgG; (3) cells were exposed to rabbit anti-TGCM serum and to conjugated sheep anti-rabbit IgG, without prior exposure of the cells to TGCM;

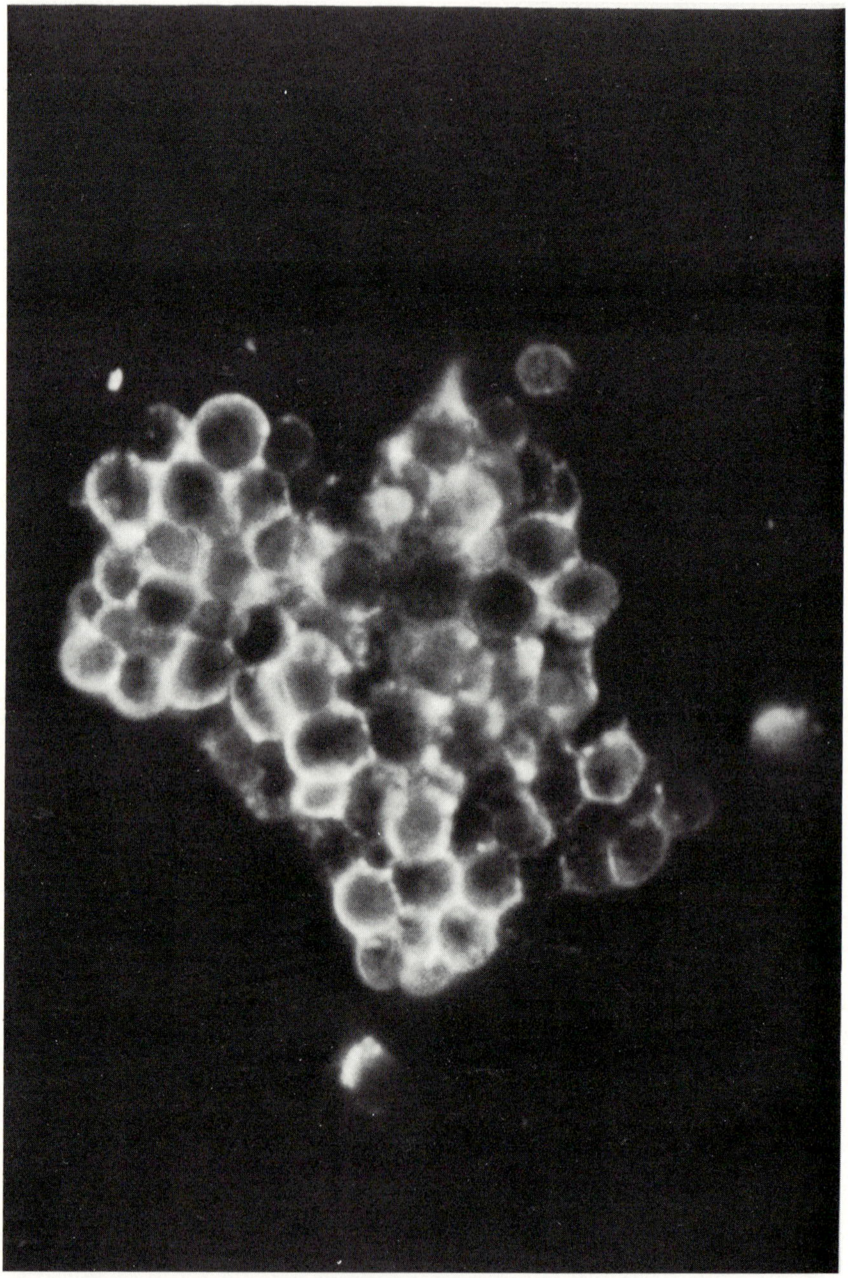

Fig. 1. Immunofluorescence of human blood lymphocytes treated with TGCM, rabbit anti-TGCM serum, and fluorescein-conjugated goat anti-rabbit IgG (×540).

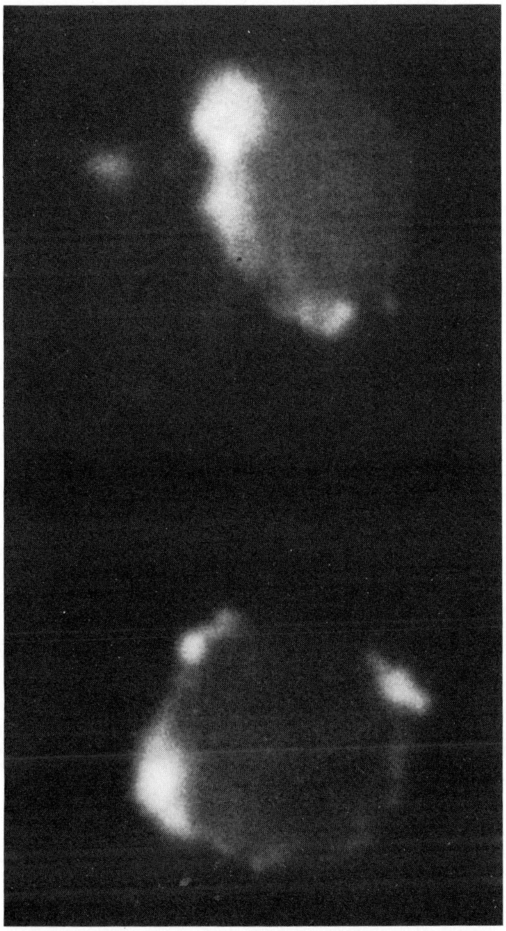

Fig. 2. Patchy ring formation and capping pattern of immunofluorescence of human blood lymphocytes treated with TGCM, rabbit anti-TGCM serum, and fluorescein-conjugated goat anti-rabbit IgG (× 1000).

(4) cells were exposed to TGCM and to rabbit anti-TGCM serum and were treated with *unconjugated* sheep anti-rabbit IgG prior to the addition of the conjugated sheep anti-rabbit IgG (blocking control).

RESULTS

When lymphocytes were incubated with TGCM, exposed to rabbit anti-TGCM serum, and then washed and resuspended in a sheep anti-rabbit IgG serum coupled with fluorescein isothiocyanide, there was a significant degree of cell aggregation, although a good number of free individual cells were also seen. Intense fluorescence was detectable on the surface of 80 to 90% of the cell preparations (Fig. 1). This immunofluorescence was relatively homogenous, covering the entire surface of cells in the aggregates and also the individual cells. Separate experiments indicated by the dye exclusion test (eosin) that the majority of the cells were viable at the time of examination. Two cells separate from a central aggregate in Fig. 1 show typical cap formation of the fluorescent antibody complexes. Similar cap and patch formation occurred on the surface of the majority of the single nonaggregated cells shown in Figs. 2 and 3. Incubation of cells from the same donors with bovine glycoprotein instead of TGCM, use of normal rabbit serum instead of anti-TGCM serum, or use of anti-TGCM serum and conjugated sheep anti-rabbit IgG without prior exposure of the cells to TGCM gave consistently negative results. Treatment with unconjugated sheep anti-IgG blocked the binding capacity of conjugated sheep anti-rabbit IgG to the cell surfaces and gave no evidence of immunofluorescence.

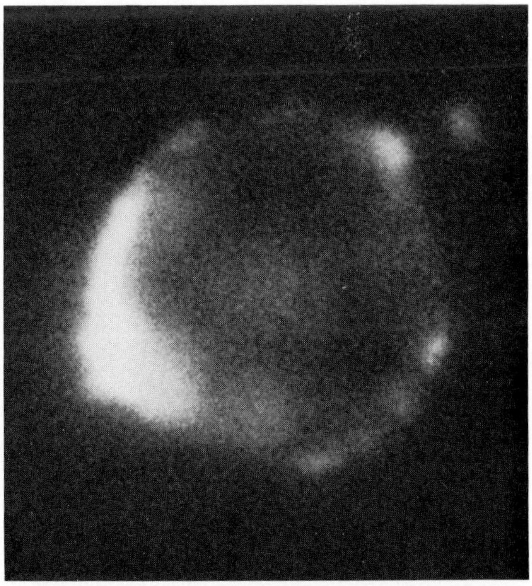

Fig. 3. Patchy ring formation and capping pattern of immunofluorescence of human blood lymphocytes treated with TGCM, rabbit anti-TGCM serum, and fluorescein-conjugated goat anti-rabbit IgG (× 1000).

DISCUSSION

Earlier studies have provided evidence for the presence on the surface of normal human blood lymphocytes of binding sites for a soluble glycoprotein extract of membranes extracted from a nephritogenic strain of Group A Type 12 streptococci.[8] Incubation of the lymphocytes with TGCM followed by exposure of the cells to rabbit anti-TGCM serum and testing with isothiocyanide-coupled sheep anti-rabbit IgG produced a specific and intense fluorescence over the surface of approximately 80 to 90% of the cells treated at 37°C. Although many of the cells became agglutinated, their viability was demonstrated through the dye exclusion test. A typical redistribution of the fluorescent antibody complexes at the cell surface, with patch and cap formation, occurred in a majority of the single cells, where agglutination did not restrict cell surface movements.

As noted earlier, a number of molecular structures have been shown to be mobile in similar fashion on the lymphocyte membrane surface.[1-3] It is of particular interest, however, that while other authors have observed that only approximately 40% of human peripheral blood lymphocytes could exhibit this redistribution phenomenon (for example, if HL-A-specific antisera were used[2]), a much higher percentage of ligand-induced displacement of lymphocyte surface molecules occurred after exposure to TGCM and anti-TGCM antisera. In this regard, since it is generally agreed that at least 80% of human peripheral lymphocytes are T cells,[13] it would appear that it may have been mainly such cells that were involved in the observed reactions. There is at present a certain degree of disagreement in the literature with regard to the origins and nature of immunoglobulins on the surface of T cells.[14-16] Convincing evidence has been brought forth, however, to support the possibility that the immunoglobulins that have been shown to be present on the surface of T cells are actually tightly bound cytophilic antibodies and are not active metabolic products of T cells.[17] In view of the high incidence of human host exposure and sensitization to streptococcal antigens,[7] the possibility exists that a high proportion of these cells may bear on their surfaces cytophilic antibodies with a strong affinity for soluble streptococcal extracts. Such an interpretation might aid in explaining the high incidence of TGCM binding observed in the present study, although it does not rule out the possibility that the corresponding binding sites may be similar in nature to lymphocyte binding sites for plant lecithins.

A sandwich-type immunofluorescence reaction (i.e., rabbit anti-TGCM antibody plus sheep anti-rabbit IgG) was used during this study. It has been suggested that the theoretical maximum span of an antibody combined with another antibody is 420 Å.[3] Since lattice formation by ligands on lymphocytes appears to be a prerequisite for the displacement and movement of the resulting molecular complexes on the cell surface,[1,3] the results suggest that the distance between TGCM-binding molecules on the lymphocyte surface may not exceed this same value, i.e., 420 Å. This result may be of relevance to earlier data indicating close spatial relationships between HL-A, species-specific, and TGCM binding sites on the surface of the human lymphocyte.[18]

REFERENCES

1. Taylor RB, Duffus PH, Raff MC, de Petri S: Nature [New Biol] 233:225, 1971

2. Kourilsky FM, Silvestre D, Neauport-Saute C, et al: Eur J Immunol 2:249, 1972

3. Unanue ER, Perkins WD, Rarnovsky MJ: J Exp Med 136:885, 1972

4. Rapaport FT, Markowitz AS: Fed Proc 31:234, 1972

5. Markowitz AS, Horn D, Aseron C, et al: J Immunol 107:504, 1971

6. Rapaport FT, Markowitz AS, McCluskey RT, et al: Transplant Proc 1:981, 1969

7. Rapaport FT: in Reisfeld R, Kahn B (eds): Markers of Biological Individuality. New York, Academic, 1972, p 182

8. Rapaport FT, Bachvaroff R, Markowitz AS, J Immunol 110:1058, 1973
9. Markowitz AS, Lange CF Jr: J Immunol 92:565, 1964
10. Wood BT, Thompson SH, Goldstein G: J Immunol 95:225, 1965
11. Boyum A: Scand J Clin Lab Invest 21:1, 1968
12. Mishell RI, Dutton RW: J Exp Med 126:423, 1967
13. Good RA, Biggar WD, Park BH: in Amos B (ed): Progress in Immunology. New York, Academic, 1971, p 699
14. Greaves MF, Hogg NM: in Amos B (ed): Progress in Immunology. New York, Academic, 1971, p 111
15. Marchalonis JJ, Cone RE, Atwell JL: J Exp Med 135:956, 1972
16. Hämmerling J, Rajewsky K: Eur J Immunol 1:447, 1971
17. Sprent J: Transplant Proc 5:1725, 1973
18. Bachvaroff R, Rapaport FT: Transplantation 15:586, 1973

Demonstration of Specific T-Lymphocyte Membrane Antigens Associated With Antibodies Inhibiting the Mixed Leukocyte Culture in Man

By Peter Wernet* and Henry G. Kunkel

T LYMPHOCYTES are responsible for various cell-mediated immune reactions such as delayed hypersensitivity, graft rejection, and graft-vs.-host reactivity. The mixed lymphocyte culture (MLC) serves as an in vitro model of the recognition aspect of homograft reactions in vivo.[1] It has been established that the reactive cells in the MLC belong predominantly or perhaps exclusively to a thymus-dependent population of antigen-sensitive lymphocytes.[2] Recent findings have suggested that the correlation between the serologically defined (SD) HL-A antigens and lymphocyte-defined (LD) reactivity[3] with respect to MLC is not as absolute as the initial studies suggested.[4,5] Separate inheritance of HL-A antigens and the determinant eliciting clear MLC has been demonstrated by Eijsvoogel et al.: this indicates independence of this MLC system from both the first (LA) and second (Four) loci.[6] However, the biochemical nature of the hypothetical T-lymphocyte receptors involved in the MLC interaction still remains unknown.[7]

On the other hand, a number of different human sera have been found that strongly inhibit the MLC reaction.[8-10] The in vitro study of the mode of action of such blocking sera and antibodies against lymphocyte membrane antibodies may help in understanding the mechanism of immunosuppression. This has been particularly evident for sera from patients with systemic lupus erythematosus (SLE).[11,12] Cytotoxic antibodies to T cells have also been described in the sera of patients with SLE.[13,14] In order to define specific membrane antigens via homologous antibodies associated with MLC suppression, the present study has employed enzymatic surface radioiodination of lymphocytes.[15] Using carefully absorbed MLC-blocking SLE sera, one surface structure on T cells was identified by this technique, which appeared particularly relevant.

MATERIALS AND METHOD

Unidirectional mixed leukocyte cultures (MLC) have been performed in a microsystem following the method of Hartzman et al.[16] Briefly, lymphocytes are isolated by Ficoll-Hypaque flotation, and triplicates of 0.30×10^6 mitomycin-treated stimulating cells and 0.15×10^6 responding cells are mixed in the wells of Falcon microtiter plates. Each culture is set up in triplicate and consists of the cells in 0.2 ml of RPMI-1640 medium supplemented with antibiotics and 20% inactivated (1-hr 56°C) normal or SLE serum. Incubation is generally allowed for 6 days at 37°C in a humidified 5% CO_2 atmosphere, and 16 hr before harvesting 2 μCi of ^{3}H-thymidine is added. The lymphocytes are harvested from each well by suction and are processed for liquid scintillation with Aquasol (New England Nuclear). HL-A typing and cytotoxic antibody activity determination were performed in a two-stage technique and will be discussed elsewhere.

Absorptions of normal and SLE sera were carried out routinely at two temperatures: 4 ml of heat-inactivated serum were incubated with an equal volume of packed ABO red cells at 4°C, and then the supernatant was incubated with another 4 ml of packed cells at 37°C. In addition, certain SLE sera were absorbed further in the same fashion with isolated and pooled lymphocytes from patients with chronic lymphocytic leukemia (CLL) having high peripheral blood counts, then absorbed with packed platelets pooled from 10 different donors in order to remove antibodies possibly directed against the Four and LA loci; in a last step the absorption was completed with allogeneic kidney cells. Beyond that a few sera were absorbed with allogeneic thymus or spleen cells or with buffy coat cells.

The sera were fractionated by gel chromatography on Sephadex G200 or pevikon-block electrophoresis.

*Recipient of grant We 505/3, Deutsche Forschungsgemeinschaft.

From the Rockefeller University, New York, N.Y.

This investigation has been supported by USPHS grants AM 34761, RR-102, and AI 10811.

Anti-human immunoglobulin sera were raised in rabbits by using isolated IgM, IgG, and light-chain preparations, as well as Bence Jones proteins. Anti-rabbit immunoglobulin antiserum was raised in a goat.

For the enzymatic surface radioiodination (SRI), a modification of the method described by Baur et al.[15] using lactoperoxidase (Sigma) to radioiodinate the lymphocyte membranes was applied. For this procedure the lymphocyte populations were first kept in short-term culture, which resulted in shedding of the autoantibodies coated on the cells in vivo as antigen–antibody complexes. The lymphocytes are able to reconstitute their surface antigens in vitro without loss of viability.[11] Lymphocytes were purified further by passage through Sephadex G10 columns for 30 min at 37°C to remove phagocytic cells. This was followed by a latex-particle ingestion test.[12]

The radioiodinated lymphocytes were solubilized with the nonionic detergent NP-40 (Shell). In a first step with rabbit anti-human Ig and subsequent goat anti-rabbit Ig antibodies in excess, all lymphocyte-derived immunoglobulin molecules were precipitated out by this sandwich technique. The remaining supernatant was incubated first with a normal or SLE or anti-HL-A serum or its IgG fraction and subsequently with the goat anti-human Ig antiserum. The formed specific precipitate was solubilized and run on a 5% polyacrylamide gel containing 0.1% SDS. The radioactive bands obtained represent antigen targets on the lymphocyte surface identified by specific antibody present in the lupus sera. Figure 1 illustrates this technique. As markers, the following radiolabeled proteins were used and are included in Figs. 3 and 4: IgG with molecular weight (MW) of about 150,000 dalton, γ-chain with MW of about 50,000 dalton, light-chain (L) with MW of 24,000 dalton, and beta-2-microglobulin (β_2M) of 11,500 dalton.

RESULTS

The response of different normal and SLE lymphocytes to constant stimulator cells in MLC reactions was compared in the presence of normal vs. SLE sera. Marked suppression was noted with certain SLE sera. In some cases this was maximal when the SLE cells were used as responders in the presence of the corresponding sera. Figure 2 illustrates one series of representative experiments. The upper curve shows the normal kinetics with the peak response at day 6, including a pronounced standard deviation. The middle curve shows the reactivity of one SLE patient's lymphocytes (Go) against a normal stimulator A in the presence of normal AB-serum-supplemented medium. The same experiment performed in SLE-serum Go-supplemented medium resulted in a complete suppression of the MLC, which is demonstrated in the bottom curve.

By testing 34 SLE patients in a similar fashion, it was found that 19 out of these showed an impaired MLC reactivity, and 7 out of the 19 gave a complete inhibition of

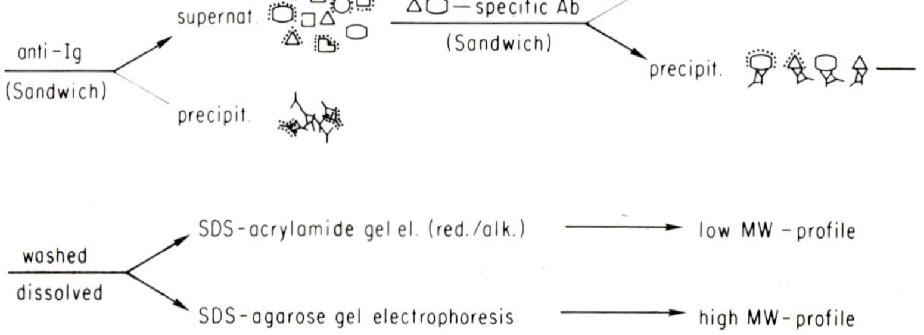

Fig. 1. Illustration of enzymatic lymphocyte surface radioiodination for characterization of membrane antigens via specific antibodies.

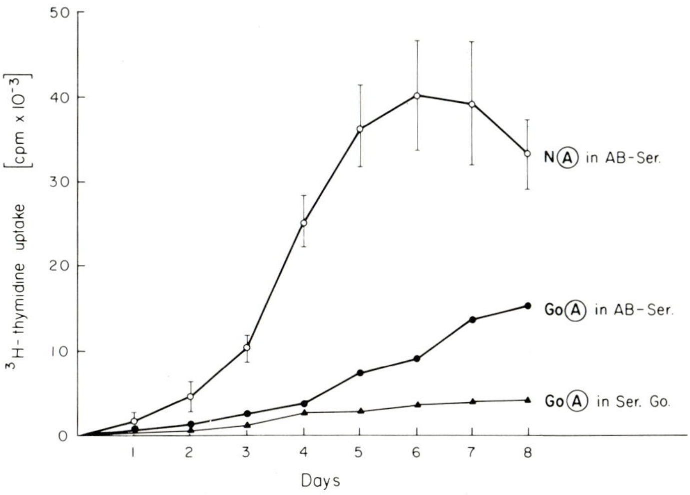

Fig. 2. Reactivity and kinetics of unidirectional MLC reactions all triggered by the same stimulating lymphocyte population A. Upper curve represents normal responder lymphocytes N in normal AB serum; middle curve is for SLE responder cells (Go) in normal AB serum; lower curve is for SLE responder cells (Go) in SLE serum Go. Complete suppression is noted in the latter case.[12]

the MLC. The SLE sera involved primarily in this suppression of cell-mediated immunity were also able to block a number of allogeneic lymphocyte combinations of normal persons. In comparing the blocking capacity and the cytotoxic potential of the lupus sera tested, a discrepancy between these two functions became apparent in vitro when some sera showed a strong MLC-suppressive but no lymphocytotoxic effect. Considerable evidence was obtained by gel filtration of the SLE sera on Sephadex G200 and by pevikon-block electrophoresis indicating that the main blocking activity in the MLC reaction was due to antibodies of the IgG class.

Information regarding the nature of the sites with which these antibodies combine on the lymphocyte membrane was obtained by using surface radioiodination procedures. In Table 1 the amount of total acid-precipitable surface radioactivity is compared with the percentage of acid-precipitable counts per minute, which have been obtained by specific immunoprecipitation using different SLE sera. These were able to block the MLC reactivity of their autologous lymphocytes as stimulators or responder population up to various dilutions. Compared to the figures for surface immunoglobulins, the amounts of SLE-antibody-mediated precipitates are in general much lower. As expected, the normal AB serum, which is a pool from six healthy

Table 1. Precipitation of Radiolabeled Surface Protein From Human Lymphocytes

Lymphocyte Origin	Total Acid-precipitable Radioactivity (c.p.m.)	Percentage Acid-precipitable Radioactivity Immunoprecipitated: By anti-Ig	By SLE Sera*: Har	Har 7S IgG	Har abs.	Esp	Don	Ham	Control AB Serum
Normal P.Bl.	7.2×10^6	4.4	2.1	1.8	1.2	2.5	1.8	5.3	0.3
Normal thymus	19.8×10^6	0.1	2.1	1.7	1.1	3.7	3.1	1.6	0.1
B-cell CLL:									
P.Bl.	20.4×10^6	3.0	2.8	2.6	0.2	3.1	2.9	7.0	0.1
SLE P.Bl.†									
Har	5.2×10^6	4.1	2.0	1.4	1.3	1.5	n.d.	3.6	0.2
Esp	3.0×10^6	5.3	2.2	1.4	0.8	3.2	1.2	2.5	n.d.
Don	1.3×10^6	5.9	1.6	n.d.	0.5	1.1	1.3	1.7	n.d.
Ham	0.8×10^6	4.0	2.3	n.d.	1.1	2.0	6.0	6.6	0.4

*All SLE sera listed block the MLC with the exception of Ham.

†SLE lymphocytes were all labeled after 24-hr short-term culture (see reference 11).

n.d. = not done.

male donors and is not MLC-inhibitory, does not cause a convincing radioprecipitate. The AB serum pool was heat-inactivated and passed through a 0.22-μ millipore filter like the SLE sera prior to incubation with the radiolabeled and solubilized cell surfaces. The pevikon-block-isolated 7S IgG fraction of SLE serum Har contained most of the specific membrane-precipitable activity of the original unabsorbed serum Har, whereas absorption of this serum with red cells, CLL lymphocytes, platelets, and kidney cells removed considerable amounts of antimembrane activities.

In other experiments, anti-HL-A2 and anti-HL-A7 sera were used to precipitate radiolabeled histocompatibility antigens from HL-A2- and 7-positive donor lymphocytes and gave similar percentages as found for the absorbed SLE serum. A mean of 1.3% of acid-precipitable specific immune precipitate was found for these two histocompatibility antigens. This suggested the possible presence of similar amounts of non-HL-A but MLC-associated antigens on the lymphocyte surface. Surface radioiodination patterns obtained for SD and LD determinants, however, seem to be different, as illustrated in Figs. 3 and 4. Figure 3A illustrates the lymphocyte surface profile obtained from the peripheral blood lymphocytes of SLE patient Har on SDS acrylamide electrophoresis using the autologous serum as the reactive antiserum. Four different targets can be identified as separate peaks with the SLE serum Har that do not appear with the control serum, which was nonsuppressive in the MLC system. From these experiments the impression was gained that active SLE sera contain a whole group of different antibodies directed against different lymphocyte surface structures. In order to get information on a SLE antibody target concerning T-cell-mediated MLC, certain SLE sera were absorbed as described above with lymphocytes from two CLL patients, with a pool of platelets from 10 different donors, and with kidney cells. The absorbed sera were still strongly suppressive in the MLC when the autologous lymphocytes were used as the responder population. Direct evidence against involvement of HL-A antibodies was shown by the continued blocking effect of absorbed SLE serum Har using an HL-A-identical but MLC-reacting lymphocyte population from an unrelated donor as stimulator cells. Figure 3B shows that this absorbed serum localized primarily one labeled surface structure at about fraction number 50. As can be calculated from the approximative

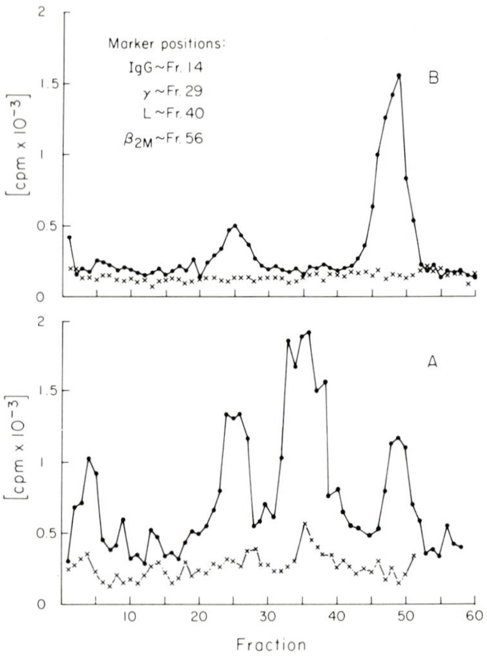

Fig. 3. SDS polyacrylamide gel patterns, representing target-surface radioiodination profiles obtained from membranes of SLE peripheral blood lymphocytes using the corresponding SLE serum as the antiserum to precipitate the membrane components. The lower curve A shows the pattern with the unabsorbed antiserum; the upper curve B is that for the SLE serum absorbed with B cells, platelets, etc., as described in the text. The absorbed serum that still strongly inhibits the MLC reaction shows a major low-MW component and a minor one of higher MW; control sera (x—x—x), not inhibitory in MLC and used in the same fashion, did not show these components. The relative positions of various marker proteins are indicated ($\beta_2M = \beta_2$ microglobulin).[12]

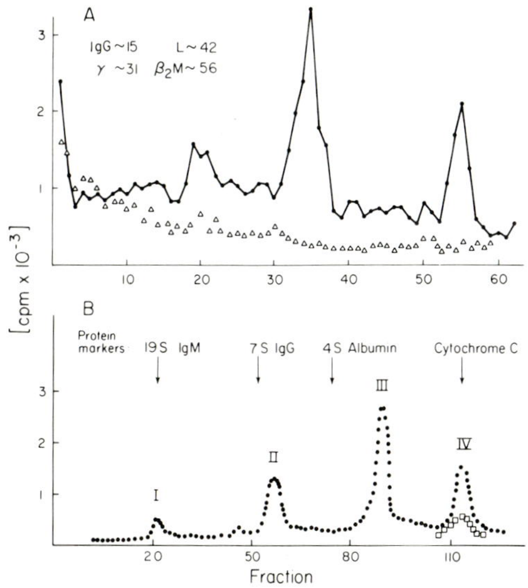

Fig. 4. (A): SDS polyacrylamide gel electrophoresis pattern of human lymphocytes We (HL-A2,12,13) using the anti-HL-A2 serum "La Porta." Marker positions are included as in Fig. 3. The HL-A antigen profile consists of one minor and two major peaks. (B) shows the gel chromatographic pattern of the solubilized radioactive HL-A–anti-HL-A complex on Sephadex G200 at pH 2.8 using a 0.1-M citrate, 0.2-M phosphate buffer (dotted line). The radioactivity of peak IV is precipitated out at pH 7.4 with an anti-β_2 microglobulin serum (squares).

positions of included marker proteins, this peak corresponds to a molecular weight of about 15,000 dalton. With the exception of a minor peak at fraction 25, all the other antibody activities were absorbed out.

Two other SLE sera that showed strong inhibition of MLC gave similar results with specific reactivity for the low-molecular-weight component. This was not observed for a limited number of sera that failed to inhibit the MLC reaction.

On the other hand, Fig. 4A shows the radioiodinated HL-A2 antigen profile obtained from We lymphocytes (HL-A2,12,13) using a monospecific anti-HL-A2 serum ("La Porta", received as a gift from Dr. M. Fotino, New York Blood Center). Three different peaks are shown on this SDS gel electrophoresis. One minor peak in fraction 19 and two major targets in fractions 35 and 55 have been identified by this anti-HL-A2 serum. The latter two components with MW of ~ 42,000 and 11,500 daltons appear constantly, but with variable ratios, whereas the high molecular peak (~ 140,000 daltons) is less frequently seen. The surface iodination profiles differ clearly from those obtained with SLE sera; both, however, contain a small-molecular-weight component. For HL-A antigens, such a small fragment of 11,000 daltons has been described recently.[17,18] A possible relationship between these two components was tested by dissolving part of the radioactive immunoprecipitate and subsequent column chromatography on Sephadex G200 at pH 2.8, including Cytochrome C as a colored MW marker (~ 12,500 daltons). Figure 4B shows the radioactive HL-A peaks obtained in relationship to the effluent volumes for several proteins. Peak IV, which contained also the Cytochrome C, was concentrated and dialysed against PBS, pH 7.4. After incubation with rabbit anti-β_2 microglobulin serum and subsequent goat anti-rabbit Ig serum, the formed precipitate contained most of the radioactivity, thus showing structural similarity of this small-MW peak of HL-A antigens to β_2 microglobulin. In the same experimental design, performed however with the small-molecular-weight component derived from SLE sera, the anti-β_2 microglobulin serum failed to precipitate down the radioactivity of that peak. Further evidence was obtained against the possibility that the small-MW molecule, identified by the MLC-blocking SLE sera, was β_2 microglobulin, but experiments are continuing on this question and will be reported in detail elsewhere.

DISCUSSION

It appears from the above experiments that human T-lymphocyte membrane preparations possess a low-molecular-weight surface constituent to which antibodies are sometimes found in human sera. Although most of the work was carried out on SLE sera, similar antibodies were found in sera from certain individuals with other conditions, including arthritis and malignancy, as well as during pregnancy and following multiple blood transfusions. All the sera showing reactivity against this material also blocked strongly the responder cells in the MLC reaction; various control sera that did not block the MLC failed to show such specificity. It should be emphasized, however, that further sera need to be studied to firmly establish this apparent association. Absorption of these antisera with B cells, platelets, and a variety of other cells failed to remove either the MLC blocking effect or the reactivity for the low-molecular-weight surface constituent. Absorption with thymocytes or spleen cells removed both effects.

A number of the absorbed sera that showed MLC inhibition showed a small higher molecular weight component along with the larger constituent described above. This peak, however, was not consistently present, and certain sera showed only the single low-molecular-weight component after reaction with the labeled surface antigens. The presence of just the single component associated with MLC inhibition also suggested a relationship. However, the possibility still remains that the blocking antibodies react with a constituent that is not solubilized by the ionic detergent utilized. Current efforts are directed toward the preparative isolation of the low-molecular-weight component so that its effect on the blocking antibodies can be determined directly. If this is successful, it appears possible that the low-molecular-weight component participates in the recognitive phase involved in the MLC reaction.

Our conclusions are that certain unabsorbed SLE sera contain antibodies directed against different lymphocyte surface components. These antibodies are not always cytotoxic, as judged by the microcytotoxicity assay with complement. Using this method we were not able to detect antibodies directed against one of the known HL-A antigens, yet the presence of these antisera on the lymphocyte surface interfered with the HL-A typing. This blockage of HL-A antigens may be significant in evaluating HL-A typing surveys.[11] One of the higher MW peaks identified on the B- and T-cell membranes (compare Figs. 3A and 4A) may well represent HL-A loci products that are not detectable by cytotoxicity. The experiments using HL-A-absorbed sera for blocking of MLC reactions exclude the immediate involvement of this antigen group in the MLC and support earlier findings by Yunis and Amos[4] that HL-A antigens are not the primary factors involved in the cell-mediated component of allotransplantation. For the absorbed SLE sera, another possibility that requires consideration is that the antibodies that inhibit the MLC reaction, even if they are directed to the low-MW component, are blocking because of reactivity to a site close to or adjoining the receptor site or via a nonspecific alteration of the lymphocyte surface. At any rate, irrespective of these various possibilities, the low-MW antigen clearly represents, in association with MLC inhibition, a good candidate for an otherwise lymphocyte-defined (LD) antigen in man.[3] Figure 4 demonstrates that the small-MW fragment of the HL-A antigen is homologous to β_2 microglobulin, whereas the low-MW component identified by the MLC response blocking SLE sera does not show such structural relationship and also appears to be a somewhat larger molecule than β_2 microglobulin. More data have to be obtained on the complex relationship between the genetic loci of the major histocompatibility complex in man and on the structural expression as well as on the functional activities of these molecules in order to understand the mechanism of the immune response. So far it is even unclear whether MLC gene products would have a relationship with the postulated Ir gene product.

In inbred guinea pigs, such Ir gene products are expressed on the T-cell surface in close relationship with the histocompatibility molecules enclosed on the same chromosome.[19] It will be of interest to study MLC and other antigen-sensitive T cells inhibiting antisera by the methods described above for possible reactivity with a component analogous to the low-MW antigen.

SUMMARY

Surface radioiodination of lymphocytes by the lactoperoxidase procedure has permitted the demonstration of an assortment of different membrane molecules which represent a part of the structural equivalent of the major histocompatibility complex. The use of mixed leucocyte culture blocking human sera as antisera (primarily from patients with systemic lupus erythematosus) exposed mainly a small-molecular-weight component on the lymphocyte surface of T cells. This target structure proved of special interest because it appeared to be associated with inhibition of certain responder cells in the mixed leucocyte culture reaction. The possible relation of this antigen to lymphocyte receptors such as HL-A antigens and β_2 microglobulin, which appear to share antigenic determinants, and to products of immune-response genes is discussed.

ACKNOWLEDGMENT

We would like to thank Dr. Marilena Fotino for the generous gift of anti-HL-A antiserum and Dr. M. D. Poulik likewise for the use of some of his anti-β_2 microglobulin serum.

REFERENCES

1. Van Rood JJ, Koch CT, van Hoff JP, et al: Transplant Proc 5:409, 1973

2. Sørensen SF: Acta Pathol Microbiol Scand [B] suppl 230, 1972

3. Bach FH, Widmer MB, Bach ML, Klein J: J Exp Med 136: 1430, 1972

4. Yunis EJ, Amos DB: Proc Natl Acad Sci USA 68:3031, 1971

5. Ceppellini R: in Amos DB (ed): Progress in Immunology. New York, Academic, 1971, p 973

6. Eijsvoogel VP, du Bois MJGJ, Melief CMJ, et al: Histocompatibility Testing. Copenhagen, Munksgaard (in press)

7. Crone M, Koch C, Simonsen M: Transplant Rev 10:36, 1972

8. Ceppellini R, Bonnard DG, Coppo F, et al: Transplant Proc 3:58, 64, 1971

9. Revillard JP, Robert M, Beutel H, et al: Transplant Proc 4:173, 1972

10. Brooks WH, Netsky MG, Normansell DE, Horwitz DA: J Exp Med 136:1631, 1972

11. Wernet P, Fotino M, Thoburn R, et al: Arthritis Rheum (abstract) 16:137, 1973

12. Wernet P, Kunkel HG: J Exp Med 138:1021, 1973

13. Terasaki PI, Mottironi VD, Barnett EV: N Engl J Med 283:724, 1970

14. Lies RB, Messner RP, Williams RC Jr: Arthritis Rheum 16:369, 1973

15. Baur S, Vitetta ES, Sherr CJ, et al: J Immunol 106:1133, 1971

16. Hartzman RJ, Segall M, Bach ML, Bach FH: Transplantation 11:268, 1971

17. Tanigaki N, Katagiri M, Nakamuro U, et al: Fed Proc 32:1017, 1973

18. Cresswell P, Turner MJ, Strominger JL: Proc Natl Acad Sci USA 70:1603, 1973

19. Green I, Paul WE, Benacerraf B: J Immunol 109:457, 1972

AUTHOR INDEX

a
4 b
5 c
6 d
7 e
8 f
9 g
0 h
1 i
8 2 j